# Minimally Invasive Therapies for Endocrine Neck Diseases

Celestino Pio Lombardi • Rocco Bellantone
Editors

# Minimally Invasive Therapies for Endocrine Neck Diseases

Springer

*Editors*
Celestino Pio Lombardi
Chief of Endocrine Surgery Unit
Policlinico Gemelli – CIC
Università Cattolica del Sacro Cuore
Rome
Italy

Rocco Bellantone
Chief of Istituto Semeiotica Chirurgica
Chief of Endocrine and Metabolic
Surgery Unit
Policlinico Gemelli
Università Cattolica del Sacro Cuore
Rome
Italy

ISBN 978-3-319-20064-4 ISBN 978-3-319-20065-1 (eBook)
DOI 10.1007/978-3-319-20065-1

Library of Congress Control Number: 2015950618

Springer Cham Heidelberg New York Dordrecht London


Printed on acid-free paper

Springer International Publishing AG Switzerland is part of Springer Science+Business Media (www.springer.com)

# Preface

The diagnostic and therapeutic approach to endocrine diseases of the neck have undergone tremendous change during the past decade owing to important research findings and technological advances. New tools and methods have been introduced into clinical practice that are capable of improving diagnosis and enabling selection of candidates for a specific interventional approach. At the same time, various minimally invasive techniques have been developed with a view to offering optimal treatment in each individual case. The consequence is that endocrinologists, pathologists, and neck and endocrine surgeons now have at their disposal a large armamentarium of possible techniques with which to study and treat the patient.

We have used minimally invasive surgical approaches in patients with endocrine diseases of the neck since 1997. We are now proud to present this book, which is based on our own longstanding experience and is supported by the expertise of leading authorities in the field, who have kindly collected and discussed their results. The aim is to allow clinicians seeking a better grasp of the indications for and the technical details of the different techniques to orient themselves in this complex field and to equip them to select diagnostic and therapeutic options appropriately, thereby tailoring care to meet the needs of the individual patient.

Rome, Italy — Celestino Pio Lombardi
Rome, Italy — Rocco Bellantone

# Contents

# Part I

# Ultrasound Imaging

# 1 Ultrasound Features of Thyroid, Parathyroid, Neck Lymph Nodes: Normal and Pathologic Pattern

Piero Maceroni

## 1.1 Thyroid

### 1.1.1 Normal Neck Anatomy and Standard Ultrasound Examination

The normal thyroid is a "H" or "U" shaped gland placed on trachea in anterior cervical neck, formed from two elongated lateral lobe connected by median isthmus. Each lobe is approximately 4.0–5.0 cm in length, 1–2 cm wide and 1–2 cm in thickness and is commonly asymmetric in size. Anterior to the thyroid are the strap muscles. Anterior and more lateral to the strap muscles is the sternocleidomastoid muscle which divides the neck in anterior and posterior triangles. Posterior to the thyroid is the longus colli muscle which is in contact with the posterior side of thyroid capsule. Laterally to the borders of thyroid are the common carotid artery (CCA) and the internal jugular vein (IJV). Behind the centrally located trachea is the esophagus; ultrasound do not trespass the trachea and so the visualization of esophagus is not allowed but, in the inferior portions, the esophagus is commonly visualized posteriorly to the thyroid because of its lateral position to the trachea. In patients who underwent thyroidectomy the empty thyroid loggia allows the visualization of esophagus on both sides of trachea. The real time observation of esophageal peristalsis during swallowing permits its correct identification.

On ultrasound examination the thyroid parenchymal echoes are fine, uniform and hyperechoic compared to adjacent muscles; the echogenic capsule is clearly visualized and helps to differentiate thyroid nodule from extrathyroidal lesions.

P. Maceroni
Dipartimento di Diagnostica per Immagini, Istituto Chirurgico Ortopedico Traumatologico "Sapienza" University of Rome,
Via Franco Faggiana, 1668, Latina 04100, Italy
e-mail: piero.maceroni@gmail.com



C.P. Lombardi, R. Bellantone (eds.), *Minimally Invasive Therapies for Endocrine Neck Diseases*, DOI 10.1007/978-3-319-20065-1_1

The connective tissues in the neck are more echogenic than thyroid parenchyma and muscles, contrariwise, are hypoechogenic.

Arterial supply to thyroid gland is granted by superior and inferior thyroid arteries; the former is the first anterior branch of external carotid artery and runs superficially on anterior border of lateral lobe, the latter arises from thyrocervical trunk, a branch of subclavian artery, and ascends vertically then curves medially to enter tracheoesophageal groove. Venous drainage of thyroid gland is constituted of three pairs of veins arising from venous plexus on surface of gland (superior and middle veins drains into internal jugular vein, inferior vein drain into brachiocefalic vein)

A standard examination requires transverse scans from upper to the lower poles to determine anatomical relationship and echogenicity of the gland; each image should include at least a part of CCA and, if possible, the IJV. Images should be labeled with bodymark to provide information regarding location and orientation. The transverse measurements are performed at the level of mid portions (the lateral caliper should include thyroid tissue extending beyond the CCA and the medial caliper should be located at the lateral side of trachea). The anteroposterior dimension should be measured preferably in the sagittal plane and the line should be at the right angle to the upper-lower line. In most pathologic patients, the thyroid lobes will longer than the length of the probe; to get an image of the entire lobe the split screen function, the extended field of view or the trapezoidal scan should be utilized. Utilizing the ellipsoid formula the volume of each lobe and of course the volume of entire gland should be calculated; if the thickness of the isthmus is less than 5 mm, its measure is irrelevant to the calculation of the total volume [1, 2].

### 1.1.2 Diffuse Thyroid Enlargement

*Chronic lymphocytic thyroiditis* is the most frequent form of diffuse enlargement of thyroid in countries with adequate iodine intake in the diet. The presence of TPO autoantibodies is estimated to 10 % of overall population and 25 % of women over 62 years; this condition predicts future thyroid dysfunction [3, 4]. The ultrasound hallmark of CLT is the *hypoechogenicity* which is linked to the presence of lymphocytic infiltrate (allows a better sound transmission than intact follicles). The degree of hypoechogenicity has been correlated to the risk of subsequent hypothyroidism. Another common feature of CLT is the *inhomogeneity* with different pattern:

1. *Hypoechogenic and inhomogeneous:* areas of lymphocytic infiltration have few internal interfaces and are therefore extremely hypoechoic compared to normal thyroid parenchyma and have an echogenicity similar to strap muscles.
2. *Micronodular:* if areas of inflammation are of small size, the reduced echogenicity appear more discrete with a pseudo micronodular pattern that mimic the presence of true small nodules.

3. *Macronodular:* when areas of flogosis are more larger they resemble pseudo macronodules which are confluent with little normal intervening parenchyma.
4. *Severely hypoechogenic:* when parenchyma is completely replaced by lymphocytes the overall echogenicity in severely low, equal to or lower than adjacent muscles (d.d. diffuse lymphoma).
5. *Fibrosis:* fibrosis develops later in the progression of CLT. The hyperechogenic fibrous band separate area of hypoechogenicity.
6. *Punctate:* multiple hyperecogenic spots are scattered through the parenchyma with an appearance of microcalcifications; this punctate densities do not generate acoustic shadow and are similar to the hyperechogenic spots seen in colloid nodules.

*Grave's Disease* – The typical sonographic pattern of Grave's disease is similar to that of autoimmune Hashimoto disease although hypoechogenicity is of lower degree. There is a diffuse hypervascularization ("thyroid inferno") and this can differentiate Grave's disease from thyrotossicosis due to thyroiditis. Perhaps there is some overlapping on the amount of flow in these two conditions and so the gold standard remains radioiodine uptake.

*Painless Thyroiditis* – The painless thyroiditis is a form of transient autoimmune thyroiditis; it may occur in asymptomatic women aged 30–50 years with level of autoantibody lower than Hashimoto disease (silent thyroiditis) or in women within 1 year after parturition (postpartum thyroiditis). The typical ultrasound pattern is diffuse hypoechogenicity similar to the other form of autoimmune thyroid disease.

*Lymphoma* – The basic requisite to the development of lymphoma is autoimmune thyroiditis because the thyroid contains no native lymphoid tissue. The diffuse form is the most frequent appearance of thyroid lymphoma, instead the focal pattern mimic a cystic lesion and only the color Doppler examination, showing the internal vascularization, can prove that is a solid lesion.

*Subacute Thyroiditis* – Subacute thyroiditis (ST) is a thyroid inflammatory disease occurring after a viral upper respiratory infection. There are three different phases: thyrotoxic, hypothyroid and recovery. The thyrotoxic phase is due to the disruption of follicles with secondary release of stored hormones. Typical sonographic pattern are ill-defined focal areas of huge hypoechogenicity which shows no internal vascularization. These areas develop along the thyroid force line (oriented with long-axis). These areas correspond to the area of tenderness and may be uni or bilateral, migrate overtime from upper to the lower pole or to the contralateral lobe.

*Suppurative Thyroiditis* – The high blood flow, iodine content, hard capsule and excellent lymphatic drainage make the thyroid resistant to infection; for this reason the suppurative thyroiditis is a rare disease. In the early phase is present a thin hypoechoic layer around the thyroid parenchyma; later are present patchy areas of ill-defined hypoechogenicity.

*Riedel's Thyroiditis* – This disease is characterized by intense macrophage and eosinophil infiltration of thyroid parenchyma with extension into adjacent anatomical structures. The ultrasound shows a diffuse enlargement of thyroid which appears hypoechogenic and hypovascularized with emphasis on fibrous septa. Fibrosis increases parenchymal hardness which is well demonstrated by elastography. Neighbouring anatomical structures may be encased by inflammatory process. Stiffness is increased at sonoelastography.

### 1.1.3 Focal Enlargement

The "nodule" can be described as a focal enlargement of thyroid parenchyma definable in all three spatial planes. The role of ultrasound is to confirm the presence and study the characters of palpable nodules and to detect the presence of nodules in the thyroid glands found to be normal on clinical examination in patients with a previous radiation to the head and neck or with a family history of thyroid cancer. The task of ultrasound, however, is not only to identify, locate and measure the nodules but to identify "suspicious" nodules to select those to be submitted to aspiration cytology. Table 1.1 lists the sonographic characters that are reported as being associated with thyroid cancer [5–9].

#### 1.1.3.1 Echogenicity

The echogenicity is the capacity to produce echoes and is proportional to the interfaces present in tissue, more interfaces more echogenicity. A rich cell structure contains less interfaces than a tissue with various components (colloid, cells, etc.) and this is the reason because the more aggressive malignant histotype (solid) appear more hypoechoic than those, more differentiated histotype, in which are present the follicular structures. The determination of echogenicity is usually carried out by comparison with the adjacent parenchyma but in some situations this comparison is rather difficult: in Hashimoto's thyroiditis parenchyma is diffusely hypoechoic. New softwares are developing to quantify natural echogenicity.

**Table 1.1** Gray scale sonographic features reported to be associated with thyroid cancer

| | Median sensitivity (range) (%) | Median specificity (range) (%) |
|---|---|---|
| Hypoechoic vs. surrounding parenchyma | 81 % (48–90 %) | 53 % (36–92 %) |
| Hypoechoic vs. strap muscles | 41 % (27–59 %) | 94 % (92–94 %) |
| Absence of Halo | 44 % (26–53 %) | 89 % (69–98 %) |
| Microcalcifications | 10 % (2–17 %) | 94 % (84–98 %) |
| Macrocalcifications | 66 % (33–100 %) | 43 % (30–77 %) |
| Irregular, microlobulated margins | 55 % (17–84 %) | 80 % (62–85 %) |
| Solid consistency | 86 % (78–91 %) | 48 % (30–58 %) |
| Taller than wide shape on transverse view | 48 % (33–84 %) | 92 % (82–93 %) |

From "*Thyroid Ultrasound and ultrasound-guided FNA*" ed. Baskin, Duik & Levine 2013 Springer

#### 1.1.3.2 Calcifications

There are different categories of calcifications:

1. *Microcalcifications* are small echogenic foci without posterior acoustic shadowing and it is hypothesized that are the ecographic equivalent of psammoma bodies (laminate calcific spherule) that are typical of papillary cancer but occasionally found in Hashimoto diseases or benign nodules. Often in ultrasound reports are described microcalcifications within nodules but in fact these small hyperechoic foci are related to the presence of dense colloid within microcysts associated with the reinforcement of the distal wall (Fig. 1.1).
2. *Macrocalcifications* are larger than 2 mm and causes posterior acoustic shadowing. They may occur either in benign or malignant lesions within areas of fibrosis, tissue degeneration or necrosis.
3. *Peripheral calcifications ("egg shell")* indicate benign lesions in majority of cases but the interruption of peripheral rim may be a sign of cancer invasion [10].

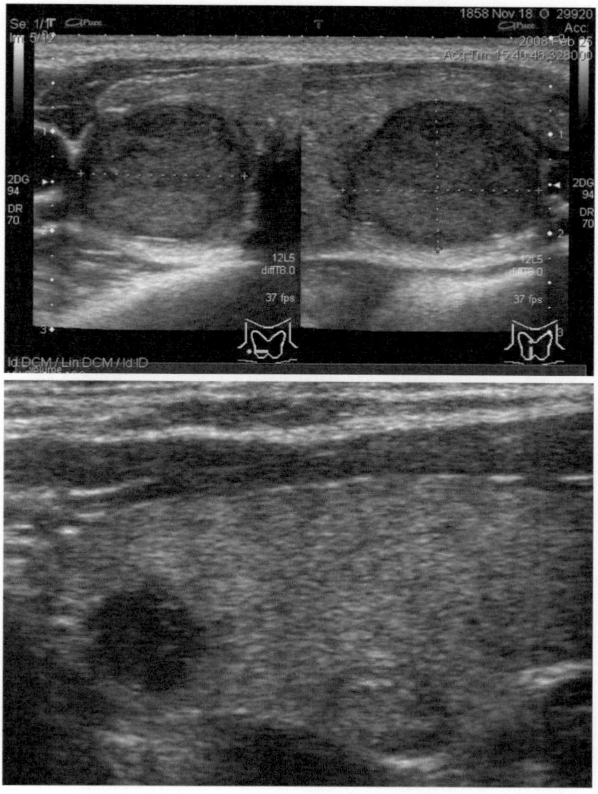


**Fig. 1.1** Benign and malignant nodule. (*Top*) Benign nodule: definite margins with thin and regular hypoechogenic halo (*Bottom*) Malignant nodule: irregular and ill-defined margins without peripheral halo

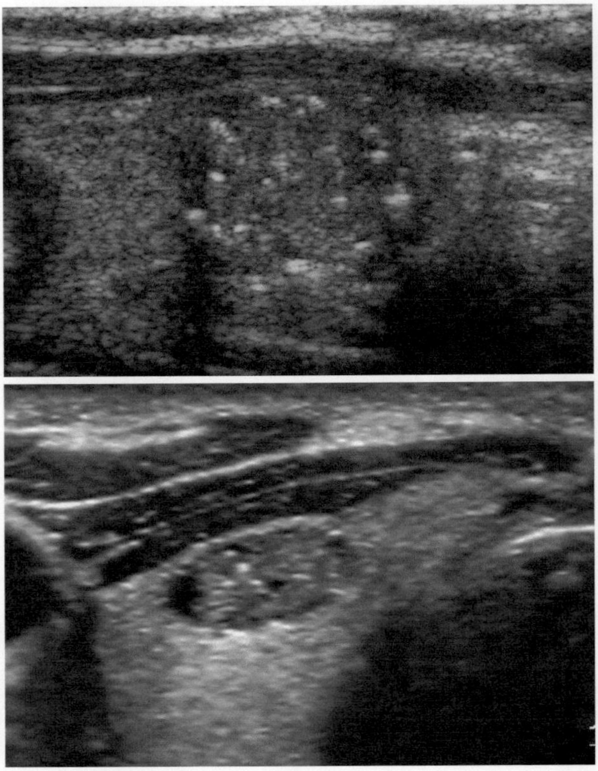

**Fig. 1.2** (*Top*) True microcalcifications. (*Bottom*) Linear hyperechogenic spots due to dense colloid content in microcysts simulating microcalcifications

#### 1.1.3.3 Margins

The new technologies for the transducers (high frequency broad band probes) allow a superb definition of margins of thyroid nodules. The presence of ill-defined margins or microlobulated borders is the sign of infiltrating neoplasia (Fig. 1.2). However, may be present indistinct margins in small hyperplastic nodules that should be not confused for infiltrative.

#### 1.1.3.4 Halo

Halo is hypo-anechoic rim that surrounds a nodule and is commonly interpreted as the image equivalent of compression of perinodular vessels e/o peripheral edema. Hyperplastic nodules grow very slowly and so displace the surrounding thyroid parenchyma bundling blood vessels in the peripheral portions, as demonstrated by color Doppler. Thin peripheral halo is present in about half of benign lesions but is less common in malignant nodules. Thick irregular halo corresponds to the capsule in benign neoplastic nodules.

#### 1.1.3.5 Vascularization

Initially the amount of intralesional vascularity was associated with malignant nodules but the most recent studies have demonstrated, in small papillary cancer, poor intralesional vascularization and a possible explanation of this discrepancy should be related to the specific pattern of neoangiogenesis in this histological type (anarchical texture, tortuous vasa and A/V shunts). Instead the follicular cancer may be more frequently associated with evident intralesional vascularity. The best method to study the internal vascularization of thyroid nodules is the broadband color Doppler because the "normal" color Doppler tends to overwrite the vascular signal giving the impression of a greater intralesional vascularity than the real one; alternatively you can use the power Doppler. Currently are available volumetric probe that allow the real time tridimensional study of parenchymal vascularization: this method demonstrates the real vascular network inside the thyroid nodule avoiding treated as internal vessels those taken enfilade at the outer edge of the nodule.

#### 1.1.3.6 Taller Than Wide

The ratio between anteroposterior and transverse diameter in thyroid nodules (measured on axial scan) may be indicator of malignancy as in the sonographic evaluation of breast carcinoma. The disproportionate growth in the anteroposterior dimension may be interpreted as an aggressive growth pattern across rather than within normal tissue force lines. The benign nodules that can mimic this pattern are respectively meta-hemorrhagic cyst and outcomes of focal thyroiditis.

#### 1.1.3.7 Stiffness

The malignancy is often associated with stiffness. The US elastography is a novel method that evaluates the tissue elasticity through analysis of radiofrequency shift during manual compression. The stiffness alone is not an indicator of malignancy but is an additional tool along with other ultrasound parameters. Ueno has codified a subjective scale with arbitrary color to differentiate benign from malignant lesions: different degrees of tissue elasticity can be color-coded in parametric images making suspicious tissue changes visible in the ultrasonic image. Recently are disposable semiquantitative and quantitative methods to classify the stiffness of a thyroid nodule. The most promising tool is acoustic radiation force impulse (ARFI) that analyzes the velocity of transmission of shear waves through a discrete lesion determining his stiffness in kilopascal (kP).

#### 1.1.3.8 Associated Features

Evidence of pathological lymph node at cervical level and interruption of thyroid capsular profile are ultrasound features that, if associated with the presence of thyroid nodules, may be diagnostic for malignancy.

## 1.2 Neck Lymph Node

The ATA's guidelines for Patients with thyroid nodules and differentiated thyroid cancer has incorporated the neck sonography for the evaluation of patients who undergoing surgery for thyroid cancer as well as for the follow-up after thyroidectomy for thyroid cancer. This comes from the fact that ultrasound has been shown to have good ability to differentiate benign from malignant lymph node [9].

*Benign lymph nodes* have an ovoid shape (short/long axis ratio <0.5), constant and symmetric cortical thickness, homogeneous parenchymal structure and low parenchymal echogenicity with hyper-echoic hilum (due to presence of fat and lymphatic/blood vessels); the parenchymal vascularization seems to be quite regular with arborous pattern [11].

*Malignant lymph nodes*, instead, have a rounded shape (short/long axis ratio >0.5), cortical focal thickening, inhomogeneous parenchymal structure (often with "ground glass" pattern) with absent hilar line; parenchymal vascularization with power Doppler (preferred to color Doppler for its greater sensitivity to arteriolar low velocity blood flow) seems to be anarchic for recruitment of peripheral cortex microscopic vessels. Strong evidence for malignancy is the presence of any type of calcifications (either micro or macro-calcifications with acoustic shadowing). The parenchymal echogenicity is equal to that of native thyroid parenchyma. Cystic necrosis areas inside the lymph node are commonly associated with malignancy. More frequent localization of papillary cancer metastatic lymph-node is the internal jugular chain that occurs between carotid artery and jugular vein; consequently any divergence of these vessels may be an indicator of occult metastatic lymph-node presence; in addition metastatic lymph-node can cause a partial vein obstruction and so color Doppler is the better method to demonstrate slowdown of venous flow. It is noteworthy to point out that some characters of thyroid nodules which are indicators of malignancy may not apply to lymph node (echogenicity, margins etc.). It is crucial to detect macroscopic metastatic lymph-node as their preoperative presence heavily modifies the risk of recurrence while microscopic nodal disease does not affect this risk. The preoperative study of central compartment is difficult for the presence of the thyroid gland that may obscure even macroscopic lymph node but this survey is less important because many endocrine surgeons routinely perform central compartment dissection during total thyroidectomy for cancer. After surgery the follow-up is best performed with association of neck ultrasound and Tg assay; the WBS is an unsatisfactory tool for monitoring patients with thyroid cancer [12–14].

## 1.3 Parathyroid

Primary hyperparathyroidism (PHPT) has an apparent increasing incidence due to the wide availability and high accuracy of multichannel analyzer for routine testing. The majority of patients are well being without clinical symptoms and/or end organ damage. Presence of a solitary adenoma is the most frequent cause of PHPT. Accurate detection and localization of adenoma enables minimally invasive direct parathyroidectomy (MIDP) to be performed in 1-day surgery or with short hospitalization, with reduced local postoperative soreness and better aesthetic results.

*Normal* – The majority of patients have four glands but the presence of supernumerary glands may be considered. The normal parathyroid gland (PTG), as well described for the first time by Sir Richard Owen in 1852 when performed the postmortem examination of a Rhynoceros [15], is ovoid or bean shaped, normally measures approximately 6 mm length, 3–4 mm tranverse and 1–2 mm in anteroposterior diameter; PTGs have a fibro-fatty capsule and his vascular supply is independent from that of the thyroid. Normal parathyroid are not visualized at ultrasound despite the use of high frequency/high resolution probe. When visible they appear as small, well-circumscribed, hypoechoic nodule posterior to thyroid gland separated from echogenic thyroid capsule. Superior PTGs are more constant in position as compared to inferior PTGs; they lie on posterior border of middle 1/3 of thyroid 75 % of time, 25 % found behind upper and lower 1/3 of thyroid, 7 % found below inferior thyroidal artery. Inferior PTGs are more variable in location; they lie lateral to lower pole of thyroid gland (50 %), within 1 cm of inferior poles (15 %) and anywhere from angle of mandible to lower anterior mediastinum (35 %). Understanding of normal anatomical localization and their variations is fundamental to localize pathological parathyroid gland that causes PHTP. Ultrasound study for preoperative localization of parathyroid adenoma must start, with transverse scan, above the thyroid at the angle of mandibole and move downwards through the thyroid to level of clavicle [16].

A simple and reliable description of the exact locations of pathologic parathyroid glands is necessary for unambiguous communications between surgeons and other specialists. A novel system of classification was elaborated by Perrier et al. [17] on the most frequent localization of pathologically enlarged glands. A type A parathyroid gland is a gland that arises from a superior pedicle, lateral to the recurrent laryngeal nerve compressed within the capsule of the thyroid parenchyma. A type B gland is a superior gland that has fallen posteriorly into the tracheoesophageal groove and lies in the same plane as the superior portion of the thyroid lobe. A type C gland is a gland that has fallen posteriorly into the tracheoesophageal groove and lies at the level of or below the inferior pole of the thyroid gland. A type D gland lies in the mid region of the posterior surface of the thyroid parenchyma, near the junction of the recurrent laryngeal nerve and the inferior thyroid artery or middle thyroidal vein; because of this location, dissection is difficult. A type E gland is an inferior gland near to the inferior portions of the thyroid lobe. A type F gland is an inferior gland that has descended into the thyrothymic ligament or superior portions of the thymus and it seems to be "ectopic" within the superior mediastinum. A type G gland is an intrathyroidal parathyroid gland.

*Pathological* – Parathyroid adenomas have some peculiar sonographic character: (1) they have an extra thyroidal location with an hyperchogenic line of demarcation with respect to thyroid parenchyma (due to summation of thyroid capsule and fibro-fatty parathyroid capsule); (2) they have an homogeneous structure with extremely low echogenicity in relation to thyroid parenchyma; (3) they have an independent vascular supply with peculiar unipolar vessel (typically a branch off the inferior thyroidal artery which enters the parathyroid gland at one of the poles; internal vascularity is also commonly seen in a peripheral distribution), less frequent is evident the "vascular arch" sign (the feeding artery tends to branch around the periphery of the gland before penetration giving a characteristic arc or rim of vascularity) and diffuse intralesional vascularization [18, 19]; parathyroid adenomas conform the shape on anatomy of surrounding structures (thyroid, tracheo-esophageal groove, neurovascular bundle) and this must take into account during study of localization to distinguish adenomas from neck lymph nodes or esophitic thyroid nodules [20, 21, 22, 23].

## References

1. Ahuja AT, Evans RM (eds) (2000) Practical head and neck ultrasound. Greenwich Medical Limited, London
2. AIUM (1999) Standards for performance of the thyroid and parathyroid ultrasound examination (AIUM Standard, approved 1998). American Institute of Ultrasound in Medicine, Laurel
3. Livolsi VA (1994) The pathology of autoimmune thyroid disease: a review. Thyroid 4(3): 333–339
4. Anderson L, Middleton W et al (2010) Hashimoto thyroiditis: Part 2, sonographic analysis of benign and malignant nodules in patients with diffuse Hashimoto thyroiditis. AJR Am J Roentgenol 195:216–222
5. Gharib H, Papini E, Paschke R, et al. American Association of Clinical Endocrinologists, Associazione Medici Endocrinologi, and European Thyroid Association. Medical guidelines for clinical practice for the diagnosis and management of thyroid nodules: executive summary of recommendations. Endocr Pract. 2010;16:468–75.
6. Mazzaferri EL (1993) Management of solitary thyroid nodule. N Engl J Med 328:553–559
7. Papini E, Guglielmi R, Bianchini A et al (2002) Risk of malignancy in non palpable thyroid nodules: predictive value of ultrasound and color Doppler features. J Clin Endocrinol Metab 87:1941–1946
8. Langer JE, Mandel SJ (2011) Thyroid nodule sonography: assessment for risk of malignancy. Imaging Med 3:513–524
9. Rago T, Vitti P, Chiovato L et al (1998) Role of conventional ultrasonography and color-flow Doppler sonography in predicting malignancy in "cold" thyroid nodules. Eur J Endocrinol 138:41–46
10. Taki S, Terahata S, Yamashita R et al (2004) Thyroid calcifications: sonographic pattern and incidence of cancer. Clin Imaging 28:268–271
11. Ahuja A, Ying M (2002) An overview of neck node sonography. Invest Radiol 37:333–342
12. Ahuja A, Ying M, Phil M, King A, Yuen HY (2001) Lymph node hilus – gray scale and power Doppler sonography of cervical nodes. J Ultrasound Med 20:987–992
13. Ahuja A, Ying M, Yuen H, Metrewely C (2001) Power Doppler sonography of metastatic nodes from papillary carcinoma of thyroid. Clin Radiol 56:284–288
14. Wang TS, Dubner S et al (2004) Incidence of metastatic well-differentiated thyroid cancer in cervical lymph nodes. Arch Otolaryngol Head Neck Surg 130(1):110–113
15. Owen R (1862) On the anatomy of the Indian Rhinoceros (Rh. Unicornis L.). Trans Zool Soc Lond 4:31–58
16. Gilmore JR (1938) The gross anatomy of parathyroid glands. J Pathol 46:133
17. Perrier ND, Edeiken B, Nunez R, Gayed I, Jimenez C, Busaidy N, Potylchensky E, Kee S, Vu T (2009) A novel nomenclature to classify parathyroid adenomas. World J Surg 33(3):412–416
18. Kamaya A, Quon A, Jeffrey RB (2006) Sonography of abnormal parathyroid gland. Ultrasound Q 22(4):253–262
19. Lane MJ, Desser TS, Weigle RJ, Jeffrey RB (1998) Use of color and power Doppler sonography to identify feeding arteries associated with parathyroid adenomas. AJR Am J Roentgenol 171(3):819–823
20. Andre V, Andre M, Dreff P, Granier H, Forlodou P, Garcia JF (1999) Intrathyroidal parathyroid adenoma. J Radiol 80(6):591–592
21. Wang C (1976) The anatomic basis of parathyroid surgery. Ann Surg 183(3):271–275

22. Frasoldati A, Pesenti M, Toschi E, Azzarito C, Zini M, Valcavi R (1999) Detection and diagnosis of parathyroid incidentalomas during thyroid sonography. J Clin Ultrasound 22(10): 796–799
23. Pesenti M, Frasoldati A, Azzarito C, Valcavi R (1999) Parathyroid incidentaloma discovered during thyroid ultrasound imaging. J Endocrinol Invest 22(10):796–799

# 2 Fine Needle Aspiration Biopsy

Pietro Locantore, Francesca Ianni, and Alfredo Pontecorvi

Thyroid nodules are frequent among general population, although the rate of malignancy is frequently low, ranging from 3 to 7 % [1]. For such reason it is necessary to select the appropriate nodules for which surgery is required. Fine needle aspiration biopsy (FNAB) is a diagnostic test routinely used in the evaluation of thyroid nodule disease and it is crucial to stratify the risk of malignancy. Furthermore, FNAB can also be used to evacuate large cystic nodules and is helpful in patients with thyroid cancer to detect lymph nodes metastases [2].

Many studies have proven the efficacy of FNAB in the management of patients with thyroid nodules with a reported sensitivity of 80–98 % and specificity of 58–100 % [3].

In the past, FNAB could be performed manually only on palpable thyroid nodules, while nowadays, because of the large diffusion of ultrasonography (US), it is possible to detect also nonpalpable nodules and such technique is helpful to identify suspicious nodules. In such situations the FNAB is performed under US guidance, which is the most widely diffused technique.

The first step to examine thyroid nodules is US. US represents the first line test to assess the location of the nodule, the size, the US pattern and to detect any possible suspicious lymph node. On the basis of US findings, considering the clinical history of the patient, the biochemical tests of thyroid function and possible information coming from radionuclide scan (thyroid scintigraphy or PET), the clinician has to select which nodules are eligible for FNAB.

The clinical characteristics that suggest performing FNAB are: patients with family history of thyroid cancer, story of neck irradiation, presence of a single, growing, fix and hard nodule, especially in young patients and in the male gender.

P. Locantore (✉) • F. Ianni • A. Pontecorvi
Unit of Endocrinology, Università Cattolica del Sacro Cuore,
Largo Gemelli, 8, Rome 00168, Italy
e-mail: pietro.locantore@icloud.com; fra_ianni@yahoo.it; pontecorvi@rm.unicatt.it



C.P. Lombardi, R. Bellantone (eds.), *Minimally Invasive Therapies for Endocrine Neck Diseases*, DOI 10.1007/978-3-319-20065-1_2

US suspicious features of thyroid nodules are: solid, hypoechoic, a “taller than wider” shape, irregular margins, absence of halo sign, microcalcifications, intranodular vascular flow.

Moreover, in case of a “cold” nodule, which has a decreased uptake of radionuclide in a conventional thyroid scintigraphy with 99-technetium or 123-Iodine, or in case of a focal uptake of FDG to PET scan, FNAB is suggested in order to exclude malignancy [4].

In presence of a multinodular goiter it is important to identify the most suspicious nodule, which is not always the dominant one. In fact, patients with multiple nodules have the same risk of malignancy as those with a single nodule. Thus, the sonographic features of each nodule should be assessed independently to determine the need for FNAB. If there are multiple coalescent nodules and none have suspicious US features, FNAB of the largest nodule is reasonable. In presence of complex nodules US guidance is essential to assess the biopsy on the solid part of the lesion, to reach a diagnostic conclusion as well as in inhomogeneous nodules US guidance is essential to biopsy the most suspicious part of the nodule.

There is no consensus among the scientific societies about the size of the nodule that can undergo FNAB.

The American thyroid association (ATA) guidelines published in 2009 [5] suggest performing FNAB in nodules: larger than 5 mm in patients with high risk history, larger than 1 cm in case of suspicious US features and larger than 2 cm in absence of suspicious US features. FNAB is not indicated in case of cystic nodule.

AACE/AME/ETA guidelines [2] published in 2010 suggest performing FNAB in nodules of any size in case of high risk patients or in case of US suspicious pattern.

The latest ATA guidelines (in press, presented at ATA satellite symposium at ICE/ENDO – June 2014) suggest performing FNAB in nodules: larger than 1 cm having high-intermediate US suspicious pattern; larger than 1.5 cm having US low suspicious pattern and larger than 2 cm having US very low suspicious pattern. In case of nodules smaller than 1 cm or cystic nodules, FNAB should never be performed.

This new approach is due to the fact that in the last three decades, overdiagnosis of clinically silent thyroid nodules by the widespread use of imaging methods has brought to an increase up to threefolds in the incidence of thyroid cancer, even though the rate of mortality has not changed. Thus far we have detected and treated thyroid microcarcinomas with questionable aggressiveness [6]. For this reason, routine FNAB is not considered cost-effective and an appropriate evaluation by an expert clinician is recommended before undergoing FNAB.

## 2.1 Procedure

FNAB is an invasive procedure and it is fundamental to obtain an adequate signed consent after the patient has been fully informed [7].

The patient must be advised about the procedure, aware of potential complications (usually self-limiting intra or extranodular bleeding), must be instructed not to swallow or speak during the insertion of the needle, must be informed of the need of taking serial samples on the same nodule, the time of the cytological result and the possibility of an inadequate sample, that may require the repetition of the sampling after at least 1 month (if possible to delay the repetition, on the basis of clinical history and US features). Correct information is also adjuvant to let the patient be relaxed during the procedure.

FNAB is a safe and minimally invasive procedure with low risks and can be usually performed on an outpatient basis by experienced physicians. In the past the procedure was performed manually, only on palpable masses, while nowadays US guidance is routinely used. In fact real-time US consents the visualization of the needle within the lesion enabling to reach targets as small as 2 mm, thereby facilitating accurate biopsy of small nonpalpable nodules. Furthermore, a color Doppler evaluation just before the procedure may help the operator to identify any large vessel in the surrounding tissue and choose the best way to sample the nodule, avoiding any vascular injury.

US is performed with a conventional high frequency linear array (7.5–14 MHz). Some arrays may also include specific supports used as needle guide. Such items may be useful in case of prolonged procedures (cyst evacuation, ethanol injection) more than in routine sampling.

A review of recently published data regarding thyroid cancer detection at US-guided FNA indicates a sensitivity of 76–98 %, a specificity of 71–100 %, a false-negative rate of 0–5 %, a false-positive rate of 0–5.7 %, and an overall accuracy of 69–97 % with the use of this method [8]. The false-negative rate with palpation-guided FNA (1–3 %) was higher than that with US-guided FNA (0.6 %) [9]. The literature reveals great variability in specimen cellularity [9]. Although the rate of specimen inadequacy with US-guided FNA is lower than that with palpation-guided FNA, US-guided FNAB yields an inadequate specimen in 10–20 % of procedures, perhaps because of the absence of uniformly adopted or standardized criteria for adequacy of thyroid FNAB specimens and specimen procurement techniques [10].

It is useful to have a proper tray including materials for topical cleaning, transducer covers, coupling gel and a wide set of needles. The needles normally used may be small (25–27 gauge) or medium (21–23 gauge).

The patient is placed in a supine position with the neck slightly extended, with a pillow or a pad placed beneath the patient's shoulders. Anesthesia is not routinely performed. Some operators use topical lidocaine gel or patch, ethyl cloryde spray (that may anyway irritate the skin). In selected cases, especially for long procedures or for the use of large needles, 1–2 ml of 1 % lidocaine solution can be injected subcutaneously. The US monitor must be placed optimally for the operator's view and the US array should be covered with a sterile mean, applying a coupling gel between the array and the sterile mean. The skin in the projective area of the thyroid nodule must be cleaned with an alcoholic solution.

The needles normally used in FNAB rise from 22 to 27 gauge. There is a correlation between the gauge of the needle and the cellularity of specimen, in fact the thinner the needle used, the higher the rate of sufficiency of cytological material. Special needle which are longer may be used for posterior nodules. Each needle may be attached to a 2–20 mL syringe, with an eventual syringe holder, according to the preference of the operator.

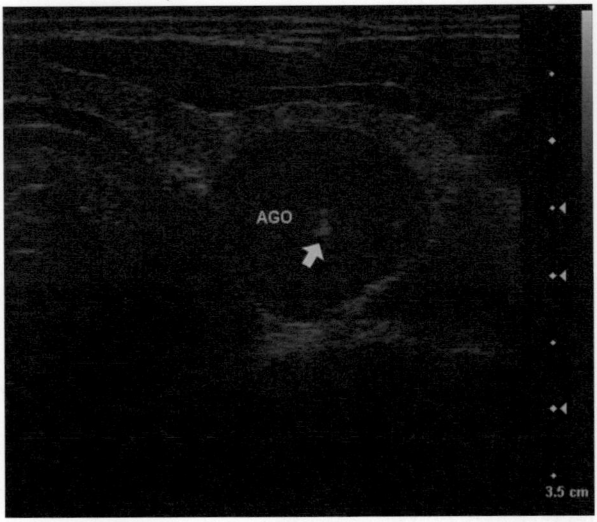


**Fig. 2.1** An US-guided FNAB with perpendicular approach. Only the tip of the needle (*AGO-arrow*) is visible within the nodule as a bright echogenic focus on the monitor

A freehand biopsy technique is the widest used technique. The syringe can be attached to the needle and placed just above the transducer. The needle may be introduced parallel or perpendicular to the transducer, and the needle tip should be carefully monitored during the procedure. All needle movements should be continuously visualized in real time. Poor needle visualization is a common difficulty. If the needle is parallel to the transducer, it will be visible in its entirety. However, if the needle is inserted at a steep angle, as it must be to reach deep lesions, or if it is inserted perpendicular to the probe, localization of its tip is more difficult (Fig. 2.1). The tip of the needle is visible only as a bright echogenic focus on the monitor as the tip bisects the scanning plane. If the needle tip is not visible, the position of the needle and transducer should be adjusted until the tip points toward the center of the lesion. When the needle reaches the target, the biopsy is performed.

Biopsy specimens may be obtained with two widely used acquisition methods. The choice between "nonaspiration" and "aspiration" is a matter of operator preference.

The "needle only" technique or "nonaspiration" technique is based on the principles of capillarity action of cellular material into the needle without aspiration. The needle is withheld with two fingers and inserted in the nodule. After that, the operator should kindly move the needle up and down for a couple of times and may perform rotations of the needle. "Nonaspiration" FNAB is less traumatic and even more rarely associated with complications. The amount of the sample is directly proportional to the time of stay of the needle inside the lesion. After the procedure, the needle is attached to a syringe to extrude the material on the smear or in the vial. Such technique should be modified in case of mixed, hemorrhagic or cystic lesions.

The "aspiration" technique or "closed suction" is characterized by the freehand introduction under US guidance of a needle with a syringe placed on it. When the needle is inside the lesion, the syringe plunger is withdrawn to create a negative pressure and induce aspiration. The needle is moved up and down, the plunger is withdrawn, inside the lesion as long as the needle is taken out of the skin. At that moment the plunger can be released. This technique is very useful to perform the aspiration of fluid lesions.

At present there is no preference between the two techniques, and the choice is based on the feeling and the experience of the operator.

It is recommended that aspiration is performed at least twice at US-guided FNAB because of the fine caliber of the needle, but the number of aspiration can range from one to five aspirations. Multiple punctures of the nodule can ensure samples from different parts of the lesion. In case of complex nodules, with large fluid parts, it is necessary to increase the number of aspirations to obtain adequate samples.

After the procedure, a firm pressure is applied to biopsy site with gauze pad. Once bleeding has stopped, a sticking plaster is placed on the puncture site, the patient is observed for a few minutes and, if there are no problems, allowed to leave. The patient should be instructed to contact hospital staff or seek the emergency room if neck swelling occurs on the way home or at home.

The material collected during FNAB can be processed in two different ways.

Conventional smear (CS) has been the standard diagnostic method for detecting thyroid lesions for many years, as it is cheap, widely codified, quick and easy to be performed. Specimen is suddenly placed on a conventional smear by depositing the needle contents onto a glass slide, then smearing the material. Each slide is then fixed with alcohol prior to staining. When the Papanicolaou staining method is used, the smears should be quickly placed in 95 % ethyl alcohol. When Diff-Quik or Giemsa stain is used, the smear should simply be allowed to air dry. Papanicolaou staining is most commonly used for cytologic analysis of thyroid specimens, and it provides the clearest depiction of nuclear chromatin, ground-glass nuclei, and nuclear groove characteristics in papillary carcinoma. Diff-Quik or Giemsa stain helps visualize the characteristics of cytoplasm and colloid.

Another method for preparing slides is to rinse the contents of the needle into a cell suspension (in the procedure room), which is then used to make liquid-based thin-layer slides, or cell block material (in the laboratory). Liquid-based thin-layer slides are stained with Papanicolaou stain and processed in a cytology laboratory. Cell block material is stained with hematoxylin-eosin stain and processed in a histology laboratory [11].

Some authors have suggested that thin prep is diagnostically superior to conventional preparation in certain nongynecologic specimens, but this technique is quite expensive, as it is necessary to have dedicated laboratory tools and pathologist who are familiar with these cytological samples.

Thin prep has many advantages compared with conventional smears, including ease of preparation by the clinician, more consistent specimen quality, uniform specimen collection, convenient transportation from remote sites, decreased needle handling, preservation of nuclear detail, decreased screening time, and the ability to perform ancillary testing. Many authors have shown that thin prep has diagnostic equivalence to conventional smears but a well-trained pathologist with the newest method is essential because cytologic findings are quite different in the two preparations with regard to amount and character of colloid, architectural disruption, background elements, and nuclear details [12].

The final cytopathologic finding is generally reported using the Bethesda criteria [13], in which a sample is considered adequate if it contains a minimum of six groups of well observed follicular cells, with at least 10 cells per group.

The increasing diffusion of liquid-based thin layer slides has increased the possibility of performing further analysis on the aspired samples to increase sensitivity and specificity of the test, especially in case of undetermined lesion. Such analysis varies from immunocytochemistry to genetic markers. In the recent years there has been a wide diffusion of new marker in thyroid cytology. As to immunocytochemistry, the most diffused markers are galectin-3, HBME-1, CK-19 and CD56, which can be used in combination.

As to molecular markers, the most used genes analyzed are BRAF, RET/PTC and RAS. In the most recent years there are at least two commercial multigene classifiers that can be applied to the FNAB samples to produce risk stratification on the basis of gene profile. Such tests still need to be proved before becoming part of a routine evaluation in the clinical practice [14, 15].

In case of inadequate samples, it can be considered to repeat the procedure no sooner than 1 month (if the US pattern of the nodule is not very suspicious), in order to prevent false-positive interpretation due to biopsy-induced reactive/reparative changes, and if available, it can be useful to have an on-site cytologic evaluation.

In case of repeated inadequate samples, other techniques have been suggested to define the diagnosis of the nodule. The most suggested technique is core-needle biopsy. The 21 gauge needle is inserted into the nodule under US guide in freehand fashion. When the tip is inside of the nodule, mandrel is removed and the needle is advanced within the nodule to obtain a tissue core. Needle is moved ahead across the nodule's margin reaching extranodular tissue. Then, the needle is removed. The obtained core sample is fixed by buffered formalin 10 % [16].

Although FNA is an established test for the evaluation of thyroid nodules with high sensitivity and accessibility, as we mentioned earlier, in some cases it does not yield sufficient diagnostic material even with repeated attempts and scant aspirates or those with borderline adequacy may be a source of diagnostic error. Core-needle biopsy provides a large histologic core of tissue, which may have a greater effect on surgical decision making than the cytologic diagnosis. For these reasons, a core-needle biopsy is considered for patients in whom FNAB produces only specimens of grossly scant-appearing cellularity after several passes or in patients who return for a repeat biopsy after a nondiagnostic initial FNAB.

FNAB is used as therapeutic procedure to evacuate large cystic lesions. After evacuation, it is necessary to monitor the lesion with US, for eventual recurrence. For those patients with subsequent recurrent symptomatic cystic fluid accumulation, surgical removal or percutaneous ethanol injection (PEI) are both reasonable strategies, based on compressive symptoms and cosmetic concerns. The PEI procedure consists in percutaneous intralesional ethanol injection, which induces dehydration followed by coagulative necrosis and vascular thrombosis and occlusion. Volumes of 0.4–2 ml of ethanol are injected, and patients may receive repeated treatments. The technique requires a well-trained staff. Transient, sometimes severe, local pain is the most frequent side effect, followed by transient fever, and occasionally transient dysphonia.

## 2.2 Contraindications

The only serious contraindication is hemorrhagic diathesis. No routine clotting screening are required before FNAB, but in case the patient is on anticoagulant drugs, these must be interrupted at least 5 days before the procedure, shifting the treatment to heparin, under medical supervision. The procedure can be performed only when the clotting parameters are normal.

The use of antiplatelet drugs is not a full contraindication to FNAB, but it increases the risk of bleeding and inadequate samples. For that the clinician should evaluate the risk of a possible interruption of such treatment 3–7 days before the procedure. In such situation it could be useful to defer the procedure and contact the referring physician of the patient to balance the risk.

In case of specific hematological disorders (such as hemophilia or thrombocytopenia), it is necessary to have a specific specialist consult before the procedure.

Furthermore, it is necessary that the patient can lay recumbent in the appropriate position for the biopsy, with an adequate neck hyperextension. In case of old patients or patients with orthopaedics, neurological, or ear disorder such limitation can be so severe that the procedure may result impossible. The patient must also be cooperative with the operator to stand still without swallowing or breathing deeply.

## 2.3 Complications

The possible complications of the procedure can be; hemorrhage, caused by accidental microvascular trauma; large hemorrhage is rare, but the risk is always high, especially in case of nodules adjacent to the vessels (carotid and jugular); pain, due to the skin, muscle and thyroid capsule innervation. Also an accidental puncture of the trachea causes an acute stinging pain. The risk of hemorrhage and pain is increased in case the patient does not stand still during the procedure.

Conventional bleeding and small hemorrhage can be dominated by compression and/or an ice pack. The operator should look for eventual internal bleeding before the patient's departure.

The risk of bacterial infection causing acute thyroiditis is very rare but it has been described in literature. For that it is important to monitor patients with higher risk of infection (AIDS, leucopenia) [17].

## 2.4 Thyroglobulin in Washout Fluid from Lymph Node FNAB

During the follow-up of patients affected by differentiated thyroid cancer (DTC), serum thyroglobulin assays and neck US are routinely recommended for the surveillance of recurrences [5]. Although the criteria for US to distinguish benign from metastatic lymph nodes have been described, its specificity is not optimal. The US criteria for possible malignant infiltration of lymph nodes included: a rounded rather than oval shape, with a long-to-short axis ratio inferior to 1.5, irregular internal echogenicity, calcifications, loss of the fatty hilus peripheral vascularity, and cystic change [5, 18].

To detect and evaluate cervical lymph nodes in patients with thyroid malignancy, US and FNAB have been standard diagnostic modalities. Although the accuracy of US diagnosis of node metastasis has improved, FNAB shows disappointing sensitivity, varying from 75 to 85 % with a high rate of nondiagnostic samples or even provide false-negative results, especially in small or cystic metastatic lymph nodes [19, 20]. To improve the diagnostic yield of FNAB, direct measurement of the concentration of thyroglobulin in the washout fluid of the needle is used in FNAB, since its first description in 1992 [19].

The measurement of thyroglobulin in the washout fluid of lymph node FNAB has been proposed to be a useful diagnostic method in detecting metastatic lymph nodes of DTC patients. Several studies have reported thyroglobulin in the washout fluid of FNAB to be more sensitive than FNAB for detecting metastasis, and the accuracy of FNAB is improved when combined with thyroglobulin in the washout fluid.

US guided FNAB is performed on suspicious lymph nodes by an experienced operator using a 21–25 gauge needle attached to a 10 mL syringe. The technique is the same as thyroid FNAB previously described. Each lesion should be aspirated at least twice. The samples can be placed on glass smears or using thin prep methods for cytological examination. The same needle and syringe must be rinsed with 0.5–1.0 ml of normal saline to a final volume of 1.0 ml and the washout submitted for measurement.

Thyroglobulin assays in the FNAB washout can be performed using electrochemiluminescence (ECLIA) immunoassay, that is conventionally standardized for serum thyroglobulin and results are expressed in "ng/mL". Results are dependent on accurate sampling and a maximum needle wash volume of not more than 1.5 ml.

However, the cutoff value of thyroglobulin in the washout fluid remains controversial on account of differences in sample treatments and thyroglobulin assays. There is no established diagnostic cut off, particularly for the latest generation of highly sensitive thyroglobulin assays [21]. Several cut off have been considered in literature both on the absolute level and as ratio respect to serum thyroglobulin (especially in case of patients with high levels of thyroglobulin on LT4). The role of thyroglobulin in the washout fluid in patients with positive antithyroglobulin antibodies is controversial. Furthermore, the use of thyroglobulin in the washout fluid in the evaluation of suspicious cervical lymph nodes is appropriate in selected patients, but interpretation may be difficult in patients with an intact thyroid gland, as diagnostic test in the preoperative phase.

The same technique can be used also to detect calcitonin in the washout fluid of FNAB of thyroid nodule suspicious for medullary thyroid carcinoma or lymph nodes FNAB in patients affected by medullary thyroid cancer [22]. The limits of the test are the same as thyroglobulin assay. The evaluation of PTH in the washout fluid of FNAB is used to identify lesions suspicious for parathyroid glands or cysts.

## References


1. Hegedus L (2004) Clinical practice. The thyroid nodule. N Engl J Med 351:1764–1771
2. Gharib H, Papini E, Paschke R, Duick DS, Valcavi R, Hegedüs L, Vitti P for the AACE/AME/ETA Task Force on Thyroid Nodules (2010) American Association of Clinical Endocrinologists, Associazione Medici Endocrinologi, and European Thyroid Association medical guidelines for clinical practice for the diagnosis and management of thyroid nodules. Endocr Pract. 16(Suppl 1):1–43
3. De Vos Toto Nederveen Cappel RJ, Bouvy ND, Bonjer HJ et al (2001) Fine needle aspiration cytology of thyroid nodules: how accurate is it and what are the causes of discrepant cases? Cytopathology 12:399–405
4. Chen W, Parsons M, Torigian DA, Zhuang H, Alavi A (2009) Evaluation of thyroid FDG uptake incidentally identified on FDG-PET/CT imaging. Nucl Med Commun 30(3):240–244
5. Cooper DS, Doherty GM, Haugen BR, Kloos RT, Lee SL, Mandel SJ, Mazzaferri EL, McIver B, Pacini F, Schlumberger M, Sherman SI, Steward DL, Tuttle RM (2009) Revised American Thyroid Association management guidelines for patients with thyroid nodules and differentiated thyroid cancer. Thyroid 19(11):1167–1214
6. Brito JP, Morris JC, Montori VM (2013) Thyroid cancer: zealous imaging has increased detection and treatment of low risk tumours. BMJ 347:f4706
7. Kim MJ, Kim EK, Park SI, Kim BM, Kwak JY, Kim SJ, Youk JH, Park SH (2008) US-guided fine-needle aspiration of thyroid nodules: indications, techniques, results. Radiographics 28(7):1869–1886
8. Serna de la Saravia C, Cuellar F, Saravio Day E, Harach HR (2006) Accuracy of aspiration cytology in thyroid cancer: a study in 1 institution. Acta Cytol 50:384–387
9. Danese D, Sciacchitano S, Farsetti A, Andreoli M, Pontecorvi A (1998) Diagnostic accuracy of conventional versus sonography-guided fine-needle aspiration biopsy of thyroid nodules. Thyroid 8:15–21
10. Papanicolaou Society of Cytopathology Task Force on Standards of Practice (1997) Guidelines of the Papanicolaou Society of Cytopathology for fine-needle aspiration procedure and reporting. Diagn Cytopathol 17:239–247
11. Duncan LD, Forrest L, Law WM Jr, Hubbard E, Stewart LE (2011) Evaluation of thyroid fine-needle aspirations: can ThinPrep be used exclusively to appropriately triage patients having a thyroid nodule? Diagn Cytopathol 39(5):341–348
12. Lee SH, Jung CK, Bae JS, Jung SL, Choi YJ, Kang CS (2014) Liquid-based cytology improves preoperative diagnostic accuracy of the tall cell variant of papillary thyroid carcinoma. Diagn Cytopathol 42(1):11–17
13. Cibas ES, Ali SZ, NCI Thyroid FNA State of the Science Conference (2009) The bethesda system for reporting thyroid cytopathology. Am J Clin Pathol 132(5):658–665
14. Alexander EK, Kennedy GC, Baloch ZW, Cibas ES, Chudova D, Diggans J, Friedman L, Kloos RT, LiVolsi VA, Mandel SJ, Raab SS, Rosai J, Steward DL, Walsh PS, Wilde JI, Zeiger MA, Lanman RB, Haugen BR (2012) Preoperative diagnosis of benign thyroid nodules with indeterminate cytology. N Engl J Med 367(8):705–715
15. Nikiforov YE, Carty SE, Chiosea SI, Coyne C, Duvvuri U, Ferris RL, Gooding WE, Hodak SP, LeBeau SO, Ohori NP, Seethala RR, Tublin ME, Yip L, Nikiforova MN (2014) Highly accurate diagnosis of cancer in thyroid nodules with follicular neoplasm/suspicious for a follicular neoplasm cytology by ThyroSeq v2 next-generation sequencing assay. Cancer 120(23):3627–3634
16. Nasrollah N, Trimboli P, Guidobaldi L, Cicciarella Modica DD, Ventura C, Ramacciato G, Taccogna S, Romanelli F, Valabrega S, Crescenzi A (2013) Thin core biopsy should help to discriminate thyroid nodules cytologically classified as indeterminate. A new sampling technique. Endocrine 43(3):659–665
17. Nishihara E, Miyauchi A, Matsuzuka F, Sasaki I, Ohye H, Kubota S, Fukata S, Amino N, Kuma K (2005) Acute suppurative thyroiditis after fine-needle aspiration causing thyrotoxicosis. Thyroid 15(10):1183–1187

18. Schlumberger M, Pacini F, Wiersinga WM, Toft A, Smit JW, Sanchez Franco F, Lind P, Limbert E, Jarzab B, Jamar F, Duntas L, Cohen O, Berg G (2004) Follow-up and management of differentiated thyroid carcinoma: a European perspective in clinical practice. Eur J Endocrinol 151(5):539–548
19. Pacini F, Fugazzola L, Lippi F et al (1992) Detection of thyroglobulin in fine needle aspirates of nonthyroidal neck masses: a clue to the diagnosis of metastatic differentiated thyroid cancer. J Clin Endocrinol Metab 74:1401–1404
20. Frasoldati A, Toschi E, Zini M et al (1999) Role of thyroglobulin measurement in fine-needle aspiration biopsies of cervical lymph nodes in patients with differentiated thyroid cancer. Thyroid 9:105–111
21. Snozek CL, Chambers EP, Reading CC, Sebo TJ, Sistrunk JW, Singh RJ, Grebe SK (2007) Serum thyroglobulin, high-resolution ultrasound, and lymph node thyroglobulin in diagnosis of differentiated thyroid carcinoma nodal metastases. J Clin Endocrinol Metab 92(11): 4278–4281
22. Boi F, Maurelli I, Pinna G, Atzeni F, Piga M, Lai ML, Mariotti S (2007) Calcitonin measurement in wash-out fluid from fine needle aspiration of neck masses in patients with primary and metastatic medullary thyroid carcinoma. J Clin Endocrinol Metab 92(6):2115–2118

# Cytology of Thyroid Lesions

# 3

Guido Fadda and Esther Diana Rossi

## 3.1 Introduction

Fine-needle aspiration cytology (FNAC) represents one of the most important diagnostic tools for evaluating thyroid lesions. It has a worldwide application because of its simplicity, safety and cost-effectiveness, leading to a correct diagnosis in more than 70 % of cases and to a correct clinical approach in more than 90 % of cases [1–4].

Numerous studies have shown that more than 70 % of all thyroid lesions result in a benign histology, between 5 and 10 % are reported as "malignant" and the remaining 20–25 % represents the so-called gray zone in which different benign and malignant entities are included and may result in a high number of unnecessary surgical operations [1–13].

The core-needle biopsy (CNB) is a procedure alternative to FNAC which involves the use of needles slightly larger than those adopted for that technique (18–21 G). The advantages of CNB are represented by a larger amount of cells which may decrease the rate of inadequate diagnoses and the possibility to obtain tissue samples useful for the application of special investigations. The disadvantages of CNB include the increased possibility of complications, such as hemorrhage and local pain, and the difficulty of performing multiple samplings of the lesion [12, 13].

The thin-layer or liquid-based cytology (LBC) technique, originally developed for application to gynecologic cervical smears, has progressively gained consensus after being applied to both non-gynecologic and fine-needle aspiration cytology.

This method is based on a two-step procedure: (a) the fixation of the totality of the material in an alcohol-based solution (methanol or ethanol depending on the

G. Fadda, MD, MIAC (✉) • E.D. Rossi, MD, PhD, MIAC
Division of Anatomic Pathology and Histology,
Catholic University "Agostino Gemelli" School of Medicine and Hospital, Rome, Italy
e-mail: guidofadda@rm.unicatt.it



C.P. Lombardi, R. Bellantone (eds.), *Minimally Invasive Therapies for Endocrine Neck Diseases*, DOI 10.1007/978-3-319-20065-1_3

technique – see below); (b) the automated processing of the material to obtain a thin layer of representative cells. A computer-assisted device transfers the fixed and partially disaggregated cells onto a single slide. The two most popular methods for LBC processing use an alcohol-based fixative solution. In the first (ThinPrep2000™, and ThinPrep5000™ Hologic Co., Marlborough, MA), the cells are aspirated from a methanol-based solution (Cytolit™) then filtered and transferred onto a positively charged slide with a gentle positive pressure. In the second (PrepStain LBC™, TriPath Imaging, Burlington, VT), the cells are collected in an ethanol-based solution (CytoRich™), centrifuged twice then slowly sedimentated onto a poly-L-lysinated slide and eventually stained with a specific hematoxylin-eosin stain. The final result for both methods is a glass slide for each lesion where the cells are concentrated onto the central area of the slide measuring 20 square mms for ThinPrep and 13 square mms for PrepStain LBC [12].

The LBC method enables the storage of a variable amount of cells in a preservative solution for up to 6 months after the biopsy. The remaining material can be used for the application of ancillary techniques such as immunocytochemistry and molecular biology [11, 14–17].

## 3.2 Non-neoplastic Lesions

A cytological sample must be adequate in terms of amount of cellularity and satisfactory in terms of quality. The definition of unsatisfactory smears implies difficulties in fixation, smearing, or staining artifacts which might impair the interpretation of the final slide. A slide is non-representative when cellularity does not represent the true components of the lesion (e.g., insufficient amount of follicular cells) [18]. In the first instance the inadequacy of the sample could be attributed to an incorrect technique, and in the latter the characteristics of the lesion do not allow a definitive cytological diagnosis [19–21]. The adequacy criteria are met when at least 6 clusters of 10–20 well-preserved cells are observed [19–21]. When using LBC preparations a second slide can be prepared with the residual preservative cells in order to meet the above mentioned adequacy criteria. In this perspective up to 18 % of cases diagnosed as inadequate with the first slide can be reclassified as adequate with the second slide. The evidence of this result is more significant than the data by Hasteh who dismiss as expensive and useless the preparation of a second ThinPrep slide [23, 24]. The LBC ThinPrep-processed slides may present scant ill-preserved cells at the periphery due to the positive pressure which may be responsible of cellular artifacts [24]. On the other hand, SurePath, according to Geers and Bourgain showed 25 % inadequacy rate on thyroid FNAC which can probably be an effect of the low sedimentation rate of the colloid droplets which might hamper their inclusion in the final slide [25].

In the category of non-neoplastic lesions we should include also cystic lesions which are another frequent responsible of inadequate results [17]. We need to distinguish a true pseudo-cystic lesion (lacking follicular cells in its wall) from the more frequent cystic or hemorrhagic regression of a nodule which might turn out to

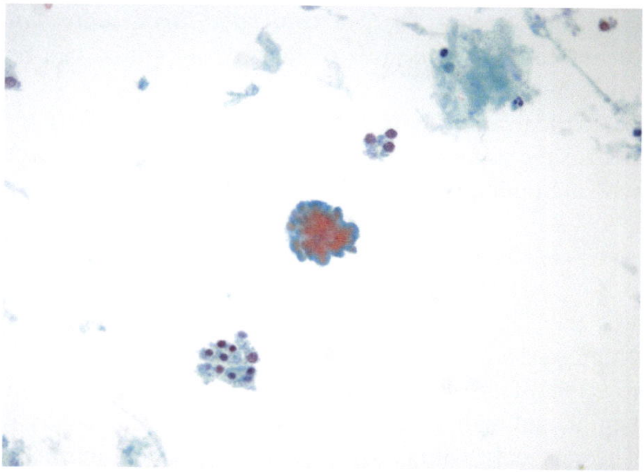

**Fig. 3.1** A colloid goiter showing a colloid droplet and clusters of typical follicular cells (LBC, Pap, 300×)

be benign or malignant after repeated samplings. In our studies cystic/hemorrhagic lesions accounted for about 7 % of all cases of our series which is in agreement with the general acceptance [9–14]. In the non-diagnostic category repetition of the FNA is recommended under US-guidance after at least 1 month. US-guided CNB may be considered in case of repeatedly non-diagnostic FNA samples [17].

A benign diagnosis is the most common cytological finding accounting for about 70 % of all cases in the majority of the series. Most benign lesions arising in the thyroid gland are classified in one the following groups: (1) nodular goiter; (2) thyroiditis; (3) Graves Disease.

The FNA of a *colloid goiter* is characterized by a wide range of morphological patterns reflecting different stages of the disease including also the detection of secondary changes such as oxyphilic metaplasia, hemorrhagic and/or cystic changes, granulation tissue, fibrosis, and calcifications. The morphological features of a colloid nodule are composed by a large amount of colloid, benign follicular cells, and some macrophages repleted of colloid material (foamy cells) (Fig. 3.1).

The cytological findings of a nodular lesion in *Graves's disease* is not specific similar to a benign goiter sometimes with the presence of lymphocytes and oncocytes in the background. The keystone feature is the presence of flame cells characterized by marginal cytoplasm vacuoles with red frayed edges.

*Chronic lymphocytic (Hashimoto's) thyroiditis* is characterized by a variable amount of lympho-monocytic cells in the background admixed with oxyphilic cells. When a thyroiditis is suspected, the detection of lympho-epithelial clusters in an inflammatory background is the pivotal clue for the diagnosis on LBC slides [15, 22–25]. Oxyphilic hyperplastic nodules in a thyroiditis should not be surgically removed because they represent the functional replacement of the parenchyma infiltrated by the inflammatory cells. Thus, the identification of oxyphilic cells in a background of inflammatory cells virtually does rule out an oxyphilic neoplasm and warrants a simple follow-up for the patient [15, 17].

*Granulomatous De Quervain's and Riedel's thyroiditis* are less common variants of inflammatory diseases of the thyroid which can be encountered in the routine practice [26, 27].

Clinical and US follow-up are suggested for non-neoplastic nodules. Repeat FNA is recommended in case of nodule growth or structural changes, and in patients who are undergoing ablative treatments [17].

## 3.3 Indeterminate Lesions

Numerous studies demonstrated that indeterminate lesions (IL) may account for up to 20 % of cytological diagnoses and they represent a "gray zone" in which both benign and malignant entities are included, especially PTC and its variants [28, 29]. The surgical treatment of IL results in a high number of unnecessary thyroidectomies which may cause additional morbidity and increase of health care costs [28–30]. The impossibility to evaluate any capsular or vascular invasion, which is the cornerstone of the diagnosis of differentiated carcinoma, represents a major limit of morphology and decreases the overall diagnostic accuracy of FNAC.

An articulate debate on this IL category has emerged in a number of new classification systems for reporting thyroid cytopathology leading to a division in subcategories with different risks of malignancy [28–31]. The Bethesda Reporting System for Thyroid Cytology (TBRSTC) subclassified IL in three categories: (1) atypia of undetermined significance and follicular lesions of undetermined significance (AUS/FLUS); (2) follicular neoplasms or suspicious for follicular neoplasm (FN/SFN); and (3) suspicious for malignancy (SM). The two published European classifications, with different definitions, have kept the distinction of IL in three categories [17, 30, 31].

The diagnosis of IL is based upon the identification of microfollicles made up of medium-sized thyrocytes in a background with scant colloid (Fig. 3.2).

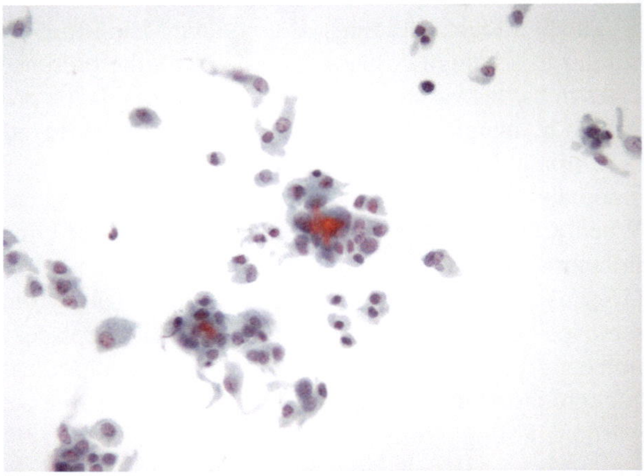

**Fig. 3.2** Microfollicular aggregates of thyroid cells from a follicular neoplasm (LBC, Pap, 300×)

In this category there is an almost complete agreement in the different classification systems in terms of malignancy risk (between 15 and 30 %). A general consensus was evident in the therapeutic action of the surgical removal of the lesion, preferably after a collegial discussion. At histology an indeterminate lesion may correspond to both a follicular adenoma or an adenomatous nodule in a goiter (70–80 % of cases) although on a morphological basis a follicular carcinoma or a follicular variant of a papillary carcinoma cannot be ruled out.

An advantage of the LBC technique in IL is the possibility to apply additional investigations (immunocytochemistry, flow cytometry, molecular biology) to the cells left in the vial and these procedures are particularly helpful in defining the malignant risk of the lesion (see below) [11, 32–34]. Our recent experience involving an immunocytochemical panel made up of HBME-1 and Galectin-3 pointed to an 81 % overall diagnostic accuracy in discriminating between low and high risk of malignancy in follicular proliferations, which increased to 92 % when a concordant positive panel was applied [11, 33, 34].

TBRSTC includes, in the IL category, the "follicular lesion with undetermined significance (FLUS)" or "atypical cells of undetermined significance (ACUS or AUS)." The morphological criteria for diagnosing AUS/FLUS of TBRSTC was based on smears with cells showing architectural and/or nuclear atypia that are not sufficient to be classified as suspicious for follicular neoplasm [28, 29, 35–37]. The reasons for enclosing a case in this category are briefly three: (1) technical problems including poor preservation or drying, artifact; (2) some atypical features but the amount of material is scant for a diagnosis; (3) atypia may be architectural or cytologic [28]. The low malignant risk indeterminate category has been only recently included in the European classifications although some papers concerning the efficacy of the AUS/FLUS category of the Bethesda system underline some difficulties in a correct definition of this category and that some studies have reported malignancy rates similar to the follicular neoplasm category [22].

The same diagnostic criteria and therapeutic actions are applied to indeterminate lesions composed mostly by oxyphilic (or Hurthle) cells (see Sect. 3.3). Smears of an oxyphilic lesion are categorized as "Oxyphilic or Hurthle cell neoplasm" when more than 90 % of the component are oxyphilic cells. These cells may feature nuclear enlargement and pleomorphism which are clinically irrelevant since they can be found in benign neoplasms or even in hyperplastic lesions [15, 38–40].

Recent studies support the idea that the majority of oxyphilic neoplasms histologically represent oxyphilic adenomas thus these nodules might be only followed-up instead of being surgically removed [40].

The clinical recommendation for IL of low malignant risk (FLUS/AUS, Thy 3f, TIR 3A) is follow-up in most cases. During the follow-up repeat FNA is recommended (after 6 months in the Bethesda classification) [17, 28, 31, 41]. Surgery is the recommended option for IL of high malignant risk and oxyphilic neoplasms (FN/SFN, HCN/SHCN, Thy 3a, TIR 3B). Frozen section examination is generally not recommended [17, 28, 31, 41].

## 3.4 Suspicious for Malignancy

This category is one of the three subgroups of IL [17, 28, 31, 41]. These cases exhibit some features consistent for a diagnosis of papillary carcinoma but lack the presence of the major criterion (nuclear pseudoinclusions or "Orphan Annie's eye"). These cases bear a risk of malignancy ranging between 60 and 80 %. With a diagnosis of SM the surgical consultation is strongly recommended. The intraoperative frozen section examination may be considered. Repeat FNA may be performed either in cases with poor cellularity or in those needing additional techniques for a better characterization.

## 3.5 Malignant Neoplasms

Thyroid malignancy represents 4–8 % of all FNAC and the majority of them (90 %) are papillary thyroid carcinoma. The diagnostic accuracy of FNAC is at about 96–100 % [28, 42–45]. This tumor type and its variants (follicular variant of PTC, Tall cell PTC, macrofollicular PTC) show evidence of follicular differentiation with the typical distinctive nuclear features.

The most important and common malignant tumor which should be appropriately identified is *papillary thyroid carcinoma (PTC)*. This entity accounts for 80 % of all cancers. The LBC diagnosis of PTC is straightforward when the nuclear pseudo-inclusions (major criterion) are detected even within tridimensional clusters of cells with nuclear elongation and clearing (Fig. 3.3) [28, 29]. Papillary structures, multinuclear giant cells, typical "chewing-gum" colloid, and psammoma bodies are seldom identified.

In this group we can include also the *cystic variant of PTC* in which the cytological smear includes also histiocytes, watery fluid, and macrophages. The diagnosis is based on the evidence of convincing nuclear features of PTC [28].

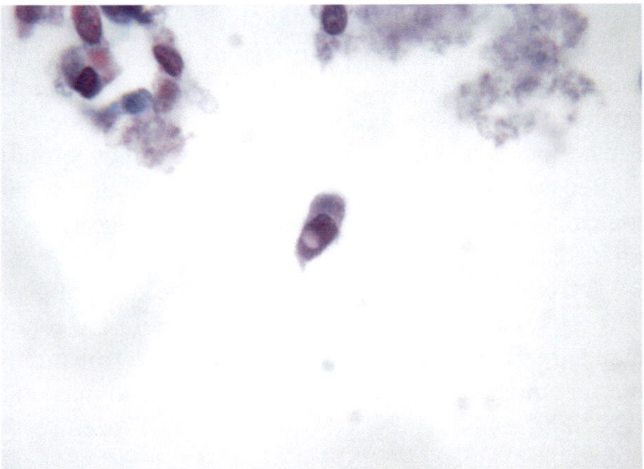

**Fig. 3.3** In the center a PTC cell with the distinctive nuclear inclusion (Orphan Annie's eye) (LBC, Pap, 500×)

Major difficulties might be encountered in the diagnosis of a *follicular variant of PTC (FVPC)* because of the lack of the typical parameters. The major misleading parameter is the absence of papillary structures and the bland nuclear features which may fall short of a correct diagnosis. All the morphological parameters are subtler than on classical PTC smear.

The variants of PTC include either tumor types which share the same prognosis and therapeutical options of the two most important variants presented above (macrofollicular, oncocytic, and cystic variants) and a few histotypes which pursue a more aggressive course (tall cell, columnar cell, and diffuse sclerosing variants). Regardless of the prognostic outlook, all these tumors show the same nuclear features of PTC so that the diagnosis is virtually always possible in the preoperative phase [42–45].

The *poorly differentiated category* of malignant neoplasm was proposed by Carcangiu as an intermediate malignancy between differentiated follicular neoplasms and anaplastic carcinomas [46, 47]. This category shows a variety of different degree of pleomorphic features.

*Anaplastic thyroid carcinoma (ATC)* is a rare and extremely aggressive thyroid carcinoma. It accounts for less than 5 % of all thyroid carcinoma with a very poor outcome and most of the patients succumb in a period of 1 year. This entity is an uncommon finding in thyroid cytology as this tumor presents a rapid growth which frustrates the attempts to plan a surgical strategy [48]. Cytological smears are composed of variable cellularity made up of large undifferentiated polygonal or spindle cells mixed with necrotic debris. The aggregation of these cells and their large cytoplasms help in distinguishing ATC from large-cell non-Hodgkin malignant lymphoma, which represents, from a clinical and morphologic viewpoint, the most important differential diagnosis.

*Medullary thyroid carcinoma (MTC)* represents 7 % of all thyroid carcinomas and can appear as a sporadic (75 %) or familiar disease (25 %) with a dominant autosomal mode of inheritance [49, 50]. The cytological diagnosis of MTC relies on the identification of a population of both plasmacytoid and spindle cells with variable nuclear pleomorphism. The typical amyloid substance with dense, amorphous texture may be present. Although the diagnosis of MTC can be suggested by morphology alone, it is advisable to confirm it by the immunocytochemical evaluation which offers the opportunity to identify calcitonin and CEA in the neoplastic cells [49–51].

A *miscellaneous* group may include both benign and malignant conditions. One of the most controversial is hyalinizing trabecular tumor (HTA) which is a rare follicular derived neoplasm which shows trabecular pattern, intratrabecular hyalinization, and some nuclear features of PTC. For this reason, some authors consider it as a variant of PTC with a benign course [51].

Primary thyroid lymphomas account for 5 % of all thyroid tumors and 2.5–7 % of all extrathyroid lymphomas [52].. Both Hodgkin's disease and non-Hodgkin lymphoma may affect the thyroid gland although the latter outnumbers the first entity. Several papers report that diffuse large-cell lymphomas, extranodal marginal zone B-cell lymphoma or mixed patterns are the most frequent types. Other types have also been reported including follicular and Burkitt's lymphoma.

The smear is cellular with prevalence of round non-cohesive lymphocytes. Their nuclei show coarse chromatin with prominent nucleoli and in some types, large basophilic cytoplasms may be detected (diffuse large B-cell lymphoma). The use of immunocytochemical markers for lymphoid lineage (LCA, CD20, bcl-6, and others) reveals a monoclonal phenotype and is helpful in the correct diagnosis. The main difficult differential diagnosis is with Hashimoto's thyroiditis and anaplastic carcinoma. The combining evaluation of morphology and application of ancillary techniques represent the keystone for the correct diagnosis.

Other primary rare entities include salivary gland carcinomas, neural tumors, parathyroid adenomas, thymomas, liposarcomas, and metastatic neoplasms from lung, breast, kidney, and laryngeal primaries [53–55].

## 3.6 Reporting Systems for Thyroid Cytology

The need of a clarity of communication led to some classification systems in order to obtain a succinct, unambiguous, and clinically useful interpretation of the FNAC [17, 22, 28–31, 56].

An articulate debate was delivered for the follicular neoplasm category as emerged in a number of new classification systems for reporting thyroid cytopathology which led to a division in subcategories with different risks of malignancy [17, 19, 21, 28–31, 41].

In this regard several classifications with different tiered schemes were discussed including the proposals of the Papanicolaou Society, the American Thyroid Association, the American Association of Clinical Endocrinologists and the British Thyroid Association [28–31]. As discussed in the FN section, a conclusion was reached by the National Cancer Institute (NCI) State of the Science conference in which the Bethesda System of Reporting Thyroid Cytopathology proposed three subcategories of the follicular/indeterminate neoplasms including (1) follicular lesions of indeterminate significance or atypia of undetermined significance (AUS); (2) follicular neoplasms and hurtle cell neoplasms (FN); (3) suspicious for malignancy (SM). The stratification of cancer risk for each of these categories ranged from 5 to 75 % [23, 24, 32]. However, as emerged by several papers, one of the limit of this subclassification of FN is the difficult reproducibility of the criteria even among expert cytopathologists [17, 19, 21, 28–31, 41].

Recently, some authors and also Bongiovanni in a meta-analytical article underlined the high overall accuracy of the Bethesda System for Reporting Thyroid Cytopathology which can be reckoned as a valid and reliable system [22].

Concerning the European scenario, except for the United Kingdom and Italy, no European country has a reporting system. The British Thyroid Association/Royal College of Pathologists subclassified follicular neoplasms (FN) into the two subgroups of Thy3a-AUS of undetermined significance and Thy3f-Follicular neoplasm with a good diagnostic agreement among British cytopathologists. In their system, any case categorized as Thy3a, Thy3f, Thy4, or Thy5 is reviewed by a multidisciplinary team in order to establish a correct management [31, 41]. Although the current Italian classification includes a single category of FN group with 20 % cancer risk, a new classification with a subdivision of the Follicular Neoplasm category in two subgroups TIR 3A (corresponding to AUS/FLUS of the Bethesda system to the Thy3f of the BTA/RCPath) and TIR 3B (corresponding to the FN/SFN of Bethesda and Thy3a of the BTA/RCPath) has been recently published [17]. As discussed in a recent paper by Cochand-Priollet, although the idea to extend the Bethesda unique project in Europe was supported by translations in the native language of some countries, some discrepancies and disagreement regarding the use of the Bethesda system occurred in the categories of AUS/FLUS and FN [56]. Furthermore, one of the problems, which need to be solved, is the comparison of data from different reporting systems.

## References


1. Fadda G, LiVolsi VA (1999) Histology and aspiration cytology of benign thyroid lesions. Rays 24:182–196
2. Galera-Davidson H, Gonzalez-Campora R (2008) Chapter 23: Thyroid. In: Bibbo M, Wilbur D (eds) Comprehensive cytopathology, vol 3. Saunders Elsevier, Philadelphia, pp 633–670
3. Bishop-Pitman M, Abele J, Ali SZ, Duick D, Elsheikh TM, Brooke Jeffrey R, Powers CN, Randolph G, Renshaw A, Scoutt L (2008) Techniques for thyroid FNA: a synopsis of the National Cancer Institute thyroid fine-needle aspiration state of the science conference. Diagn Cytopathol 36:407–424
4. Ghofrani M, Beckman D, Rimm DL (2006) The value of onsite adequacy assessment of thyroid fine-needle aspirations is a function of operator experience. Cancer Cytopathol 108: 110–113
5. Na DG, Kim JH, Sung JY, Baek JH, Jung KC, Lee H, Yoo H (2012) Core-needle biopsy is more useful than repeat fine-needle aspiration in thyroid nodules read as nondiagnostic or atypia of undetermined significance by the Bethesda system for reporting thyroid cytopathology. Thyroid 22:468–475
6. Samir AE, Vij A, Seale MK, Desai G, Halpern E, Faquin WC, Parangi S, Hahn PF, Daniels GH (2012) Ultrasound-guided percutaneous thyroid nodule core biopsy: clinical utility in patients with prior nondiagnostic fine-needle aspirate. Thyroid 22:461–467
7. Nasrollah N, Trimboli P, Guidobaldi L, CicciarellaModica DD, Ventura C, Ramacciato G, Taccogna S, Romanelli F, Valabrega S, Crescenzi A (2013) Thin core biopsy should help to discriminate thyroid nodules cytologically classified as indeterminate. A new sampling technique. Endocrine 43:659–665
8. Rossi ED, Fadda G (2008) Thin-layer liquid-based preparation of exfoliative non-gynaecologic and fine-needle aspiration biopsy cytology. Diagn Histopathol 14:563–570
9. Rossi ED, Raffaelli M, Zannoni GF, Pontecorvi A, Mulè A, Callà C, Lombardi CP, Fadda G (2009) Diagnostic efficacy of conventional as compared to liquid-based cytology in thyroid lesions. Evaluation of 10,360 fine needle aspiration cytology cases. Acta Cytol 53:659–666
10. Fadda G, Rossi ED, Raffaelli M, Mulè A, Pontecorvi A, Miraglia A, Lombardi CP, Vecchio FM (2006) Fine-needle aspiration biopsy of thyroid lesions processed by thin-layer cytology: one-year institutional experience with Histologic correlation. Thyroid 16:975–981
11. Rossi ED, Raffaelli M, Minimo C, Mule' A, Lombardi CP, Vecchio FM, Fadda G (2005) Immunocytochemical evaluation of thyroid neoplasms on thin-layer smears from fine-needle aspiration biopsies. Cancer Cytopathology 105:87–95
12. Gharib H (2004) Changing trends in thyroid practice: understanding nodular thyroid disease. Endocr Pract 10:31–39
13. Yassa L, Cibas ES, Benson CB, Frates MC, Doubilet PM, Gawande AA, Moore FD Jr, Kim BW, Nosè V, Marqusee E, Reed Larsen P, Alexander EK (2007) Long-term assessment of a multidisciplinary approach to thyroid nodule diagnostic evaluation. Cancer 111:508–516

14. Fadda G, Rossi ED (2011) Liquid based cytology in fine needle aspiration biopsies of the thyroid gland. Acta Cytol 55:389–400
15. Rossi ED, Zannoni GF, Lombardi CP et al (2012) Morphological and immunocytochemical diagnosis of thyroiditis: comparison between conventional and liquid based cytology. Diagn Cytopathol 40:404–409
16. Linder J (1998) Recent advances in thin-layer cytology. Diagn Cytopathol 18:24–32
17. Nardi F, Basolo F, Crescenzi A, Fadda G, Frasoldati A, Orlandi F, Palombini L, Papini E, Zini M, Pontecorvi A, Vitti P (2014) Italian consensus for the classification and reporting of thyroid cytology. J Endocrinol Invest 37(6):593–599
18. Haider AS, Rakha EA, Dunkley C et al (2011) The impact of using defined criteria for adequacy of fine needle aspiration cytology of the thyroid in routine practice. Diagn Cytopathol 39:81–88
19. Baloch ZW, Cibas ES, Clark DP et al (2008) The National Cancer Institute thyroid fine needle aspiration state of the science conference: a summation. Cytojournal 5:6
20. Chow LS, Gharib H, Goellner JR et al (2001) Nondiagnostic thyroid fine needle aspiration cytology: management dilemmas. Thyroid 11:1147–1151
21. Guidelines of the Papanicolaou Society of Cytopathology for the examination of fine needleaspiration specimens from thyroid nodules: the Papanicolaou Society of Cytopathology Task Force on Standards of Practice (2007) Diagn Cytopathol 15:84–89
22. Bongiovanni M, Spitale A, Faquin WC et al (2012) The Bethesda system for reporting thyroid cytopathology: a meta-analysis. Acta Cytol 56:333–339
23. Rossi ED, Morassi F, Santeusanio G et al (2010) Thyroid fine-needle aspiration cytology processed by thin prep: an additional slide decreased the number of inadequate results. Cytopathology 5:21–26
24. Hasteh F, Pang Y, Pu R, Michael CW (2007) Do we need more than one ThinPrep to obtain adequate cellularity in fine needle aspiration? Diagn Cytopathol 35:740–743
25. Geers AJ, Bourgain C (2011) Liquid based FNAC of the thyroid: a 4 year survey with SurePath. Cancer Cytopathol 119:58–67
26. Lu CP, Chang TC, Wang CY et al (1997) Serial changes in ultrasound guided fine needle aspiration cytology in subacute thyroiditis. Acta Cytol 41:238–243
27. Harigopal M, Sahoo S, Recant WM et al (2004) Fine needle aspiration of Riedel's disease: report of a case and review of the literature. Diagn Cytopathol 30:193–197
28. Cibas ED, Ali S (2001) The Bethesda system for reporting thyroid cytopathology. Am J Clin Pathol 32:658–665
29. The Papanicolaou society of cytopathology task force on standards of practice. Guidelines of the Papanicolaou society of cytopathology for the examination of fine needle aspiration specimens from thyroid nodules (1996) Mod Pathol 9:710–15.
30. Fadda G, Basolo F, Bondi A et al.; SIAPEC-IAP Italian Consensus Working Group (2010) Cytological classification of thyroid nodules. Proposal of the SIAPEC-IAP Italian consensus working group. Pathologica 102:405–408
31. Lobo C, McQueen A, Beale T et al (2011) The UK royal college of pathologists thyroid fine-needle aspiration diagnostic classification is a robust tool for the clinical management of abnormal thyroid nodules. Acta Cytol 55:499–506
32. Fadda G, Rossi ED, Raffaelli M et al (2011) Follicular thyroid neoplasms can be classified as low and high risk according to HBME-1 and Galectin 3 expression on liquid based fine needle cytology. Eur J Endocrinol 165:447–453
33. Correia-Rodrigues HG, Nogueira De Pontes AA et al (2012) Use of molecular markers in samples obtained from preoperative aspiration of thyroid. End J 59:417–424
34. Rossi ED, Martini M, Capodimonti S et al (2013) Diagnostic and prognostic value of immunocytochemistry and BRAF mutation analysis on liquid based biopsies of thyroid neoplasms suspicious for carcinoma. Eur J Endocrinol 168:853–859
35. Nayar R, Ivanovic M (2009) The indeterminate thyroid FNA: experience from an academic center using terminology similar to that proposed in the 2007 NCI Thyroid Fine needle aspiration state of the science conference. Cancer Cytopathol 117:195–2002

36. Faquin WC, Cibas ED, Renshaw AA (2005) Atypical cells in fine needle aspiration biopsy specimens of benign thyroid cysts. Cancer 105:71–79
37. Mahajan A, Lin X, Nayar R (2013) Thyroid Bethesda reporting category, suspicious for papillary thyroid carcinoma, pitfalls and clues to optimize the use of this category. Cytopathol 24:85–91
38. Giorgadze T, Rossi ED, Fadda G et al (2004) Does the fine needle aspiration diagnosis of "Hurthle cell neoplasm/follicular neoplasm with oncocytic features" denote increased risk of malignancy? Diagn Cytopathol 31:307–312
39. Renshaw A (2002) Hurthle cell carcinoma us a better gold standard than Hurthle cell neoplasm for thyroid fine needle aspirates: defining more consistent and specific cytologic criteria. Cancer 96:261–266
40. Rossi ED, Martini M, Straccia P et al (2013) The cytological category of oncocytic [Hurthle] cell neoplasm mostly includes low-grade risk lesions at histology: an institutional experience. Eur J Endocrinol 169:649–655
41. British Thyroid Association (2007) Guidelines for the management of thyroid cancer, 2nd edn. Royal College of Physicians [in association with] British Thyroid Association, London
42. Solomon A, Gupta PK, LiVolsi VA et al (2002) Distinguishing tall cell variant of papillary thyroid carcinoma from usual variant of papillary thyroid carcinoma in cytologic specimens. Diagn Cytopathol 27:143–148
43. Chung D, Ghossein RA, Lin O (2007) Macrofollicular variant of papillary carcinoma: a potential thyroid FNA pitfall. Diagn Cytopathol 35:560–564
44. Odashiro D, Nguyen GH (2006) Diffuse sclerosing variant papillary carcinoma of the thyroid: report of four cases with fine needle aspirations. Diagn Cytopathol 34:247–249
45. Moreira AL, Waisman J, Cangiarella JF (2004) Aspiration cytology of the oncocytic variant of papillary adenocarcinoma of the thyroid gland. Acta Cytol 48:137–141
46. Carcangiu ML, Zampi G, Rosai J (1984) Poorly differentiated [insular] thyroid carcinoma. A reinterpretation of Langhans "Wuchernde struma". Am J Surg Pathol 8:655–668
47. Bongiovanni M, Bloom L, Krane JF et al (2009) Cytomorphologic features of poorly differentiated thyroid carcinoma. A multi institutional analysis of 40 cases. Cancer Cytopathol 117:185–194
48. Brooke PK, Hameed M, Zakowski MF (1994) Fine needle aspiration of anaplastic thyroid carcinoma with varied cytologic and histologic patterns. Diagn Cytopathol 11:60–63
49. Green I, Ali SZ, Allen EA et al (1997) A spectrum of cytomorphologic variations in medullary thyroid carcinoma. Fine needle aspiration findings in 19 cases. Cancer 81:40–44
50. Rossi ED, Raffaelli M, Mule A et al (2008) Relevance of immunocytochemistry on thin layer cytology in thyroid lesions suspicious for medullary carcinoma: a case-control study. Appl Immunohistochem Mol Morphol 16:548–553
51. Filie AC, ASA SL, Geisinger KR et al (2008) Utilization of ancillary studies in thyroid fine needle aspirates: a synopsis of the national cancer institute thyroid fine needle aspiration state of the science conference. Diagn Cytopathol 36:438–441
52. Sangalli G, Serio G, Zampatti C et al (2001) Fine needle aspiration cytology of primary lymphoma of the thyroid: a report of 17 cases. Cytopathology 12:257–263
53. Vazquez Ramirez F, Otal Salaverri C, Argueta Manzano O et al (2000) Fine needle aspiration cytology of high grade mucoepidermoid carcinoma of the thyroid. A case report. Acta Cytol 44:259–264
54. Rossi ED, Mule A, Zannoni GF et al (2004) Asymptomatic intrathyroidal parathyroid adenoma. Report of a case with a cytologic differential diagnosis including thyroid neoplasms. Acta Cytol 483:437–440
55. Papi G, Fadda G, Corsello SM et al (2007) Metastastes to the thyroid gland: prevalence, clinicopathological aspect and prognosis: a 10-year experience. Clin Endocrinol 66:565–571
56. Cochand-Priollet B, Schmitt FC, Totsch M et al (2011) The Bethesda terminology for reporting thyroid cytopathology: from theory to practice in Europe. Acta Cytol 55:507–517

# 4 Molecular Markers in Thyroid Fine-Needle Aspiration Biopsies

Maria Chiara Zatelli, Efisio Puxeddu, Elisa Menicali, Ettore degli Uberti, and Sebastiano Filetti

The incidence of thyroid nodules is increasing, representing a malignant neoplasm only in 5–15 % of cases. Preoperative, ultrasonographically guided fine-needle aspiration biopsy (FNAB) is the cornerstone of thyroid-nodule evaluation. Most diagnostic FNAB are read as cytopathologically benign or malignant, but 15–30 % remain indeterminate [1]. The Bethesda System for Reporting Thyroid Cytopathology (BSRTC) classification defines indeterminate cytology as either atypical cells of undetermined significance/follicular lesion of undetermined significance (AUS/FLUS) or follicular neoplasm (FN)/suspicious for a follicular neoplasm (SFN) [2]. Patients with cytologically indeterminate nodules are often referred for diagnostic surgery, though most of these nodules prove to be benign postoperatively [3].

In this context genetic markers may be useful as diagnostic tools, complementing and integrating the information provided by cytology and improving preoperative risk stratification especially for indeterminate nodules.

Currently available tests have a limited sensitivity in excluding cancer, but may offer additional useful information to improve initial surgical indication and clinical management.

M.C. Zatelli • E. degli Uberti
Department of Medical Sciences, University of Ferrara, Ferrara, Italy

E. Puxeddu • E. Menicali
Department of Medicine, University of Perugia, Perugia, Italy

S. Filetti (✉)
Department of Internal Medicine and Medical Specialties, Policlinico Umberto I, University of Rome, Viale del Policlinico, 155, Rome 00161, Italy
e-mail: sebastiano.filetti@uniroma1.it



C.P. Lombardi, R. Bellantone (eds.), *Minimally Invasive Therapies for Endocrine Neck Diseases*, DOI 10.1007/978-3-319-20065-1_4

## 4.1 FNAB Material Retrieval, Conservation, Work-Up

To obtain biological material suitable for molecular markers evaluation fine needle aspiration biopsy (FNAB) procedures should be performed with the same modalities followed for cytological purposes. Sampling can be carried out by employing a 22 Gauge caliber on a 5–10 ml syringe, applying manual aspiration, under ultrasound (US) guidance. Usually, 1–3 needle passes provide enough material for both cytology and molecular analysis. However, in particular circumstances, more tissue may be necessary (Fig. 4.1).

For DNA studies, a dedicated FNAB material can be smeared on a microscope glass slide and air-dried or can be collected in a dedicated tube. Reliable results can be obtained also by washing out the needle with 3–5 ml normal saline in a collection tube after having prepared the smear for cytology [4]. The samples can be stored at room temperature for up to 12 h, but should be preferentially centrifuged, suspended in a small volume of normal saline (0.5–1 ml) and kept frozen at -20 °C until processed for DNA isolation.

For RNA studies, material from one dedicate FNAB must be collected in solutions that preserve RNA integrity, suspended in RNAse-free buffers, stored frozen, and processed as quickly as possible for RNA isolation. Samples collected for RNA studies can also be used for DNA studies, dividing the samples before nucleic acids isolation takes place.

## 4.2 Assessment of Molecular Abnormality in Cytological Sample

### 4.2.1 MicroRNA

MicroRNAs (miRNAs) are small non-coding 19–25 nucleotides long highly conserved RNAs that potently modulate gene expression by inhibiting mRNA transcription or translation [5, 6], possibly acting as oncogenes or tumor suppressor

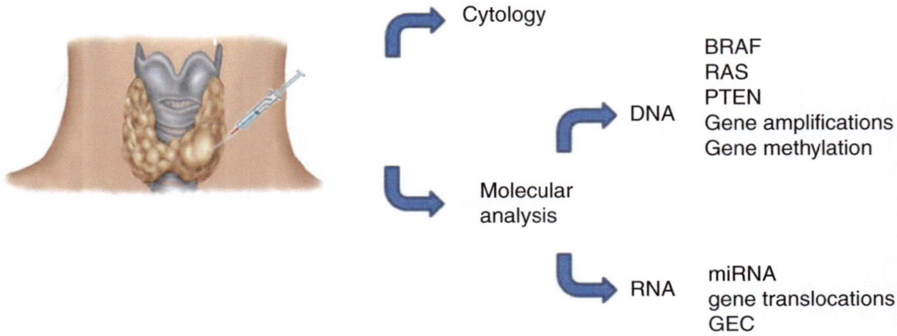


**Fig. 4.1** Workflow of molecular diagnostics from thyyroid nodules FNAB

genes [7]. miRNAs can be isolated from formalin-fixed paraffin embedded (FFPE) tissues, with good yield and quality levels [8, 9], and from FNAB material, achieving suboptimal yield and quality but comparable results [10]. Differential miRNA expression profiles have been characterized in thyroid cancers, benign thyroid lesions, and normal thyroid tissue [11], indicating that miRNA profiles may effectively become useful in differentiating benign from malignant lesions. Indeed, upregulation of several miRNAs, such as miR-146b, miR-187, miR-221, and miR-222, has been shown in papillary thyroid cancers (PTC) [12, 13] while others, such as miR-197 and miR-346, are over-expressed in follicular thyroid cancer (FTC) [14]. miRNA expression has been found to differentiate between benign and malignant lesions with variable accuracy in cases of indeterminate cytology [15, 16].

Most of miRNA studies have been performed on frozen or FFPE tissues that warrant higher yield and better miRNA quality as compared to FNAB samples. Therefore, the results should be regarded with caution and need to be validated in large, prospective, blinded, multicenter studies.

### 4.2.2 Gene Mutations

The identification of somatic point mutations in FNAB material represents a powerful method to rule in thyroid malignant nodules, being feasible in routine air-dried smears or in syringe wash out material from FNAB. *BRAF* and *RAS* somatic heterozygous mutations are indeed identified by several different methods starting from FNAB-derived DNA with good sensitivity and accuracy [1, 17–29].

*BRAF* gene, located on chromosome 7q, encodes a serine/threonine kinase belonging to the family of RAF proteins, taking part to the MAPK transduction pathway [30]. *BRAF* mutations, the most common mutations in PTC, are associated with constitutive activation of MAPK pathway and lead to follicular thyroid cell transformation. Their prevalence depends on the evaluated population, varying from 14 to 83 % of PTCs [31–34]. The *BRAF* V600E mutation at exon 15 is highly specific, since it almost always coincides with the presence of a PTC, representing a molecular marker for PTC and PTC-derived cancers. This mutation has been found to associate with recurrent disease, aggressive behavior and reduced iodide up-take [35], indicating a poorer prognosis [36, 37]. However, further investigation highlighted that *BRAF* V600E mutation is more frequent in older patients, may be found in metastatic lymph nodes but not in primary tumors [38], suggesting that BRAF mutations are not the main determinant for PTC morbidity and mortality. This aspect has been addressed in retrospective studies [39, 40], but prospective studies are still lacking.

*RAS* genes encode for a family of G-proteins participating in the MAPK and PI3K/AKT signaling pathways. The most common somatic mutations occur at codon 12 and 13 of the *N-RAS* and *K-RAS* isoforms and at codon 61 of the *H-RAS* isoform, being more frequently associated with FTC, follicular adenomas and, more rarely, with follicular variant of PTC [37]. The false-positive rate is high, since *RAS* mutations have been found in thyroid nodules that turned out to be benign lesions at final histology. Therefore, the diagnostic sensitivity of FNAB for thyroid cancer is often not improved by *RAS* mutation analysis [41]. However, *RAS* mutations may associate with malignant transformation of follicular adenomas into FTC, pushing mutated thyroid cells towards dedifferentiation and aggressive behavior [42].

### 4.2.3 Gene Translocations

Gene translocations can be investigated in FNAB material, after isolation of total RNA from the sample. Therefore, accurate and reliable analysis requires carefully collected and stored samples.

The *RET* gene, an acronym for REarranged during Transfection, is located on chromosome 10q11.2 and encodes for a tyrosine kinase receptor, which, in turn, is involved in the regulation of several cellular key functions [43]. Several chromosomal rearrangements involving the 3′ end of *RET*, corresponding to the C-terminal kinase domain, and the 5′ end of unrelated genes, leading to a constitutive activation of the kinase, have been described [44]. Among *RET/PTC* rearrangements, the most common are *RET/PTC1* and *RET/PTC3*, the latter being more frequent in radiation-induced PTC [45]. The presence of a *RET/PTC* rearrangement does not invariably predict the presence of a cancer, since these rearrangements can be detected also in benign lesions, with a prevalence of 13.9–52.4 % in benign neoplasms, 10–20 % in PTC and ~20 % in follicular variant of PTC, while they have not been reported in FTC [46]. Therefore, the diagnostic value of *RET/PTC* rearrangement in FNAB material is limited, even though it has been reported that it might be helpful in the settings of FNAB with indeterminate cytology [24, 47]. A meta-analysis showed that *RET/PTC* rearrangement testing has a low sensitivity and an average accuracy [48], therefore, *RET/PTC* rearrangements detection does not improve the high diagnostic accuracy for malignancy of *BRAF* mutation testing. Indeed, the latter has a very high positive predictive value, even in indeterminate samples, which is not enhanced by simultaneous testing for both *RAS* mutations and *RET/PTC* rearrangements. On the other hand, in indeterminate lesions corresponding to atypia of undetermined significance the lack of alterations in all these three genetic markers corresponds to a very low cancer risk, thereby indicating a very high negative predictive value for the combination of the three molecular investigations [49].

Many differentiated functions of thyrocytes such as those mediated by thyroglobulin, sodium-iodide symporter and TSH receptor are profoundly influenced by the paired box gene 8 (*PAX8*), located at chromosome 2 [50, 51]. Peroxisome proliferator-activated receptor gamma (*PPARγ*), an orphan nuclear hormone receptor, is involved in the regulation of carbohydrate and lipid metabolism and is transcribed from a gene located on chromosome 3. The chromosomal translocation t(2;3)(q13;p25) results in the fusion of the two genes, called *PAX8/PPARγ* rearrangement, which encodes for a fusion protein that, in turn, activates the PI3K/AKT pathway and is involved in thyroid tumorigenesis [52]. However, the presence of this rearrangement is not diagnostic for cancer, being identified also in benign lesions (range 0–13 %), possibly characterizing evolutive lesions [53], on the contrary a higher frequency has been detected and associates with a more favorable prognosis in FTC (up to ~40 %) [54, 55]. The *PAX8/PPARγ* rearrangement has not been described in PTCs. Therefore, this test may be useful when assessing cytologically indeterminate lesions, in that, when the rearrangement is detected, an accurate evaluation of the nodule capsule and vessels by the pathologist is suggested [54]. Testing for *PAX8/PPARγ* rearrangements, therefore, is burdened by a low sensitivity, but seems to have a high positive predictive value [48].

### 4.2.4 Gene Amplifications

Among the potential molecular biomarkers that can be assayed on FNAB material for diagnostic purposes, also gene amplifications should be considered. An exemplification is represented by *PI3KCA* gene amplification. Indeed, in addition to activating mutations, *PI3KCA* gene amplification has also been implicated in cancer, for example, in ovarian and cervical cancers [56, 57]. The copy number gain is associated with increased cell growth and decreased apoptosis. The frequency of *PI3KCA* mutations and gene amplification was investigated in thyroid carcinomas and appeared to be higher in follicular and in anaplastic thyroid carcinoma, rather than in papillary thyroid carcinoma [58–61]. Significantly higher expression levels of *PI3KCA* gene were detected in cytological samples of the PTC group in comparison with the nontoxic multinodular goiter group ($P<0.05$) [62]. Wu and colleagues described a strong association between *PI3KCA* copy number gain and high-risk clinic-pathological features in thyroid tumor, suggesting a potential role of that amplification in thyroid cancer progression [63]. Indeed, further investigations are needed to determine the definitive role of *PI3KCA* gene in thyroid cancer pathogenesis and progression and to clarify its role of molecular biomarker in nodule diagnostic procedures.

### 4.2.5 Gene Expression Variation

Unnecessary thyroid surgery could be avoided with a more accurate preoperative diagnosis of nodules based on the analysis of gene expression profile variations.

Real-time PCR (RT-PCR), as well as microarray studies have been employed to assess different gene expression profiles in benign and malignant lesions. For instance, after demonstrating the usefulness of six marker genes for the molecular distinction of benign and malignant thyroid tumors at the surgical specimen level, Karger and colleagues performed RT-PCR for *ADM3*, *HGD1*, *LGALS3*, *PLAB*, *TFF3*, and *TG* in cytological material in a prospective series of cancers with proven histological result, to investigate whether these markers could be applied for the differential preoperative diagnosis. *HGD1* and *TFF3* expression levels were significantly lower in FNAB of thyroid cancers compared with those of benign nodules and normal thyroid tissue. Conversely, *ADM3* and *LGALS3* expression levels were significantly higher in FNAB of thyroid cancers compared with benign lesions. Using two-marker gene sets, it was possible to distinguish between benign and malignant thyroid cancers with a negative predictive value (NPV) of up to 78 % and a positive predictive value (PPV) of up to 84 % [64].

Similarly, the mRNA expression level of other 9 genes (*KIT*, *SYNGR2*, *C21orf4*, *Hs.296031*, *DDI2*, *CDH1*, *LSM7*, *TC1*, *NATH*) was tested in cytological specimen. A computational model was developed (i.e., Neural Network Bayesian Classifier) and a multiple-variable analysis was performed to assess the correlation among the markers. *KIT*, *CDH1*, *LSM7*, *C21orf4*, *DDI2* expression levels were significantly different between benign and malignant tumors ($P<0.05$) and the neural network classifier, constituted by the markers used in the most predictive model along with *BRAF* mutational status, achieved a predictive power of 88.8 % [65].

### 4.2.6 Aberrant Gene Methylation

Among the potential molecular biomarkers that can be assayed on FNAB material for diagnostic purposes, also DNA methylation should be considered. Indeed, gene promoter methylation is one of the most common epigenetic alterations in human cancers, including thyroid carcinoma [66]. It is known that promoter hypermethylation usually occurs in cancer cells in order to inactivate tumor suppressor genes [67].

In a recent paper, Zhang and coworkers demonstrated the feasibility of DNA methylation assay in FNAB material and defined specificity and sensitivity of a panel of methylation markers for evaluating thyroid nodules. In detail, they performed quantitative methylation-specific PCR (Q-MSP) to determine differences between PTC and benign nodules in the methylation levels of five genes, including *CALCA*, *DAPK1*, *TIMP3*, *RAR-beta*, and *RASSF1A*. These genes were selected based on their documented relevance in thyroid cancer [68]. They found that in PTC methylation level of *DAPK1* was significantly higher than that in benign samples ($P<0.0001$). Conversely, in PTC methylation level of *RASSF1A* was significantly lower than that in benign samples ($P<0.003$). However, their diagnostic specificity and accuracy were low. The authors also investigated the relationship between *BRAF* mutation and gene methylation levels. *BRAF* mutation was significantly associated with *DAPK1* methylation ($P=0.0009$), as well as with absence of *RASSF1A* methylation ($P=0.026$). Moreover, combined analysis of *BRAF* mutation and methylation markers increased the diagnostic sensitivity, accuracy and also specificity of the molecular test [69].

DNA methylation markers alone, therefore, appear to have a limited usefulness in the diagnosis of thyroid cancer; however, by exploiting together with other molecular markers could improve the diagnostic accuracy of FNAB.

### 4.2.7 Veracyte Afirma Gene Expression Classifier (GEC): Analytical and Clinical Value

The search for tools to predict benignity of cytological indeterminate thyroid nodules and to potentially avoid surgery on these nodules, has elicited the development of a gene expression classifier (GEC) test (Afirma®, Veracyte, Inc., South San Francisco, CA) that can be run on the FNAB sample. The Afirma GEC is an RNA-based assay designed to evaluate the gene expression profile of a given thyroid nodule by comparing it with the panel of 167 mRNA expression patterns (derived from 142 genes identified originally from the Affymetrix Human Exon Array) associated with benign nodules. It is characterized by a high sensitivity (90 %) in indeterminate cytology lesions to identify the signature of a benign thyroid nodule with 95 % NPV: that is similar to the risk of malignancy in a resected thyroid nodule with a preoperatively benign FNA cytopathology diagnosis [3, 70]. Specificities of the test were low, as expected, at 53 % for AUS/FLUS and 49 % for FN/SFN. NPV drops to 85 % in the case of a suspicious for malignancy cytology. Veracyte currently requires 2 sets of FNA samples: one for cytological evaluation and one for running the gene expression profiling (the Afirma GEC test). The patient's FNA sample is subjected to standardized cytological evaluation by the company's independent cytopathology examination at the thyroid cytopathology partners (TCP; Austin, TX). Cytological results are based on the Bethesda classification. FNA samples with Bethesda categories of benign, malignant or suspicious for malignancy do not undergo further evaluation with Afirma GEC and only the cytological diagnosis is forwarded to the ordering physician. For cytological samples with the diagnosis of AUS/FLUS/FN/SFN, clinicians should expect to receive a 2-part report from Veracyte: cytological evaluation and the GEC test result. The Afirma GEC sample undergoes RNA extraction and nucleic acid amplification. Processed Afirma GEC samples are hybridized to a custom Afirma Thyroid Microarray and analyzed with a classification algorithm using linear support vector machine logic [71]. The GEC test result is binary and reported as benign or suspicious if the samples were adequate. The genetic material is first put through 6 different cassettes before applying the final benign versus malignant classifier. The first 6 cassettes act as filters for rare subtypes of thyroid cancer and nonfollicular cell-derived tumors (malignant melanoma, renal cell carcinoma, medullary thyroid cancer, and parathyroid tissue), which prevent the material from being scored by the main thyroid classifier. The test has a false-negative rate of 5–15 % and, therefore, a new assessment is important if the nodule enlarges or clinical suspicions arise. Furthermore, a PPV for a suspicious test result is only 38 %. Two prospective multicenter studies evaluated the negative predictive value (NPV) for the Afirma GEC, which is the key diagnostic performance metric used to make a decision to monitor patients in lieu of referral for diagnostic thyroid surgery [3, 70]. Both studies utilized diagnosis of the surgical pathology specimen by a central panel of blinded academic endocrine histopathologists as the reference standard for clinical validation [71]. In one of these studies, the rate of malignancy was nearly equivalent in AUS/FLUS and FN/SFN (24 % vs. 25 %) [3]. This rate is not representative of the general risk of malignancy observed for AUS/FLUS lesions (5–15 %). Thus, the AUS/FLUS groups in the studies may not have been representative of the general population. This observation opens the issue of the need for more studies aimed at extending the evaluation of the analytical performance of Afirma GEC on much larger population layers in an international setting. Moreover, the high rate of false-positive results and not the negligible rate of false negatives narrows the indications of the test, cutting away the suspicious for malignancy cytology, burdened by a too high risk of malignancy making a false-negative rate of 5–15 % unacceptably high, and the nonsuspicious AUS/FLUS, where the risk of malignancy (5–15 %) is equivalent to the false-negative rate and the high false-positive rate may confound the evaluation and management of benign nodules [2].

## 4.3 Impact on Diagnosis

The availability of molecular markers has improved the diagnostic performance of FNAB in many settings. The major diagnostic contribution is expected in the group of cytological indeterminate nodules, where the available tests may be helpful in ruling in (mutation panels) or ruling out (GEC) thyroid cancer. This approach should ideally allow to avoid surgery in nodules that are benign, and to indicate therapeutic (and not diagnostic) surgery when the nodule is malignant. However, the currently available molecular tests have failed to offer both high sensitivity and high specificity. GEC demonstrated high sensitivity and high negative predictive value in samples having a low risk of malignancy (the "rule out" option). This approach would allow applying a conservative follow up and avoid diagnostic lobectomy for nodules, which are very likely to be benign follicular hyperplastic nodules, sparing resources and securing patients quality of life. On the other hand, this approach has a low specificity, and therefore is not optimal for identifying cancer. Conversely, mutation panels have a high specificity and positive predictive value (the "rule in" option) for cancer, allowing identifying malignant nodules to be addressed to therapeutic surgery. However, a negative test does not correspond to the absence of cancer, indicating the need for diagnostic surgery in the presence of an indeterminate cytology [72]. Ideally, both "rule in" and "rule out" testing should be performed when cytology is not informative, but the cost of this approach may override the clinical benefit for the patient.

Molecular testing has also been demonstrated to increase diagnostic sensitivity and accuracy for thyroid cancer in cytological benign nodules [4, 18], allowing anticipating the diagnosis of thyroid cancer through the detection of malignant lesions at a lower disease stage [49]. Most of the gathered experience is related to the *BRAF* mutation, whose detection by solid and validated techniques is strongly associated with PTC. Several reports indicate that diagnosis of thyroid cancer can be significantly improved by simultaneous testing for multiple mutations, as stated above, such as *BRAF* and *RAS* mutations as well as *RET/PTC* and *PAX8/PPARγ* rearrangements [47, 72, 73]. The identification of one of these genetic derangements may help in characterizing the risk of malignancy of a thyroid nodule, allowing a more accurate risk stratification for the patient and assisting the clinician in choosing patient management, especially in the settings of a nodule with indeterminate cytology. However, it must be underlined that more recent evidence indicates that *BRAF* analysis is superior to other mutation tests, such as *RAS* mutations and *RET/PTC* rearrangements, even when performed in combination [49], for the diagnosis of PTC. These discrepancies may be due to the different inclusion criteria employed in the sample selection (i.e., the investigated thyroid nodules) in the different studies, which are linked to a different pre-test probability of being a cancer.

The diagnostic impact of genetic derangements needs to be validated by prospective multicenter clinical studies, also assessing analytic validity and clinical utility as well as cost-effectiveness.

## 4.4 Impact on Surgical Choice

Molecular markers assayed on FNAB material might also harbor a prognostic significance and be useful to define the more appropriate surgical strategy according to the estimated aggressiveness of the lesion.

In particular, genetic markers – including mutations in *RAS*, *PIK3CA*, *AKT1*, *PTEN*, *p53*, *CTNNB1*, *ALK*, and *TERT* genes – show promise [74, 75]. However, the best-defined prognostic marker for thyroid carcinomas, namely PTC, is *BRAF* mutation [39, 40, 76–81].

The high NPV for recurrence of a *BRAF* negative test has suggested its use in clinical practice, especially in the preoperative planning where it can help to determine the extent of initial surgery [74].

In the absence of clinical and sonographic lymph node involvement, the accomplishment of a prophylactic central compartment lymph node dissection in all thyroid cancer surgeries is controversial [82]. Several studies have shown that prophylactic central compartment lymph node dissection reduces postoperative thyroglobulin levels and may decrease local regional recurrences. However, no study has demonstrated a reduction in disease-specific mortality [83–86]. Moreover, prophylactic central compartment lymph node dissection has been associated with a higher rate of postsurgical hypoparathyroidism and laryngeal nerve damage even when the procedure was performed by high volume surgeons [85]. In PTC, *BRAF* mutation has appeared as a significant predictor of central compartment lymph node metastasis on both univariate (OR 8.4, $P=0.01$) and multivariate (OR 9.7, $P=0.02$) analyses [87, 88]. Thus, preoperative *BRAF* mutation detection has been suggested to be one way to identify PTC patients who would best benefit from prophylactic central compartment lymph node dissection [75]. Several studies have also reported that *BRAF* mutation positive papillary thyroid microcarcinomas (PTMC) are characterized by higher rates of extrathyroidal tumor extension and cervical lymph node metastasis [89, 90]. Although the majority of PTMC are indolent, a subset of these tumors can behave aggressively leading to recurrence and mortality. Very recently, Niemeier and coworkers developed a molecular-pathological (MP) score for PTMC that included *BRAF* status and three histopathological features: superficial tumor location, intraglandular tumor spread/multifocality, and tumor fibrosis. This risk stratification model appeared a good predictor of extrathyroidal tumor spread and tumor aggressiveness measured as lymph node metastases or tumor recurrence [91]. In this context, a positive preoperative testing for *BRAF* mutation in a PTMC might induce a change in the surgical strategy moving from the American Thyroid

Association-recommended lobectomy to a more radical total thyroidectomy [74]. However, there is still no prospective evidence that this approach will favorably change the outcome of these low-risk patients.

## 4.5 Future Perspectives

FNAB is the most reliable preoperative test to diagnose thyroid cancer. Although FNAB is able to classify thyroid nodules as benign or malignant in the majority of cases [1], nondiagnostic or indeterminate cytological results occur in up to 30 % of thyroid FNAB specimens, underlying the need for molecular biomarkers that help to increase its diagnostic accuracy.

In the last decades, several efforts have been made in the development of molecular tests for cancer diagnosis in thyroid nodules. Panels of gene expression markers [92], as well as somatic mutation panels [73, 93] have improved the preoperative diagnostic accuracy for patients with indeterminate cytology, and will become an important tool for diagnosis in the future.

Significant progress in the understanding of thyroid cancer genetics, as well as advances in high-throughput technologies have contributed to molecular test improvement. Recent results from The Cancer Genome Atlas (TCGA) project provided a comprehensive genomic profile of thyroid cancer [94]. New driver mutations were identified in PTC, either entirely novel (*EIF1AX*) or novel alterations of known drivers (*RET*, *BRAF*, and *ALK* fusions). These discoveries have substantially decreased the "dark matter" of the PTC genome. PTC cases with unknown genetic driver have been reduced from 25 % to less than 4 %, which should improve molecular diagnosis. The current availability of targeted Next-Generation Sequencing (NGS) offers a convenient and cost-effective technique for detection of most of TCGA driver alterations also in those challenging samples like FNA specimens. The sensitivity, speed, and reduced cost per sample make it an attractive method compared to other available clinical tests.

Beyond their diagnostic role, molecular markers in FNAB specimens are expected to have an enormous impact on cancer prognosis. Pre-surgical identification of more aggressive tumors should facilitate optimal management of thyroid cancer patients, and their stratification into clinically meaningful categories. Indeed, predictive factors will guide the extent of initial thyroid surgery, select treatment options, and determine eligibility for clinical trials. The prognostic value of *BRAF* mutation has long been debated. TCGA study indicates that *BRAF*-mutated PTC represents a heterogeneous group of tumors, consisting of different molecular subtypes, with variable grade of thyroid differentiation. This may explain the uncertainty regarding the prognostic role of *BRAF* mutation [39, 40] and support the conclusion that it cannot be used alone as prognostic marker. Otherwise, the presence of several driver mutations in thyroid cancer may indicate a more aggressive tumor behavior. Co-occurrence of *BRAF* or *RAS* mutation with *TP53, PIK3CA,* or *AKT1* has been observed in poorly differentiated, anaplastic thyroid cancers [58, 59, 95], as well as in aggressive PTCs [94]. In this context, targeted NGS-based approaches are particularly useful to detect more variations at the same time in small samples, increasing sensitivity and negative predictive value of the test. Moreover, *TERT* promoter mutations have been found in thyroid cancer, with higher prevalence in aggressive, less differentiated thyroid carcinoma [94, 96, 97], suggesting its role as prognostic molecular marker for cancer in thyroid nodule.

As demonstrated in thyroid TCGA study, multi-level approaches involving mutational analysis as well as miR/mRNA expression profiling may help to define clinically relevant subclasses of thyroid tumors. Combined methods will offer multiple markers for cancer diagnosis in FNA specimens, increasing positive predictive value (i.e., in *RAS*-mutated cases) or preoperatively identifying subset of aggressive cancers.

Additional studies will be needed to define molecular signature useful for the pre-surgical management of patients. Through these advances, molecular diagnostics will improve thyroid patient care.

## References

1. Cooper DS, Doherty GM, Haugen BR et al (2009) Revised American Thyroid Association management guidelines for patients with thyroid nodules and differentiated thyroid cancer. Thyroid 19(11):1167–1214
2. Parangi S, Suh H (2014) The role of genetic markers in the evaluation and management of thyroid nodules. Surg Clin North Am 94(3):515–528
3. Alexander EK, Kennedy GC, Baloch ZW et al (2012) Preoperative diagnosis of benign thyroid nodules with indeterminate cytology. N Engl J Med 367(8):705–715
4. Rossi M, Buratto M, Bruni S et al (2012) Role of ultrasonographic/clinical profile, cytology, and BRAF V600E mutation evaluation in thyroid nodule screening for malignancy: a prospective study. J Clin Endocrinol Metab 97(7):2354–2361
5. Bartel DP (2004) MicroRNAs: genomics, biogenesis, mechanism, and function. Cell 116(2): 281–297
6. Filipowicz W, Jaskiewicz L, Kolb FA et al (2005) Post-transcriptional gene silencing by siRNAs and miRNAs. Curr Opin Struct Biol 15(3):331–341
7. Zhang B, Pan X, Cobb GP et al (2007) MicroRNAs as oncogenes and tumor suppressors. Dev Biol 302(1):1–12
8. Hui A, How C, Ito E et al (2011) Micro-RNAs as diagnostic or prognostic markers in human epithelial malignancies. BMC Cancer 11:500
9. Zhang X, Chen J, Radcliffe T et al (2008) An array-based analysis of microRNA expression comparing matched frozen and formalin-fixed paraffinembedded human tissue samples. J Mol Diagn 10(6):513–519
10. Chen YT, Kitabayashi N, Zhou XK et al (2008) MicroRNA analysis as a potential diagnostic tool for papillary thyroid carcinoma. Mod Pathol 21(9):1139–1146
11. Lodewijk L, Prins AM, Kist JW et al (2012) The value of miRNA in diagnosing thyroid cancer: a systematic review. Cancer Biomark 11(6):229–238
12. He H, Jazdzewski K, Li W et al (2005) The role of microRNA genes in papillary thyroid carcinoma. Proc Natl Acad Sci U S A 102(52):19075–19080
13. Nikiforova MN, Tseng GC, Steward D et al (2008) MicroRNA expression profiling of thyroid tumors: biological significance and diagnostic utility. J Clin Endocrinol Metab 93(5): 1600–1608
14. Weber F, Teresi RE, Broelsch CE et al (2006) A limited set of human microRNA is deregulated in follicular thyroid carcinoma. J Clin Endocrinol Metab 91(9):3584–3591

15. Vriens MR, Weng J, Suh I et al (2012) MicroRNA expression profiling is a potential diagnostic tool for thyroid cancer. Cancer 118(13):3426–3432
16. Keutgen XM, Filicori F, Crowley MJ et al (2012) A panel of four MicroRNAs accurately differentiates malignant from benign indeterminate thyroid lesions on fine needle aspiration. Clin Cancer Res 18(7):2032–2038
17. Pelizzo MR, Boschin IM, Barollo S et al (2011) BRAF analysis by fine needle aspiration biopsy of thyroid nodules improves preoperative identification of papillary thyroid carcinoma and represents a prognostic factor. A mono-institutional experience. Clin Chem Lab Med 49(2):325–329
18. Zatelli MC, Trasforini G, Leoni S et al (2009) BRAF V600E mutation analysis increases diagnostic accuracy for papillary thyroid carcinoma in fine-needle aspiration biopsies. Eur J Endocrinol 161(3):467–473
19. Xing M, Clark D, Guan H et al (2009) BRAF mutation testing of thyroid fine-needle aspiration biopsy specimens for preoperative risk stratification in papillary thyroid cancer. J Clin Oncol 27(18):2977–2982
20. Nikiforov YE, Steward DL, Robinson-Smith T et al (2009) Molecular testing for mutations in improving the fine needle aspiration diagnosis of thyroid nodules. J Clin Endocrinol Metab 94(6):2092–2098
21. Jo YS, Huang S, Kim YJ et al (2009) Diagnostic value of pyrosequencing for the BRAF(V600E) mutation in ultrasound-guided fine needle aspiration biopsy samples of thyroid incidentalomas. Clin Endocrinol (Oxf) 70(1):139–144
22. Kim SK, Kim DL, Han HS et al (2008) Pyrosequencing analysis for detection of a BRAFV600E mutation in an FNAB specimen of thyroid nodules. Diagn Mol Pathol 17(2):118–125
23. Sapio MR, Guerra A, Posca D et al (2007) Combined analysis of galectin-3 and BRAFV600E improves the accuracy of fine-needle aspiration biopsy with cytological findings suspicious for papillary thyroid carcinoma. Endocr Relat Cancer 14(4):1089–1097
24. Pizzolanti G, Russo L, Richiusa P et al (2007) Fine-needle aspiration molecular analysis for the diagnosis of papillary thyroid carcinoma through BRAF V600E mutation and RET/PTC rearrangement. Thyroid 17(11):1109–1115
25. Kumagai A, Namba H, Akanov Z et al (2007) Clinical implications of pre-operative rapid BRAF analysis for papillary thyroid cancer. Endocr J 54(3):399–405
26. Sapio MR, Posca D, Raggioli A et al (2007) Detection of RET/PTC, TRK and BRAF mutations in preoperative diagnosis of thyroid nodules with indeterminate cytological findings. Clin Endocrinol (Oxf) 66(5):678–683
27. Chung KW, Yang SK, Lee GK et al (2006) Detection of BRAFV600E mutation on fine needle aspiration specimens of thyroid nodule refines cyto-pathology diagnosis, especially in BRAF600E mutation-prevalent area. Clin Endocrinol (Oxf) 65(5):660–666
28. Hayashida N, Namba H, Kumagai A et al (2004) A rapid and simple detection method for the BRAF(T1796A) mutation in fine-needle aspirate thyroid carcinoma cells. Thyroid 14(11):910–915
29. Xing M, Tufano RP, Tufaro AP et al (2004) Detection of BRAF mutation on fine needle aspiration biopsy specimens: a new diagnostic tool for papillary thyroid cancer. J Clin Endocrinol Metab 89(6):2867–2872
30. Xing M (2005) BRAF mutation in thyroid cancer. Endocr Relat Cancer 12(2):245–262
31. Brzezianska E, Pastuszak-Lewandoska D, Wojciechowska K et al (2007) Investigation of V600E BRAF mutation in papillary thyroid carcinoma in the Polish population. Neuro Endocrinol Lett 28(4):351–359
32. Oler G, Cerutti JM (2009) High prevalence of BRAF mutation in a Brazilian cohort of patients with sporadic papillary thyroid carcinomas: correlation with more aggressive phenotype and decreased expression of iodide-metabolizing genes. Cancer 115(5):972–980
33. Kim KH, Kang DW, Kim SH et al (2004) Mutations of the BRAF gene in papillary thyroid carcinoma in a Korean population. Yonsei Med J 45(5):818–821
34. Girlando S, Cuorvo LV, Bonzanini M et al (2010) High prevalence of B-RAF mutation in papillary carcinoma of the thyroid in north-east Italy. Int J Surg Pathol 18(3):173–176

35. Durante C, Puxeddu E, Ferretti E et al (2007) BRAF mutations in papillary thyroid carcinomas inhibit genes involved in iodine metabolism. J Clin Endocrinol Metab 92(7):2840–2843
36. Puxeddu E, Durante C, Avenia N et al (2008) Clinical implications of BRAF mutation in thyroid carcinoma. Trends Endocrinol Metab 19(4):138–145
37. Handkiewicz-Junak D, Czarniecka A, Jarząb B (2010) Molecular prognostic markers in papillary thyroid cancer: current status and future directions. Mol Cell Endocrinol 322(1-2):8e28
38. Baldini E, Sorrenti S, Tuccilli C et al (2014) Emerging molecular markers for the prognosis of differentiated thyroid cancer patients. Int J Surg 12(Suppl 1):S52–S56
39. Xing M, Alzahrani AS, Carson KA et al (2013) Association between BRAF V600E mutation and mortality in patients with papillary thyroid cancer. JAMA 309(14):1493–1501
40. Xing M, Alzahrani AS, Carson KA et al (2015) Association between BRAF V600E mutation and recurrence of papillary thyroid cancer. J Clin Oncol 33(1):42–50
41. Fallahi P, Giannini R, Miccoli P et al (2014) Molecular diagnostics of fine needle aspiration for the presurgical screening of thyroid nodules. Curr Genomics 15(3):171–177
42. Fagin JA (2002) Minireview: branded from the start-distinct oncogenic initiating events may determine tumor fate in the thyroid. Mol Endocrinol 16(5):903–911
43. de Groot JW, Links TP, Plukker JT et al (2006) RET as a diagnostic and therapeutic target in sporadic and hereditary endocrine tumors. Endocr Rev 27(5):535–560
44. Mitsutake N, Miyagishi M, Mitsutake S et al (2006) BRAF mediates RET/PTC-induced mitogen-activated protein kinase activation in thyroid cells: functional support for requirement of the RET/PTC RAS-BRAF pathway in papillary thyroid carcinogenesis. Endocrinology 147(2):1014–1019
45. Nikiforov YE, Rowland JM, Bove KE et al (1997) Distinct pattern of ret oncogene rearrangements in morphological variants of radiation-induced and sporadic thyroid papillary carcinomas in children. Cancer Res 57(9):1690–1694
46. Kunavisarut T (2013) Diagnostic biomarkers of differentiated thyroid cancer. Endocrine 44(3):616–622
47. Cantara S, Capezzone M, Marchisotta S et al (2010) Impact of proto-oncogene mutation detection in cytological specimens from thyroid nodules improves the diagnostic accuracy of cytology. J Clin Endocrinol Metab 95(3):1365–1369
48. Rodrigues HG, de Pontes AA, Adan LF (2012) Use of molecular markers in samples obtained from preoperative aspiration of thyroid. Endocr J 59(5):417–424
49. Rossi M, Buratto M, Tagliati F et al (2015) Relevance of BRAF(V600E) mutation testing versus RAS point mutations and RET/PTC rearrangements evaluation in the diagnosis of thyroid cancer. Thyroid 25(2):221–228
50. Macchia PE, Lapi P, Krude H (1998) PAX8 mutations associated with congenital hypothyroidism caused by thyroid dysgenesis. Nat Genet 19(1):83–86
51. Pasca di Magliano M, Di Lauro R, Zannini M (2000) Pax8 has a key role in thyroid cell differentiation. Proc Natl Acad Sci U S A 97(24):13144–13149
52. Eberhardt NL, Grebe SK, McIver B et al (2010) The role of the PAX8/PPARgamma fusion oncogene in the pathogenesis of follicular thyroid cancer. Mol Cell Endocrinol 321(1):50–56
53. Dwight T, Thoppe SR, Foukakis T et al (2003) Involvement of the PAX8/peroxisome proliferator-activated receptor gamma rearrangement in follicular thyroid tumors. J Clin Endocrinol Metab 88(9):4440–4445
54. Nikiforova MN, Biddinger PW, Caudill CM et al (2002) PAX8-PPARgamma rearrangement in thyroid tumors: RT-PCR and immunohistochemical analyses. Am J Surg Pathol 26(8): 1016–1023
55. Marques AR, Espadinha C, Catarino AL et al (2002) Expression of PAX8-PPAR gamma 1 rearrangements in both follicular thyroid carcinomas and adenomas. J Clin Endocrinol Metab 87(8):3947–3952
56. Shayesteh L, Lu Y, Kuo WL et al (1999) PIK3CA is implicated as an oncogene in ovarian cancer. Nat Genet 21(1):99–102
57. Ma YY, Wei SJ, Lin YC et al (2000) PI3KCA as an oncogene in cervical cancer. Oncogene 19(23):2739–2744

58. García-Rostán G, Costa AM, Pereira-Castro I et al (2005) Mutation of the PIK3CA gene in anaplastic thyroid cancer. Cancer Res 65(22):10199–10207
59. Hou P, Liu D, Shan Y et al (2007) Genetic alterations and their relationship in the phosphatidylinositol 3-kinase/Akt pathway in thyroid cancer. Clin Cancer Res 13(4):1161–1170
60. Wang Y, Hou P, Yu H et al (2007) High prevalence and mutual exclusivity of genetic alterations in the phosphatidylinositol-3-kinase/akt pathway in thyroid tumors. J Clin Endocrinol Metab 92(6):2387–2390
61. Xing M (2010) Genetic alterations in the phosphatidylinositol-3 kinase/Akt pathway in thyroid cancer. Thyroid 20(7):697–706
62. Wojciechowska-Durczyńska K, Krawczyk-Rusiecka K, Cyniak-Magierska A et al (2010) Relative quantification of PIK3CA gene expression level in fine-needle aspiration biopsy thyroid specimens collected from patients with papillary thyroid carcinoma and non-toxic goitre by real-time RT-PCR. Thyroid Res 3(1):5
63. Wu G, Mambo E, Guo Z et al (2005) Uncommon mutation, but common amplifications, of the PIK3CA gene in thyroid tumors. J Clin Endocrinol Metab 90(8):4688–4693
64. Karger S, Krause K, Gutknecht M et al (2012) ADM3, TFF3 and LGALS3 are discriminative molecular markers in fine-needle aspiration biopsies of benign and malignant thyroid tumours. Br J Cancer 106(3):562–568
65. Tomei S, Marchetti I, Zavaglia K et al (2012) A molecular computational model improves the preoperative diagnosis of thyroid nodules. BMC Cancer 12:396
66. Xing M (2007) Gene methylation in thyroid tumorigenesis. Endocrinology 148(3):948–953
67. Herman JG, Baylin SB (2003) Gene silencing in cancer in association with promoter hypermethylation. N Engl J Med 349(21):2042–2054
68. Hoque MO, Rosenbaum E, Westra WH et al (2005) Quantitative assessment of promoter methylation profiles in thyroid neoplasms. J Clin Endocrinol Metab 90(7):4011–4018
69. Zhang B, Liu S, Zhang Z et al (2014) Analysis of BRAF(V600E) mutation and DNA methylation improves the diagnostics of thyroid fine needle aspiration biopsies. Diagn Pathol 9:45
70. Chudova D, Wilde JI, Wang ET et al (2010) Molecular classification of thyroid nodules using high-dimensionality genomic data. J Clin Endocrinol Metab 95(12):5296–5304
71. Ali SZ, Fish SA, Lanman RB et al (2013) Use of the Afirma® Gene Expression Classifier for Preoperative Identification of Benign Thyroid Nodules with Indeterminate Fine Needle Aspiration Cytopathology. PLoS Curr 5
72. Ward LS, Kloos RT (2013) Molecular markers in the diagnosis of thyroid nodules. Arq Bras Endocrinol Metab 57(2):89–97
73. Nikiforov YE, Carty SE, Chiosea SI et al (2014) Highly accurate diagnosis of cancer in thyroid nodules with follicular neoplasm/suspicious for a follicular neoplasm cytology by ThyroSeq v2 next-generation sequencing assay. Cancer 120(23):3627–3634
74. Xing M, Haugen BR, Schlumberger M (2013) Progress in molecular-based management of differentiated thyroid cancer. Lancet 381(9871):1058–1069
75. Yip L (2015) Molecular markers for thyroid cancer diagnosis, prognosis, and targeted therapy. J Surg Oncol 111(1):43–50
76. Xing M (2007) BRAF mutation in papillary thyroid cancer: pathogenic role, molecular bases, and clinical implications. Endocr Rev 28(7):742–762
77. Elisei R, Cosci B, Romei C et al (2008) Prognostic significance of somatic RET oncogene mutations in sporadic medullary thyroid cancer: a 10-year follow-up study. J Clin Endocrinol Metab 93(3):682–687
78. Xing M (2010) Prognostic utility of BRAF mutation in papillary thyroid cancer. Mol Cell Endocrinol 321(1):86–93
79. Kim TY, Kim WB, Rhee YS et al (2006) The BRAF mutation is useful for prediction of clinical recurrence in low-risk patients with conventional papillary thyroid carcinoma. Clin Endocrinol (Oxf) 65(3):364–368
80. Frasca F, Nucera C, Pellegriti G et al (2008) BRAF(V600E) mutation and the biology of papillary thyroid cancer. Endocr Relat Cancer 15(1):191–205

81. Puxeddu E, Filetti S (2014) BRAF mutation assessment in papillary thyroid cancer: are we ready to use it in clinical practice? Endocrine 45(3):341–343
82. Carty SE, Cooper DS, Doherty GM et al (2009) Consensus statement on the terminology and classification of central neck dissection for thyroid cancer. Thyroid 19(11):1153–1158
83. Hughes DT, White ML, Miller BS et al (2010) Influence of prophylactic central lymph node dissection on postoperative thyroglobulin levels and radioiodine treatment in papillary thyroid cancer. Surgery 148(6):1100–1106
84. Popadich A, Levin O, Lee JC et al (2011) A multicenter cohort study of total thyroidectomy and routine central lymph node dissection for cN0 papillary thyroid cancer. Surgery 150(6):1048–1057
85. Wang TS, Cheung K, Farrokhyar F et al (2013) A meta-analysis of the effect of prophylactic central compartment neck dissection on locoregional recurrence rates in patients with papillary thyroid cancer. Ann Surg Oncol 20(11):3477–3483
86. Lang BH, Tang AH, Wong KP et al (2012) Significance of size of lymph node metastasis on postsurgical stimulated thyroglobulin levels after prophylactic unilateral central neck dissection in papillary thyroid carcinoma. Ann Surg Oncol 19(11):3472–3478
87. Howell GM, Nikiforova MN, Carty SE et al (2013) BRAF V600E mutation independently predicts central compartment lymph node metastasis in patients with papillary thyroid cancer. Ann Surg Oncol 20(1):47–52
88. Lee KC, Li C, Schneider EB et al (2012) Is BRAF mutation associated with lymph node metastasis in patients with papillary thyroid cancer? Surgery 152(6):977–983
89. Rodolico V, Cabibi D, Pizzolanti G et al (2007) BRAF V600E mutation and p27 kip1 expression in papillary carcinomas of the thyroid <or=1 cm and their paired lymph node metastases. Cancer 110(6):1218–1226
90. Lupi C, Giannini R, Ugolini C et al (2007) Association of BRAF V600E mutation with poor clinicopathological outcomes in 500 consecutive cases of papillary thyroid carcinoma. J Clin Endocrinol Metab 92(11):4085–4090
91. Niemeier LA, Kuffner Akatsu H, Song C et al (2012) A combined molecular-pathologic score improves risk stratification of thyroid papillary microcarcinoma. Cancer 118(8):2069–2077
92. Alexander EK, Schorr M, Klopper J et al (2014) Multicenter clinical experience with the Afirma gene expression classifier. J Clin Endocrinol Metab 99(1):119–125
93. Beaudenon-Huibregtse S, Alexander EK, Guttler RB et al (2014) Centralized molecular testing for oncogenic gene mutations complements the local cytopathologic diagnosis of thyroid nodules. Thyroid 24(10):1479–1487
94. Cancer Genome Atlas Research Network (2014) Integrated genomic characterization of papillary thyroid carcinoma. Cell 159(3):676–690
95. Ricarte-Filho JC, Ryder M, Chitale DA et al (2009) Mutational profile of advanced primary and metastatic radioactive iodine-refractory thyroid cancers reveals distinct pathogenetic roles for BRAF, PIK3CA, and AKT1. Cancer Res 69(11):4885–4893
96. Melo M, da Rocha AG, Vinagre J et al (2014) TERT promoter mutations are a major indicator of poor outcome in differentiated thyroid carcinomas. J Clin Endocrinol Metab 99(5): E754–E765
97. Xing M, Liu R, Liu X et al (2014) BRAF V600E and TERT promoter mutations cooperatively identify the most aggressive papillary thyroid cancer with highest recurrence. J Clin Oncol 32(25):2718–2726

# Part II

# Ultrasound-Guided Interventional Techniques

# Percutaneous Ethanol Injection for the Management of Thyroid Lesions

5

Rinaldo Guglielmi, Enrico Papini, Irene Misischi, Filomena Graziano, Lucilla Petrucci, Roberta Rinaldi, and Andrea Frasoldati

## 5.1 Introduction

The last 20 years have observed the proposal of several minimally invasive techniques for non-surgical treatment of thyroid nodules. This chapter describes, on the basis of our experience and of a brief literature review, the efficacy, safety, cost-effectiveness and current clinical indications of the first of these procedures: percutaneous ethanol injection (PEIT).

The injection of ethanol into the tissues induces a chemical injury of the cells and small vessels that is followed by sclerotic changes and shrinkage of the target area. Fibrosis is the final result of the process of cell dehydration and protein denaturation, and is followed by coagulative necrosis, small vessel thrombosis and haemorrhagic infarcts [1, 2]. The use of the toxic properties of ethanol for therapeutical purposes dates up to the first half of the 1980s, when PEIT was originally described for the minimally invasive treatment of hepatocellular carcinoma, renal cysts and hyperplastic parathyroid glands in patients with secondary hyperparathyroidism [3–7]. In the subsequent years, PEIT was extended to thyroid cystic lesion and autonomous functioning nodules (AFTNs) with promising results [8–12]. Currently, PEIT is acknowledged as the first-line non-surgical treatment for relapsing benign thyroid cysts [13].

R. Guglielmi, MD (✉)
Department of Endocrinology, Regina Apostolorum Hospital, Albano Laziale, Rome, Italy

Department of Endocrinology & Metabolism, Ospedale Regina Apostolorum, Albano, Rome, Italy
e-mail: rinaldo.guglielmi@alice.it

E. Papini • I. Misischi • F. Graziano • L. Petrucci • R. Rinaldi
Department of Endocrinology, Regina Apostolorum Hospital, Albano Laziale, Rome, Italy

A. Frasoldati
Endocrine Unit, Arcispedale Santa Maria Nuova, Reggio Emilia, Italy



C.P. Lombardi, R. Bellantone (eds.), *Minimally Invasive Therapies for Endocrine Neck Diseases*, DOI 10.1007/978-3-319-20065-1_5

The use of PEIT for toxic nodules and AFTNs was widely employed along the 1990s. Since then, however, this practice progressively declined, due to its controversial long-term results and low tolerability. Presently, PEIT is considered for toxic and pretoxic solid thyroid nodules only in few specific conditions [13].

## 5.2 Cytological Assessment

The first step in considering PEIT treatment for a thyroid lesion is to rule out malignancy. Hence, a repeat cytological evaluation by fine needle aspiration sonographic-guided biopsy (US-FNA) is indicated in all nodules that are considered for PEIT.

US-FNA assessment is strictly required for solid thyroid nodules before treatment with minimally invasive procedures. Its utility in purely cystic thyroid lesions is uncertain due to the low prevalence of malignancy and the low reliability of cytological sampling. In fact, because of the sparse number of follicular cells in cystic lesions sampling, FNAUS results are frequently classified as non-diagnostic [14]. In some cases, moreover, it may be difficult to distinguish the benign cyst-lining cells from those of a cystic papillary carcinoma [15]. To overrule this problem, in the recent Italian Consensus for Classification and Reporting of Thyroid Cytology [16], the non-diagnostic class (TIR 1) was divided in two subgroups. The second category (TIR 1C) is characterized by absence or rare follicular cells but presents a large amount of homogeneous colloid and is suggestive for benign cystic nodule [16].

In case of complex, mixed-structured thyroid nodules, to limit the haemorrhagic and inflammatory changes occurring within the nodule after the initial fluid aspiration [17], it is appropriate to first biopsy the solid component of the nodule. In a surgical series of 34 patients operated because of large cystic lesions, recurrent after initial aspiration, the rate of malignancy was as high as 12 % (4 cystic papillary carcinoma), and a review of the literature confirmed a high median prevalence of cancer (15 %) in cystic thyroid nodules that underwent surgery [18]. These data from surgical series, however, are flawed by selection bias. The actual rate of malignancy in the whole population of cystic nodules that are met by endocrinologists in their everyday's clinical practice is quite low, likely less than 1 % [19]. As a whole, these data recommend the routine use of US FNA to rule out malignancy in cystic thyroid nodule referred to PEIT, with a careful attention to large (>3 cm) lesions with a thick and irregular solid wall.

Cytological assessment of hyperfunctioning (hot) nodules and AFTNs is generally not recommended [13]. Nevertheless, a non-negligible rate of malignancy (3.1 %) has been reported in AFTNs in a recent revision of the literature [20]. Moreover, prediction of malignancy in hot nodules may be difficult on clinical and US basis. Monzani et al. reported a case of papillary cancer in a series of 12 patients treated with surgery because of PEIT failure [2]. Based on these considerations, FNAUS should be always considered for AFTNs that are candidate to PEIT, especially in high-risk patients, multinodular goitres, and in cases with suspicious sonographic features [20].

### 5.2.1 Technique

The patient should be placed in a supine position with the neck fully stretched by means of a low pillow under his/her shoulders. To avoid the risk of bacterial contamination of the lesion, a careful disinfection of the neck skin should be performed, a sterile sheet should be placed over the patient's chest and sterile devices and disposables (e.g. probe cover, US gel, needles and gloves) should be used during the manoeuvre. To avoid an accidental contact of ethanol with patient's eyes, glasses can be used. Local anaesthesia is necessary to prevent patient's discomfort only if large needles (<21 gauge) are required for the drainage of dense thick collections. A preliminary US examination of the thyroid gland and the neck is necessary before proceeding to PEIT to select the appropriate point of needle insertion and the needle path. Nodule diameters and volume should be assessed before treatment and a complete pretreatment set of images should be stored for comparison with the changes after treatment. US guidance and monitoring are mandatory throughout the procedure (Figs. 5.1 and 5.2).

Needle insertion may be performed according to two different approaches: using a needle pointing device (US-guided) or with a free-hand (US-assisted) technique [30]. No head-to-head studies have been carried out to compare the outcomes of

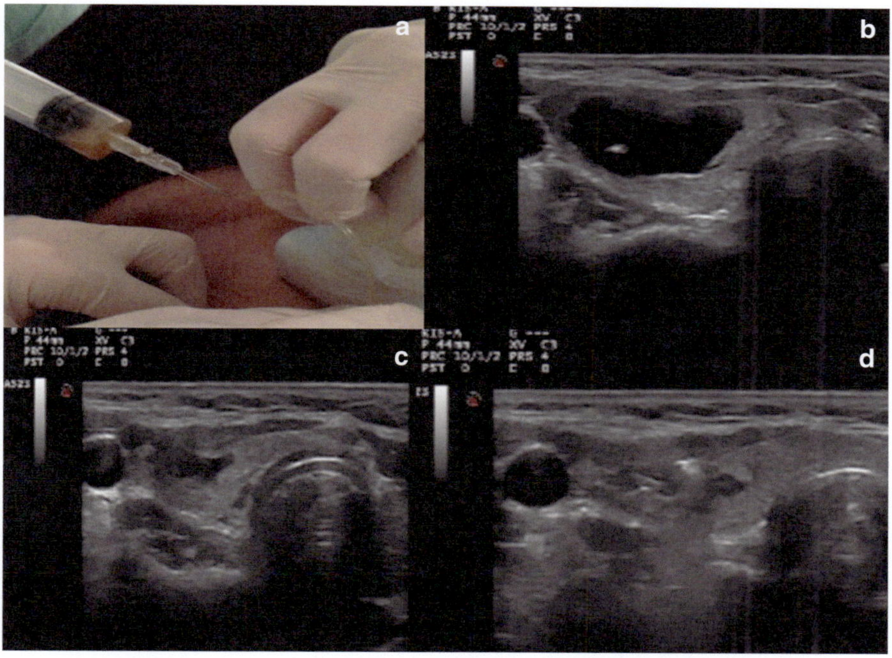


**Fig. 5.1** Percutaneous ethanol injection: procedure of treatment. (**a**) Fluid drainage. (**b**) Needle tip within the fluid area of nodule. (**c**) Near total fluid removed. (**d**) Ethanol infusion

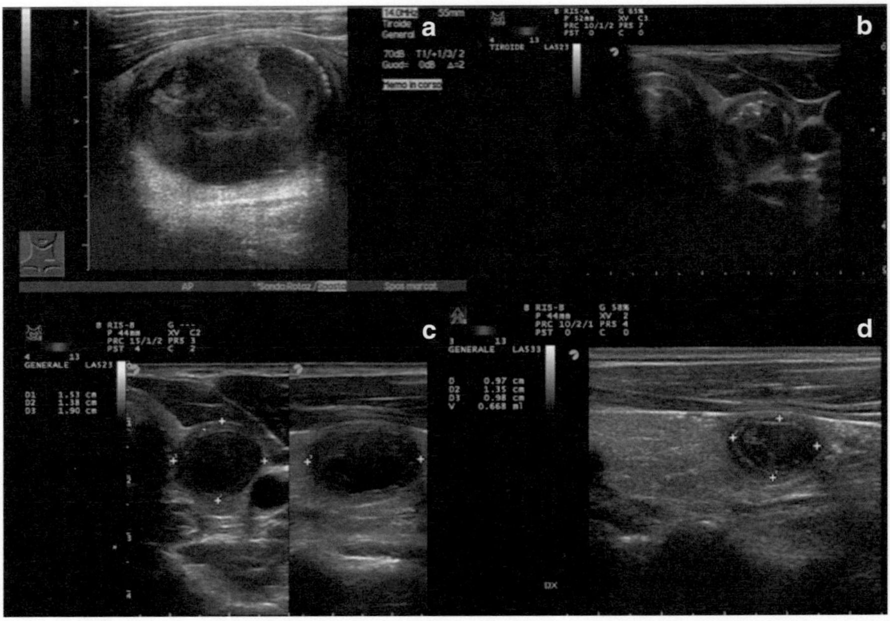

**Fig. 5.2** Long-term results of percutaneous ethanol injection treatment of a large cystic lesion of the thyroid gland. (**a**) Baseline volume: 19 cc. (**b**) Ethanol injection after fluid drainage. (**c**) 6 months after treatment nodule volume: 2.1 cc. (**d**) 24 months after treatment nodule volume: 0.6 cc

PEIT performed with either of these two approaches. US-assisted technique usually requires well-trained operators because the needle path cannot be assessed before the procedure and the progression of the needle tip toward the target lesion needs a continuous monitoring. The use of a needle pointing device allows a more rapid and safe insertion but obliges the operator to a fixed entry site and does not allows changes in needle positioning. This approach may represent a limit during the procedure, especially in case of complex cystic lesions of the thyroid, which often require a repositioning of the needle during the manoeuvre. Alternatively, after the use of the needle pointing device for guiding needle insertion, the tool may be removed from the US probe to widen the range of needle movements within the target lesion.

#### 5.2.1.1 Cystic Nodules

The first step is the near complete drainage of the fluid component from the lesion. Fluid aspiration is facilitated by the use of a syringe holder (e.g. the Cameco pistol) that makes easier to reach an effective negative pressure. After fluid extraction, the aspirating syringe is substituted with one containing 95 % sterile ethanol. Alcohol is carefully and gently injected into the remaining, near virtual, cavity of the cyst. In order to limit the risk of needle displacement during syringe changes, a 20 cm plastic tube connecting the syringe to the needle, possibly furnished with a T clamp system, can be used.

During US monitoring, the infusion of ethanol is easily visualized as a hyperechoic cloud slowly refilling the cyst cavity. The ethanol infused into the cavity of thyroid cysts can either be removed within a short period (e.g. 3–5 min) of time or may be left inside the cyst, to ensure a more protracted activity. The second option is widely adopted because re-aspiration of the injected ethanol seems not necessary for decreasing the risk of ethanol leakage and peri-thyroidal fibrosis [21]. No major differences in efficacy between the two treatment modalities are reported, while ethanol removal was reported to be associated to a higher rate of discomfort for the patient [22].

The volume of injected ethanol generally corresponds to 35–50 % of the volume of the fluid drained from the cystic lesion. Cho et al. reported a significantly better outcome when the amount of ethanol injected into the thyroid cysts was >10 ml [22]. However, the exact ethanol amount should be tailored according to the size and structure of the lesion, the operator opinion during the procedure and the patient compliance.

#### 5.2.1.2 Viscous Cystic Nodules

About 30 % of the large and about 10 % of the small-size cystic nodules are characterized by a highly viscous content [13, 14]. When the fluid collection is dense, the use of a 18-gauge needle should be considered for its drainage. If colloid material cannot be aspirated even with a 18-gauge needle, cyst decompression is very difficult to be attained and surgery remains the main therapeutic option [23]. Alternatively, in very viscous cysts, a two-step treatment has been suggested: first, a small amount of ethanol (e.g. 0.5–1.0 ml) is injected in the attempt to make the dense content more fluid. Then, 2 weeks later, a regular treatment of cystic nodule may be attempted after the occurrence of an at least partial colloid fluidification [24, 25]. This two-step PEIT procedure for viscous nodules is anedoctically reported to be effective, with results apparently comparable to those obtained in pure fluid nodules [23, 24], but no controlled trials are available. A second approach is the drainage of the dense colloid collection, after a local anaesthesia with xylocaine, by means of a large (16-gauge) needle connected to a suction pump. The injection of ethanol is postponed to 10 min, using an amount of alcohol corresponding to 50 % of the aspirated fluid. This approach was reported to attain a significant decrease of the volume of thyroid cysts with viscous component (78 % and 95 % at 1- and 6-months examinations, respectively [26].

#### 5.2.1.3 Complex Nodules

In complex thyroid lesions, PEIT procedure is similar to that employed for "pure" cystic nodules, but multiple treatments are often required because the cavity is usually multiloculated. The volume reduction appears in these cases less striking to the persistence of the solid component of the lesion.

#### 5.2.1.4 Solid Nodules

In solid lesions, a pre-existent cavity is lacking and the diffusion of the injected ethanol is erratic [30]. Hence, multiple areas of the nodule should be treated with minimal amounts (0.1–0.3 mL) of ethanol during each session. This approach is necessary to prevent the seepage of ethanol into the thyroid capsule and the surrounding cervical tissues and the consequent occurrence of sharp neck pain and of possible fibrosis. For solid cold nodules, the injection of a total ethanol dose of 20–30 % of the pretreatment nodular volume is suggested. Ethanol injection should be immediately stopped in case of uneven intranodular diffusion of alcohol, ethanol seepage outside the nodule, or complaint of severe pain during the procedure [27].

On the basis of the reported series, the volume reduction of cold nodules after PEIT is not strictly related to the amount of ethanol injected. A similar reduction (about 50 %), in fact, may be achieved in cold nodules with the injection of a volume of ethanol corresponding either to 20 %, 25 % or 50 % of the baseline nodule volume [28]. To achieve a more relevant volume reduction (up to about 75 %), Caraccio et al. used a high cumulative ethanol dose (up to 130 % of the pretreatment nodule volume) [29]. This report confirms the absence of a precise correlation between the volume of injected ethanol and the obtained nodule shrinkage. The use of high cumulative doses of ethanol to obtain an additive reduction of 25 % versus the baseline nodule volume seems questionable in clinical practice. Even if the efficacy of multiple sessions of PEIT for very large thyroid nodules has been claimed [30], in clinical practice the need of repeated PEIT sessions makes the treatment of solid thyroid lesions as scarcely cost-effective when compared to surgery.

Once the injection has been completed, the final infusion (0.5–1 ml) of saline solution or lydocaine may prevent, by flushing the needle, the transient but sometimes sharp pain that may follow the needle extraction, due to ethanol leakage into the thyroid capsule or the surrounding cervical tissues.

In skilled hands, PEIT is devoid of major side effects, provided some points of caution are accomplished: (a) the needle tip should be clearly seen along the entire phase of ethanol infusion; (b) the procedure should be immediately stopped if the needle position is not clearly defined; (c) the occurrence of progressive resistance to the injection of ethanol should stop the manoeuvre and the needle position should be verified before a further ethanol injection; (d) the occurrence of cough or pain should make immediately stop the infusion [31]. A complete patient information and his/her reassurance before the procedure are of pivotal importance for the tolerability and safety of PEIT [13]. The experience of the operators, the patients' compliance and the quality of US imaging influence the final outcome of the procedure and the risk of complications. These factors may explain the reduced rate of side effects and complications reported in more recent studies [32, 33].

### 5.2.2 Assessment of the Response to PEIT

Nodule volume reduction is the outcome more frequently reported in studies focused on PEIT treatment of thyroid lesion. The size of thyroid nodules is usually assessed by ultrasound and is calculated by means of the ellipsoid formula ($D1 \times D2 \times D3 \times 0.52$) [34] before and 6–12 months after the procedure. For pure cystic lesions, devoid of a solid component, a volume reduction from 50 to 89 % may be defined as a partial response, while a volume reduction greater than 90 % may be considered as a complete response [30, 35].

Pressure and/or cosmetic symptoms should be assessed before and 6–12 months after PEIT. Patients are asked to rate local symptoms on a ten-step visual analogue scale, while physical findings are registered by the physician on a 1–4 cosmetic score based on palpation and inspection [28, 36, 37]. Even if volume decrease is usually correlated to the amelioration of the symptoms/cosmetic scores of the patients [27], these last parameters should always be separately considered to define the actual treatment efficacy and the improvement of the quality of life.

In AFTN or "toxic" nodules, the response to PEIT may be defined as a positive if, together with the reduction of the volume and of the pressure and/or cosmetic symptoms, serum TSH and thyroid hormones (FT3, FT4) return within normal levels 6–12 months after treatment [35]. PEIT treatment may be considered "complete" when all the nodules appear perfused from the injected ethanol with no colour-Doppler signal detectable after the procedure. Anyway, in some occasions, hyperfunctioning tissue is still present at scintiscan even when colour-Doppler signals are undetectable [38]. An abundant vascularization of the nodule is a negative predictor of successful response, as it may cause a rapid drainage of ethanol ("syphon effect"), resulting in a partial neutralization of the chemical damage and a consequent lower success rate of the procedure [39]. In case of AFTN, total disappearance of the "hot" nodule and a complete recovery of extranodular uptake at scintiscan may be viewed as a complete response to PEI [30]. The failure of treatment is indicated by still undetectable TSH levels during the post-treatment follow-up [35].

### 5.2.3 Side Effects

The tolerability of PEIT is fairly good and its side effects are few and transient. Discomfort and pain are reported as similar to those experienced by patients undergoing FNAUS. Only a minority of patients treated with PEIT complain of a slight to moderate pain, lasting for several minutes after the procedure and of a subsequent local tenderness lasting 2–3 days [27].

Pain is rare when predominantly cystic lesions are treated [40]. Instead, treatment of solid nodules, especially when deeply located or close to the thyroid capsule, may be very painful because of extranodular ethanol leakage. This event may be followed by a perilesional fibrosis that could negatively influence a successive surgical treatment, if required [41]. During needle withdrawing, a small amount (0.5–1.0 ml) of xylocaine or saline solution may be injected to avoid the back-diffusion of alcohol along the needle tract and to prevent the occurrence of local pain [42]. Some authors suggested to add 1 g of oral paracetamol or salicylate to the local anaesthesia with lidocaine before ethanol injection [27], but this measure seems not to be necessary in ordinary practice.

Dysphonia is a rare adverse effect in PEIT treatment of thyroid cysts. This complication, on the other hand, is not infrequent (1–4 %) when solid nodules are treated. Dysphonia is due to the chemical injury induced to the laryngeal nerve by the extracapsular diffusion of the injected ethanol. This complication, fortunately, in most cases recover in few weeks after a short course of steroid therapy [35]. To early diagnose a potential nerve injury, the patient is asked to pronounce some words immediately after the conclusion of ethanol injection [42]. To minimize the risk of leakage, the operator should inject ethanol slowly and at a low pressure, especially in case of already treated, fibrotic lesions, and carefully monitor the location of the needle tip within the nodule. The sudden onset of intense pain or cough, in the absence of US signs of haemorrhagic swelling inside or around the nodule, may signal the extrathyroidal leakage of ethanol [31].

Two cases of injury of cervical sympathetic chain, followed by transient Horner's syndrome, have been reported after PEIT treatment of thyroid nodules [43].

In euthyroid patients, PEIT is not followed by significant changes of serum TSH and thyroid hormone levels [31]. The onset of hyper- or hypothyroidism, associated with development of serum auto-antibodies, was occasionally reported [27, 41]. A case of Graves' ophthalmopathy in a patient previously treated with PEIT was anedectotally reported. No evidence, however, demonstrates a possible relationship between ethanol injection and induction of an anti-thyroidal autoimmune response [44].

When treating toxic nodules with PEIT, a prophylactic treatment with β-blockers may be appropriate to prevent the possible exacerbation of thyrotoxic symptoms, usually caused by a transient increase in serum levels of thyroid hormones [35]. Blood pressure should be monitored after the administration of β-blockers, because hypotension, due to the combined effect of the drug and of the peripheral vasodilatation induced by metabolites of ethanol (acetaldehyde acetate), has been reported in few cases [45]. Other major side effects such as cervical haematoma, ipsilateral facial dysesthesia, jugular vein thrombosis and septic complications have been occasionally described. The most relevant complication up to now reported is a single case of chemical necrosis of the larynx combined with necrosis of cervical tissues in a patient treated with PEIT for an AFTN [46]. Severe side effects and major complications, however, are always the consequence of inappropriate modalities of treatment and surveillance of the procedure.

## 5.3 PEIT of Thyroid Cysts

### 5.3.1 Rationale

Thyroid nodules may be defined as cystic if the fluid component is >60 % of their volume. Pure cysts and, more frequently, pseudocystic lesions represent a common finding (likely 25–30 % of all thyroid nodules detected by US) in clinical practice [31]. The majority of large cystic thyroid lesions is caused by intralesional bleeding and/or degeneration of a pre-existing nodule and their fluid content is made of colloid, blood and necrotic debris. Haemorrhagic cystic lesions present suddenly with neck tenderness, pain and pressure symptoms. Their spontaneous regression is possible but most of these lesions persist, frequently grow over time, and usually recur after aspiration [47–51]. Since drainage results in a stable regression only in a minority of cases, further modalities of treatment should be considered [36]. LT4 suppression therapy was demonstrated as scarcely effective in prevent cyst recurrence in several randomized trials. Prolonged TSH suppression, moreover, may cause minor adverse effects, osteoporosis or atrial arrhythmia [52, 53]. Surgery has therefore long been viewed as the standard therapeutic approach for cystic nodules, especially if large and symptomatic [18]. In the last two decades, due to the excellent clinical results provided by a number of different studies [21, 23, 30, 35–37, 40, 50, 51, 54–57], PEIT has become the first-line treatment for thyroid cystic lesions [13, 58, 59]. Various agents have been proposed for the sclerotherapy of thyroid cysts (sodium tetradecyl sulphate, hydroxypolyaethoxydodecan, tetracycline, OK-432) [51, 60] but ethanol injection should be considered as the most cost-effective of them.

### 5.3.2 Results

PEIT treatment may be defined as successful if it results in a ≥50 % reduction of baseline cyst volume. This outcome is achieved in the vast majority (about 70–90 %) of patients, with a mean volume decrease ranging from 65 to 95 % [35]. Interestingly, a correlation between baseline and final volume is not generally observed in cystic lesions [35]. In addition to volume measurement, many studies report other parameters, like pressure or cosmetic symptoms, rated accordingly to specific scale values. Amelioration of local symptoms and cosmetic complaints usually mirrors the entity of volume decrease and is commonly observed in more than 2/3 of the treated patients [27, 36]. Stable symptoms improvement occurs more frequently after PEIT than after simple cyst drainage [35, 40, 56]. This evidence was provided by a prospective randomized study which compared the results of ethanol injection versus isotonic saline flushing, both followed by fluid aspiration. US control indicated a clear superiority (82 % vs. 48 % cure rate) of PEIT [40]. PEIT outcomes are persistent in the long term, with an exceedingly low recurrence rate (3.4 % and 6.5 % over 5 and 10 years, respectively) [23, 35].

It has long been debated if PEIT has a similar efficacy in case of large (>40–50 ml) cysts as well [30, 40]. A large initial volume, anyway, is not clearly correlated with an unsuccessful outcome [21, 23, 35, 54, 57]. According to some studies, the reduction of the lesion volume is directly correlated to the amount of drained fluid and to that of instilled ethanol [21, 51]. On the other hand, the nodule structure exerts a main impact on the final outcome. As a rule, complex cysts and "mixed" nodules with a large solid component are less susceptible of a marked and stable volume reduction as compared to (nearly) "pure" cysts. Moreover, the first ones usually require a prolonged treatment with multiple PEIT sessions [30, 35, 51, 57, 61]. Hence, when dealing with complex cysts, the best results are obtained in smaller lesions [30, 35]. Another possible obstacle to a successful PEIT procedure is the quality of the cyst content [21, 37, 51]. A high viscosity of the fluid, usually predicted by the US appearance of the colloid collection, should suggest the use of large bore needles for the drainage. The chemical and physical properties of the fluid content, however, may change and the finding of a content too viscous to be fully drained does not invariably predict a poor treatment outcome (see the technique section for further details) [24–26]

### 5.3.3 Indications for Clinical Practice

PEIT should be used as the first-line treatment for thyroid cystic lesions after the risk of malignancy has been ruled out [13, 59, 62]. The impact of this approach in clinical practice is relevant because pseudocystic lesions are frequent (25–30 % of all thyroid nodules detected by US) and are frequently growing over time [48]. In comparison with surgery, PEIT is extremely less expensive, presents a nearly negligible risk of permanent complications and is not followed by the need of lifelong substitution therapy.

## 5.4 Autonomously Functioning Thyroid Nodules (AFTNs)

### 5.4.1 Rationale

AFTNs are benign neoplasms, usually monoclonal, associated to a variable degree of thyroid hyperfunction. The disease may be classified in two subgroups according to thyroid hormone levels: (a) pretoxic nodules, when TSH is undetectable but thyroid hormone are within the normal limits, and (b) toxic nodules, when undetectable TSH is accompanied by T3 and/or T4 levels above the normal range. Classical therapeutic options are surgery or radioiodine treatment. In most cases radioiodine, although complicated by a non-negligible rate of late hypothyroidism, is the first choice of treatment but its use in young patients is controversial. Surgery is commonly indicated for toxic nodules larger than 4–5 cm (that are frequently associated to pressure symptoms) because these lesions require high activities of radioiodine and necessitate protective measures in several European countries [63, 64]. Due to the potential complications and costs of surgery and the limited effects of radioiodine treatment on nodule volume, PEIT has been proposed since 1990 as a novel treatment for AFTNs [9–11].

### 5.4.2 Results

Data published during the first 10 years of use of PEIT reported a high percentage (about 90 %) of patients completely or partially cured by PEIT [9, 11, 12, 65, 66]. A major limit of these trials was the short (usually $\leq$1 year) follow-up period and the heterogeneous criteria of enrolment and treatment. Studies based on long-term surveillance reported up to 35 % prevalence of recurrences of thyrotoxicosis [30, 33, 35]. Predictive factors of PEIT efficacy were assessed in the large multicentric Italian study. Pretoxic nodules showed better results than toxic nodules, with a cure rate of 83.4 % vs 66.5 % [65]. A more favourable outcome for pretoxic vs toxic nodules has been confirmed by subsequent trials [35]. Moreover, a ≥30 % fluid component and a ≤15 ml pretreatment volume were associated with a better outcome, independently from the baseline functional status. The best responses were observed in small nodules (≤5 mL volume) with only partial inhibition of the extranodular uptake [35]. In this, as in most studies, cure rate was inversely correlated to baseline volume. Yet, a satisfactory, even if rarer, outcome has been reported also for large (≥40 ml) toxic nodules [32, 38, 66, 67].

A complete ablation of hyperfunctioning tissue is not always obtained after PEIT. In a study on 117 patients with a median follow-up of 2.5 years, a favourable hormonal outcome was reported in 87 % of cases, but radioisotope scan revealed the effacement of the hot areas in only 10 % of patients [38]. Differences in the volume and US structure of the treated lesions and variability of PEIT procedures (e.g. number of treatment sessions, volume of ethanol injected and schedule of follow-up) may account for the inconsistency of results reported by the various authors.

PEIT was proposed in combination with radioiodine as a multi-modality therapy for large AFTNs. Zingrillo et al. treated two groups of patients with AFTNs larger than 4 cm alternatively either with radioiodine alone or with radioiodine after 2–4 preliminary sessions of PEIT. After 12 months of follow-up, nodules treated with combined therapy had the same hormonal normalization rate but a significantly higher reduction of volume and local symptoms compared with nodules treated with radioiodine alone [68]. This approach, which combines the advantages of a limited number of PEIT sessions and of a reduced $^{131}$I dose, could avoid surgery in patients with large symptomatic AFTN and might induce a lower rate of late hypothyroidism [58].

### 5.4.3 Indications for Clinical Practice

In the majority of patients with small-size "hot" thyroid nodules, PEIT may result in normal thyroid function and significant volume reduction. Unfortunately, these results are usually obtained with multiple sessions of therapy, each one associated with non-negligible discomfort and risk of side effects. Moreover, the risk of recurrence of hyperthyroidism in the long term has not been completely defined. Thus, PEIT of hyperfunctioning thyroid nodules should be considered in selected cases only: Symptomatic patients who are not candidate to traditional treatments (as pregnant women), small pretoxic AFTNs in young patients who exhibit a low progression to overt hyperthyroidism and large AFTNs as an adjunctive tool in multi-modality treatment.

## 5.5 Cold Nodules

### 5.5.1 Rationale

The assessment of the a priori risk of malignancy is the first step in the management of "cold" thyroid nodules [13] Once malignancy and abnormal thyroid function have been excluded, patients may be followed up with clinical and US surveillance unless local compression or cosmetic symptoms are present [13].

When treatment is required, long-term LT4 suppressive therapy demonstrates a limited efficacy and is associated with potential side effects [13, 69]. Hence, surgery is the traditional treatment of symptomatic or steadily growing thyroid nodules. However, due to the potential complications and costs of surgery, PEIT was the first minimally invasive US-guided ablation treatment proposed for the shrinkage of large or growing benign thyroid nodules [27].

### 5.5.2 Results

Several studies demonstrated that PEIT may induce a volume decrease from 40 to 70 % vs baseline in cold thyroid nodules [27, 28, 30, 51, 70]. Large volume seems not to be an absolute obstacle for PEIT efficacy. In a series of cold thyroid nodule larger than 10 ml, a >50 % reduction was reported in 90 % of the treated cases [71]. Similar results were reported in a second study, with a 75 % mean volume reduction that was maintained up to 36 months. Volume decrease was clinically significant (≥50 % of baseline volume) in 88.9 % of patients [30]. In a well-designed randomized, prospective study on solitary "cold" thyroid nodules treated either with PEIT or LT4 suppressive therapy, Bennendbaek et al. reported the achievement of a significantly greater nodule volume reduction (47 % vs. 9 %) in the PEIT versus the LT4 group. PEIT, moreover, resulted in a significantly higher (56 % vs. 32 %) rate of relief of pressure and cosmetic complains. The decrease of the volume of perinodular thyroid tissue (about 20 % versus baseline) was reported only in the LT4-treated group [27]. The association of PEIT with LT4 is not followed by additional volume decrease of the lesions [70]. The structure of the nodule, as assessed by the preliminary US evaluation, is a good predictor of the outcome of PEIT. Long-term decrease is remarkably lower in solid nodules as compared to complex or cystic lesions. These data indicate that a solid, densely parenchymatous structure is less successfully affected by ethanol injection than a spongiform or multiloculated tissue [51].

### 5.5.3 Indications for Clinical Practice

In "cold" benign solid thyroid nodules, PEIT is definitely less effective than in cystic lesions. Moreover, the risk of side effects or complications is higher and the schedule of treatment is more complex and time consuming. A further limit is the concern for the possible presence of an occult malignancy. False negative cytological results are infrequent but possible (from 1 to 3 % in the various series), and histological evidence of papillary thyroid cancer has been occasionally reported in patients previously treated with PEIT who finally underwent thyroid surgery [2].

On the basis of these considerations, PEIT should be considered for the management of non-functioning thyroid nodules in elderly or poor surgical risk patients who complain of pressure symptoms only when US-guided thermal ablation procedures are not accessible.

## 5.6 Cervical Metastasis of Thyroid Cancer

### 5.6.1 Rationale

The management of recurrent cervical mestatasis from well-differentiated thyroid cancer (WDTC) is a frequent problem during follow-up of thyroid cancer. Due to their often slow and indolent progression, small neck recurrences do not require an immediate surgical treatment and clinical observation may be a rational option for some of them. In a controlled series of 166 patients under post-surgical surveillance for WDTC, less than 30 % of small-size metastatic or suspicious lymph nodes showed a >3 mm increase during a period of 3.5 years. Relevant limits of the study were the absence of cytological confirmation for the majority (78 %) of lymph nodes and the potential clinical interference of the previous radioiodine ablation [72]. Surgical resection is the treatment of choice for cervical metastasis from WDTC but repeat surgery of central neck compartment is burdened by a high risk of complications (e.g. laryngeal nerve palsy and/or hypoparathyroidism) [73]. In these patients, radioiodine may be an ineffective therapeutic tool. Cervical recurrences may require multiple radioiodine doses to be cured or may be non-radioiodine-avid [74]. Due to these considerations, US-guided percutaneous ablation treatments (e.g. PEIT, laser ablation (LTA) or radiofrequency (RF)) may be considered as alterative options to surgery and radioiodine therapy.

PEIT treatment for nodal metastasis was first introduced at Mayo Clinic in the 1990s and, since then, several contributes have been produced [75, 76].

### 5.6.2 Results

All the available data, even if derived from a small number of centres, show favourable clinical results. Hay et al. reported a significant decrease in lymph node size in all the treated patients, with a mean volume reduction from 492 to 20 $mm^3$ during a 2-year follow-up [75, 76]. Similar results have been reported from Heilo et al., who reported a high frequency (84 %) of complete ablation in 109 cervical nodes treated with PEIT [77]. Both studies reported a low incidence of side effects or complications (severe neck pain, permanent hypoparathyroidism and periglandular sclerosis). At a difference with the results in thyroid nodules, the structure (solid or cystic) of neck recurrences did not significantly influence the efficacy of PEIT ablation [77–81].

### 5.6.3 Indications for Clinical Practice

PEIT may be considered as an effective therapeutic option for small-size WDTC neck recurrences when further surgery and/or radioiodine therapy are not amenable or refused. Data from studies with a more protracted follow-up period are necessary to establish the actual rate of successful treatments, the probability of relapse, and the impact on survival and quality of life, taking into account the frequently indolent behaviour of these lesions. Although LTA and RFA seem to promise better results [82, 83], a recent report based on a long-term follow-up, demonstrates a similar efficacy of PEIT when compared to RFA for the control of locoregional WDTC recurrences [84]. Current ATA Guidelines suggest a potential role in the future for non-surgical techniques able to safely remove or destroy small cervical nodal metastases, minimizing the iatrogenic harm or discomfort for the patients [59]. Due to its potential side effects and complications, PEIT treatment of WDTC neck recurrences should be performed only in centres with proved experience in US-guided interventional techniques.

## 5.7 Other Neck Lesions

PEIT was proposed for the treatment of thyroglossal duct cysts (TDC), a not infrequent congenital neck abnormality arising from the embryonic thyroglossal duct structures [85–87]. The traditional treatment of these lesions, located along the midline of the neck, is surgery [88]. Although the data are sparse and the outcomes in part controversial, Kim et al. in 2011 reported a >80 % success rate in a series of 11 patients with TDC treated with PEIT [87]. The procedure was carried out with the same technical approach used for the cystic lesions with dense viscous content (see: "Technique" section). PEIT DTC treatment was not associated with relevant side effects but mild cervical pain [85–87].

Parathyroid (PT) cysts are non-functioning lesions, usually revealed incidentally by neck US evaluation. The cystic component may be the outcome of a gradual retention of the secretions of a parathyroid adenoma. Their prevalence is probably underestimated, due to the absence of general effects [89, 90]. Like thyroid cysts, PT cysts frequently recur after drainage by means of FNA. Sclerosing agents have been proposed as an alternative to surgery and PEIT was reported as an effective and safe treatment [91–94]. PT cysts are deeply located and are sometimes close to the recurrent laryngeal nerve. Hence, an extreme care should be taken to avoid ethanol seepage outside the target lesion. Due to the high rate of relapse, PEIT is not a cost-effective therapeutic tool for the treatment of parathyroid hyperplasia in secondary or tertiary hyperparathyroidism [5, 94–96].

## 5.8 Costs

PEIT is a low-cost technique because it is rapid, performed in an outpatient setting and requires only widely available US equipments and inexpensive disposables. The cost of ethanol is low (about 5 € for a 10 ml vial of 95 % sterile ethanol). The endocrinologist and/or sonographer can perform the treatment after an appropriate training period (500 US-guided FNA procedures may represent an appropriate level of clinical practice for starting to practice PEIT).

The mean time reported to perform a single procedure is 15 min for cystic thyroid lesions and 25 min for hyperfunctioning nodules [35]. The median number of sessions needed for a complete treatment is 2 in thyroid cysts, 4 in AFTNs and 5 in toxic nodules. So, the median cumulative period required for a complete treatment may be calculated in approximately 30 min in cystic thyroid nodules, 2 h in AFTNs and 2.5 h in hyperfunctioning nodules.

The cost of PEIT, on the basis of Italian National Health Service reimbursement, is 420 € for cysts (2 day-hospital refund), 840 and 1050 € for AFTN and toxic nodule (4 and 5 day-hospital refund), respectively. The median costs for surgery and $^{131}I$ ablation are 3350 and 210 €.

## Conclusions

The majority of data on the clinical use of PEIT in thyroid lesions are derived from non-controlled studies. Furthermore, criteria for nodule selection, amount of ethanol injected and number of sessions are variable in the different series. All these factors explain the variable outcomes reported by different trials. On the basis of the available evidences and of our experience, however, PEIT can be considered as a therapeutic option for the following conditions:

- *Cystic nodules*. PEIT is the first-line non-surgical therapy for symptomatic relapsing cystic nodules. Although other sclerosing agents have been reported to be as effective as ethanol, currently alcohol injection should be considered as the standard sclerosing technique because it is safe, rapid, inexpensive and easily repeatable.
- *AFTNs and "toxic" nodules*. PEIT treatment of AFTNs should be considered only in selected cases. Its use seems appropriate in symptomatic patients who are not candidate to the traditional treatments (radioiodine and surgery), in young patients or pregnant women with small AFTN not associated with functional suppression of extranodular tissue, and as a possible adjunctive tool for a multi-modality approach to large AFTNs.
- *Cold nodules*. PEIT is effective in reducing the volume of solid "cold" thyroid nodules The procedure should be limited, in absence of more accurate procedures, in elderly patients at poor surgical risk when thermal ablation techniques are not accessible.
- *Local WDTC recurrences*. PEIT is an effective therapeutic option for neck recurrences of WDTC. This procedure may be considered, in alternative to simple follow-up, for the management of not threatening cervical metastasis in patients already submitted to neck dissection when a second surgery and/or radioiodine therapy are not appropriate or ineffective. Experienced operators are requested for the treatment of these very selected cases.

- *Other neck lesions*. PEIT may be considered as a therapeutic option in patients with TDC and parathyroid cysts when surgery is contraindicated or refused. Treatment of hyperplastic parathyroid gland is at risk of major complications (recurrent nerve injury and severe pain).

**Disclosure of Interest** None of the authors have financial or commercial interests

## References


1. Crescenzi A, Papini E, Pacella CM et al (1996) Morphological changes in a hyperfunctioning thyroid adenoma after percutaneous ethanol injection: histological, enzymatic and sub-microscopical alterations. J Endocrinol Invest 19:371–376
2. Monzani F, Caraccio N, Basolo F et al (2000) Surgical and pathological changes after percutaneous ethanol injection therapy of thyroid nodules. Thyroid 10:1087–1092
3. Bean WJ (1981) Renal cysts: treatment with alcohol. Radiology 138:329–331
4. Bean WJ, Rodan BA (1985) Hepatic cysts: treatment with alcohol. Am J Radiol 144: 237–241
5. Solbiati L, Giangrande A, DePra L et al (1985) Percutaneous ethanol injection of parathyroid tumors under US guidance: treatment for secondary hyperparathyroidism. Radiology 155:607–610
6. Livraghi T, Giorgio A, Mario G et al (1985) Hepatocellular carcinoma and cirrhosis in 746 patients: long term results of percutaneous ethanol injection. Radiology 197:101–108
7. Rossi R, Savastano S, Tommasselli AP et al (1995) Percutaneous computer tomography-guided ethanol injection in aldosterone-producing adrenal adrenocortical adenoma. Eur J Endocrinol 132:302–305
8. Rozman B, Benze-Zigman Z, Tomic-Brzac H et al (1989) Sclerosation of thyroid cysts by ethanol. Period Biol 91:1116–1118
9. Livraghi T, Paracchi A, Ferrari C et al (1990) Treatment of autonomous thyroid nodule with percutaneous ethanol injection: preliminary results. Radiology 175:827–829
10. Yasuda K, Ozaki O, Sugino K et al (1992) Treatment of cystic lesions of the thyroid by ethanol instillation. World J Surg 16(5):958–961
11. Martino E, Murtas MI, Liviselli A et al (1992) Percutaneous intranodular ethanol injection for treatment of autonomously functioning thyroid nodules. Surgery 112:1161–1165
12. Papini E, Panunzi C, Pacella CM et al (1993) Percutaneous ultrasound-guided ethanol injection: a new treatment of toxic autonomously functioning thyroid nodules? J Clin Endocrinol Metab 76:411–416
13. Gharib H, Papini E, Paschke R, Duick DS, Valcavi R, Hegedüs L, Vitti P, AACE/AME/ETA Task Force on Thyroid Nodules (2010) American Association of Clinical Endocrinologists, Associazione Medici Endocrinologi, and European Thyroid Association medical guidelines for clinical practice for the diagnosis and management of thyroid nodules: executive summary of recommendations. Endoc Pract 16(3):468–475
14. Cibas ES, Syed ZA (2009) The bethesda system for reporting thyroid cytopathology. Am J ClinPathol 132:658–665
15. Faquin WC, Cibas ES, Renshaw AA (2005) "Atypical" cells in fine-needle aspiration biopsy specimens of benign thyroid cysts. Cancer 105(2):71–79
16. Nardi F, Basolo F, Crescenzi A, Fadda G, Frasoldati A, Orlandi F, Palombini L, Papini E, Zini M, Pontecorvi A, Vitti P (2014) Italian consensus for the classification and reporting of thyroid cytology. J Endocrinol Invest 37(6):593–599
17. Braga M, Cavalcanti TC, Collaço LM, Graf H (2001) Efficacy of ultrasound-guided fine-needle aspiration biopsy in the diagnosis of complex thyroid nodules. J Clin Endocrinol Metab 86(9):4089–4091

18. Abbas G, Heller KS, Khoynezhad A, Dubner S, Sznyter SL (2001) The incidence of carcinoma in cytologically benign thyroid cysts. Surgery 130(6):1035–1038
19. Udelsman R (2001) Summary of the 22th annual meeting of the American Association of Endocrine Surgeons, Atlanta
20. Mirfakhraee S, Mathews D, Peng L, Woodruff S, Zigman JM (2013) A solitary hyperfunctioning thyroid nodule harboring thyroid carcinoma: review of the literature. Thyroid Res 6(1):7. doi:10.1186/1756-6614-6-7
21. Cho YS, Lee HK, Ahn IM et al (2000) Sonographically guided ethanol sclerotherapy for benign thyroid cysts: results in 22 patients. AJR Am J Roentgenol 174(1):213–216
22. Kim DW, Rho MH, Kim HJ et al (2005) Percutaneous ethanol injection for benign cystic thyroid nodules: is aspiration of ethanol-mixed fluid advantageous? AJNR Am J Neuroradiol 26(8):2122–2127
23. Del Prete S, Caraglia D, Vitale G, Giuberti G, Marra M, D'Alessandro AM, Lupoli G, Addeo R, Facchini G, Rossiello R, Abbruzzese A, Capasso E (2002) Percutaneous ethanol injection efficacy in the treatment of large symptomatic thyroid cystic nodules: ten-year follow-up of large series. Thyroid 12:815–821
24. Zingrillo M, Torlantano M, Ghiggi MR, D'Aloiso L, Nirchino V, Bisceglia M, Liuzzi A (1996) Percutaneous ethanol injection of large thyroid cystic nodules. Thyroid 6:403–408
25. Zieleźnik W, Kawczyk-Krupka A, Peszel Barlik M, Cebula W, Sieroń A (2005) Modified percutaneous ethanol injection in the treatment of viscous cystic thyroid nodules. Thyroid 15(7):683–687
26. Sung JY, Baek JH, Kim YS, Jeong HJ, Kwak MS, Lee D, Moon W (2008) One-step ethanol ablation viscous cystic thyroid nodules. AJR 191:1730–1733
27. Bennedbaek FN, Nielsen LK, Hegedus L (1998) Effect of percutaneous ethanol injection therapy versus suppressive doses of l-thyroxine on benign solitary sold cold nodules: a randomized trial. J Clin Endocrinol Metab 83:830–835
28. Bennendbaek FN, Hegedus L (1999) Percutaneous ethanol injection therapy in benign solitary cold thyroid nodules: a randomized trial comparing one injection with three injections. Thyroid 9:225–233
29. Caraccio N, Goletti O, Lippolis PV, Casolaro A, Cavina E, Miccoli P, Monzani F (1997) Is percutaneous ethanol injection a useful alternative for the treatment of the cold benign thyroid nodule? Five years' experience. Thyroid 7:699–704
30. Lee SJ, Ahn I (2005) Effectiveness of PEI therapy in benign nodular and cystic disease: long-term follow up experience. Endocr J 52(4):455–462
31. Valcavi R, Frasoldati A (2013) Percutaneous Ethanol Injection (PEI) in the treatment of thyroid cysts, nodules and other neck lesions. In: Baskin Sr JH, Duick DS, Levine RA. Thyroid ultrasound and ultrasound-guided FNA, 3rd edn. Springer, pp 315–346
32. Del Prete S, Russo D, Caraglia M et al (2001) Percutaneous ethanol injection of autonomous thyroid nodules with a volume larger than 40 ml: three years of follow-up. Clin Radiol 56(11):895–901
33. Yano Y, Sugino K, Akaishi J et al (2011) Treatment of autonomously functioning thyroid nodules at a single institution: radioiodine therapy, surgery, and ethanol injection therapy. Ann Nucl Med 25(10):749–754
34. Bruneton JS (1987) Ultrasonography of the neck. Springer, Berlin, p 7
35. Guglielmi R, Pacella CM, Bianchini A et al (2004) Percutaneous ethanol injection treatment in benign thyroid lesions: role and efficacy. Thyroid 14:125–131
36. Valcavi R, Frasoldati A (2004) Ultrasound-guided percutaneous ethanol injection therapy in thyroid cystic nodules. Endocr Pract 10:269–275
37. Sung JY, Kim YS, Choi H et al (2011) Optimum first-line treatment technique for benign cystic thyroid nodules: ethanol ablation or radiofrequency ablation. AJR Am J Roentgenol 196(2):W210–W214
38. Tarantino L, Francica G, Sordelli I et al (2008) Percutaneous ethanol injection of hyperfunctioning thyroid nodules: long-term follow-up in 125 patients. AJR Am J Roentgenol 190: 800–808

39. Di Lelio A, Rivolta M, Casati M, Capra M (1995) Treatment of autonomous thyroid nodules: value of percutaneous ethanol injection. AJR 164:207–213
40. Bennedbaek FN, Hegedus L (2003) Treatment of recurrent thyroid cysts with ethanol: a randomized double blind controlled trial. J Clin Endocrinol Metab 88:5773–5777
41. Bennedbaek FN, Karstrup S, Hegedüs L (1997) Percutaneous ethanol injection therapy in the treatment of thyroid and parathyroid diseases. Eur J Endocrinol 136(3):240–250
42. Raggiunti B, Fiore G, Mongia A, Balducci G, Ballone E, Capone F (2009) A 7-years follow-up of patients with thyroid cysts and pseudocysts treated with PEI: volume change and costs analysis. J Ultrasound 12:107–111
43. Pishdad GR, Pishdad P, Pishdad R (2011) Horner's syndrome as a complication of percutaneous ethanol treatment of thyroid nodule. Thyroid 21:327–328
44. Regalbuto C, Le Moli R, Muscia V et al (2012) Severe Graves' after percutaneous ethanol injection in a nontoxic thyroid nodule. Thyroid 22(2):210–213
45. Gelczer RK, Charboneau JW, Hussain S, Brown DL (1998) Complications of percutaneous ethanol ablation. J Ultrasound Med 17:531–533
46. Mauz PS, Maassen MM, Braun B, Brosch S (2004) How safe is percutaneous ethanol injection for treatment of thyroid nodule? Report of a case of severe toxic necrosis of the larynx and adjacent skin. Acta Otolaryngol 124(10):1226–1230
47. De Los Santos ET, Keyhani-Rofagha S, Cunningham JJ et al (1990) Cystic thyroid nodules: the dilemma of malignant lesions". Arch Intern Med 150:422–427
48. Sheppard MC, Franklyn JA (1994) Management of the single thyroid nodule. Clin Endocrinol 41:719–724
49. Jensen F, Rasmussen SN (1976) The treatment of thyroid cysts by ultrasonographically-guided fine needle aspiration. Acta Chir Scand 142:209–211
50. Monzani F, Lippi F, Goletti O et al (1994) Percutaneous aspiration and ethanol sclerotherapy for thyroid cysts. J Clin Endocrinol Metab 78:800–802
51. Kim JH, Lee HK, Lee JH et al (2003) Efficacy of sonographically guided percutaneous ethanol injection for treatment of thyroid cysts versus solid thyroid nodules. AJR 180:1623–1726
52. McCowen KD, Reed JW, Fariss BL (1980) The role of thyroid therapy in patients with thyroid cysts. Am J Med 68:853–855
53. Sdano MT, Falciglia M, Welge JA, Steward DL (2005) Efficacy of thyroid hormone suppression for benign thyroid nodules: meta-analysis of randomized trials. Otolaryngol Head Neck Surg 133:391–396
54. Zingrillo M, Torlontano M, Chiarella R et al (1999) Percutaneous ethanol injection may be a definitive treatment for symptomatic thyroid cystic nodules not treatable by surgery: five-year follow-up study. Thyroid 9:763–767
55. Verde G, Papini E, Pacella CM et al (1994) Ultrasound guided percutaneous ethanol injection in the treatment of cystic thyroid nodules. Clin Endocrinol 41:719–724
56. Antonelli A, Campatelli A, Di Vito A et al (1994) Comparison between ethanol sclerotherapy and emptying with injection of saline in treatment of thyroid cysts. Clin Investig 72(12): 971–974
57. Kanotra SP, Lateef M, Kirmani O (2008) Non-surgical management of benign thyroid cysts: use of ultrasound-guided ethanol ablation. Postgrad Med J 84(998):639–643
58. Pacini F (2003) Role of percutaneous ethanol injection in management of nodular lesions of the thyroid gland. J Nucl Med 44:211–212
59. Cooper DS, Doherty GM, Haugen BR et al (2009) Revised American Thyroid Association management guidelines for patients with thyroid nodules and differentiated thyroid cancer. Thyroid 19(11):1167–1214
60. Kalra N, Ahuja CK, Dutta P, Rajwanshi A, Mittal BR, Bhansali A, Khandelwal N (2014) Comparison of sonographically guided percutaneous sodium tetradecyl sulfateInjection with ethanol injection in the treatment of benign nonfunctioning thyroid nodules. J Vasc Interv Radiol. 25(8):1218–1224. pii: S1051-0443(14)00489-8
61. Kim YJ, Baek JH, Ha EJ, Lim HK, Lee JH, Sung JY, Kim JK, Kim TY, Kim WB, Shong YK (2012) Cystic versus predominantly cystic thyroid nodules: efficacy of ethanol ablation and analysis of related factors. Eur Radiol 22(7):1573–1578

62. Papini E, Pacella CM, Misischi I, Guglielmi R, Bizzarri G, Døssing H, Hegedus L (2014) The advent of ultrasound-guided ablation techniques in nodular thyroid disease: towards a patient-tailored approach. Best Pract Res Clin Endocrinol Metab 28(4):601–618
63. Hamburger JI (1987) The autonomously functioning thyroid nodules: Goetsch's disease. Endocr Rev 8:439–442
64. Gorman CA, Robertson JS (1978) Radiation dose in the selection of 131I or surgical treatment for toxic thyroid adenoma. Ann Intern Med 89:85–90
65. Lippi F, Ferrari C, Manetti L et al (1996) Treatment of solitary autonomous thyroid nodules by percutaneous etanol injection. Results of an Italian multicenter study. J Clin Endocrinol Metab 81:3261–3264
66. Monzani F, Caraccio N, Goletti O (1997) Five year follow-up of percutaneous ethanol injection for the treatment of hyperfunctioning thyroid nodules: a study of 117 patients. Clin Endocrinol 46:9–15
67. Zingrillo M, Torlontano M, Ghiggi MR et al (2000) Radioiodine and percutaneous ethanol injection in the treatment of large toxic thyroid nodule: a long-term study. Thyroid 10:985–989
68. Zingrillo M, Modoni S, Conte M, Frusciante V, Trischitta V (2003) Percutaneous ethanol injection plus radioiodine versus radioiodine alone in the treatment of large toxic thyroid nodules. J Nucl Med 44:207–210
69. Yousef A, Clark J, Clark J, Doi SAR (2010) Thyroxine suppression therapy for benign, non-functioning solitary thyroid nodules: a quality-effects meta-analysis. Clin Med Res 8(3/4):150–158
70. Caraccio N, Goletti O, Lippolos PV et al (1999) Is percutaneous ethanol injection a useful alternative for the treatment of the cold benign thyroid nodule? Five years' experience. Thyroid 7:699–704
71. Zingrillo M, Collura D, Ghiggi MR, Nirchio V, Trischitta V (1998) Treatment of large cold benign thyroid nodules not eligible for surgery with Percutaneous Ethanol Injection. J Clin Endocrinol Metabol 83(11):3905–3907
72. Robenshtok E, Fish S, Bach A, Domínguez JM, Shaha A, Tuttle RM (2012) Suspicious cervical lymph nodes detected after thyroidectomy for papillary thyroid cancer usually remain stable over years in properly selected patients. J Clin Endocrinol Metab 97:2706–2713
73. Monchik JM, Donatini G, Iannuccilli J et al (2006) Radiofrequency ablation and percutaneous ethanol injection treatment for recurrent local and distant well-differentiated thyroid carcinoma. Ann Surg 244:296–304
74. Yim JH, Kim WB, Kim EY, Kim WG, Kim TY, Ryu JS, Moon DH, Sung TY, Yoon JH, Kim SC, Hong SJ, Shong YK (2011) Adjuvant radioactive therapy after reoperation for locoregionally recurrent papillary thyroid cancer in patients who initially underwent total thyroidectomy and high-dose remnant ablation. J Clin Endocrinol Metab 96:3695–3700
75. Hay ID, Charboneau JW (2011) The coming of age of ultrasound-guided percutaneous ethanol ablation of selected neck nodal metastases in well-differentiated thyroid carcinoma. J Clin Endocrinol Metab 96:2717–2720
76. Lewis BD, Hay ID, Charboneau JW et al (2002) Percutaneous ethanol injection for treatment of cervical lymph node metastases in patients with papillary thyroid carcinoma. AJR 178:699–704
77. Heilo A, Sigstad E, Fagerlid KH, Håskjold OI, Grøholt KK, Berner A, Bjøro T, Jørgensen LH (2011) Efficacy of ultrasound-guided percutaneous ethanol injection treatment in patients with a limited number of metastatic cervical lymph nodes from papillary thyroid carcinoma. J Clin Endocrinol Metab 96:2750–2755
78. Lim CY, Yum JS, Lee J et al (2007) Percutaneous ethanol injection therapy for locally recurrent papillary thyroid carcinoma. Thyroid 17:347–350
79. Kim BM, Kim MJ, Kim EK et al (2008) Controlling recurrent papillary thyroid carcinoma in the neck by ultrasonography-guided percutaneous ethanol injection. Eur Radiol 18:835–842
80. Sohn YM, Hong SW, Kim EK et al (2009) Complete eradication of metastatic lymph node after percutaneous ethanol injection therapy: pathologic correlation. Thyroid 19:317–319
81. Vannucchi G, Covelli D, Perrino M, De Leo S, Fugazzola L (2014) Ultrasound-guided percutaneous ethanol injection in papillary thyroid cancer metastaticlymph-nodes. Endocrine 47(2):648–651

82. Papini E, Bizzarri G, Bianchini A, Valle D, Misischi I, Guglielmi R, Salvatori M, Solbiati L, Crescenzi A, Pacella CM, Gharib H (2013) Percutaneous ultrasound-guided laser ablation is effective for treating selected nodal metastases in papillary thyroid cancer. J Clin Endocrinol Metab 98(1):E92–E97
83. Baek JH, Kim YS, Sung JY, Choi H, Lee JH (2011) Locoregional control of metastatic well-differentiated thyroid cancer by ultrasound-guided radiofrequency ablation. AJR Am J Roentgenol 197:W331–W336
84. Guenette JP, Monchik JM, Dupuy DE (2013) Image-guided ablation of postsurgical locoregional recurrence of biopsy-proven well-differentiated thyroid carcinoma. J Vasc Interv Radiol 24(5):672–679
85. Fukumoto K, Kojima T, Tomonari H et al (1994) Ethanol injection sclerotherapy for Baker's cysts, thyroglossal duct cysts, and brianchial cleft cysts. Ann Plast Surg 33:615–619
86. Baskin HJ (2006) Percutaneous ethanol injection of thyroglossal duct cysts. Endoc Pract 12:355–357
87. Kim SM, Baek JH, Kim YS et al (2011) Efficacy and safety of ethanol ablation for thyroglossal duct cysts. AJNR Am J Neuroradiol 32:306–309
88. Clark OH, Okerlund MD, Cavalieri RR et al (1979) Diagnosis and treatment of thyroid parathyroid and thyroglossal duct cysts. J Clin Endocrinol Metab 48:983–988
89. Ippolito G, Fausto Palazzo F, Sebag F et al (2006) A single institution 25-year review of true parathyroid cysts. Lagenbecks Arch Surg 391:13–18
90. Frasoldati A, Valcavi R (2004) Challenges in neck ultrasonography: lymphadenopathy and parathyroid glands. Endocr Pract 10(3):261–268
91. Okamura K, Ikenoue H, Sato K et al (1992) Sclerotherapy for benign parathyroid cysts. Am J Surg 163:344–345
92. Sanchez A, Carretto H (1993) Treatment of a nonfunctioning parathyroid cysts with tetracycline injection. Head Neck 15:263–265
93. Akel M, Salti I, Azar ST (1999) Successful treatment of parathyroid cyst using ethanol sclerotherapy. Am J Med Sci 317:50–52
94. Baskin HJ (2004) New applications of thyroid and parathyroid ultrasound. Min Endocrinol 29:195–206
95. Fugakawa M, Kitaoga M, Tominaka Y et al (2003) Guidelines for percutaneous ethanol injection therapy of the parathyroid glands in chronic dialysis patients. Nephrol Dial Transplant 18(Suppl 3):31–33
96. Chen HH, Lin CJ, Wu CJ et al (2011) Chemical ablation of recurrent and persistent secondary hyperparathyroidism after subtotal parathyroidectomy. Ann Surg 253(4):786–790

# 6 Percutaneous Laser Thermal Ablation (LAT): Techniques, Indications, Experience and Complications

Enrico Papini, Irene Misischi, Antonio Bianchini, Filomena Graziano, Rinaldo Guglielmi, Marco Chianelli, and Giancarlo Bizzarri

Thyroid nodules are a frequent clinical problem in endocrine practice [1, 2]. The majority of them are benign and asymptomatic but some steadily grow and may cause pressure symptoms or concern [1]. Surgical resection is the traditional approach to thyroid lesions that, even if benign at repeated fine-needle aspiration biopsy (FNA), are symptomatic or progressively enlarging [3]. Surgery, however, carries some problems: is expensive, is associated with a low but not negligible risk of cosmetic damage or complications, and is frequently followed by the need of a substitution therapy [3]. During the last years, non-surgical, minimally invasive procedures (MIT) have been investigated for the treatment of thyroid lesions when surgery is technically difficult or is refused by the patient [4]. Bown [5] first used laser energy for the debulking of hepatic tumours and later, in the year 2000, US-guided laser ablation (LAT) was proposed for the management of benign solid thyroid nodules [6]. Currently, the procedure is increasingly used for the treatment of selected patients with thyroid lesions and its principles, outcomes, side effects and indications will be reviewed in the following chapters.

## 6.1 Principles and Technique

The expression "percutaneous laser ablation" (LAT) defines the destruction of a target lesion that is realised with the deposition of laser light energy, transmitted via an optical fibre, into the tissue [5]. Laser light is coherent and monochromatic, can be highly focused and permits the transmission of large amounts of energy with

E. Papini, MD, FACE (✉) • I. Misischi • F. Graziano • R. Guglielmi • M. Chianelli
Department of Endocrinology, Regina Apostolorum Hospital, Albano Laziale, Rome, Italy
e-mail: papinie@gmail.com

A. Bianchini • G. Bizzarri
Diagnostic Imaging, Regina Apostolorum Hospital, Albano Laziale, Rome, Italy



C.P. Lombardi, R. Bellantone (eds.), *Minimally Invasive Therapies for Endocrine Neck Diseases*, DOI 10.1007/978-3-319-20065-1_6

minimal dispersion. Light is transmitted from an external laser source into the target lesion by means of 300–400-mm optical fibres, which consists of a silica-based core surrounded by a cladding of hard polymer material. The photons released by the optic fibre scatter within the target lesion, rapidly produce heat and induce coagulative necrosis of the cells surrounding the needle tip [6, 7]. A further diffusion of heating within the tissue is due to heat conduction, influenced by blood supply, tissue characteristics and the occurrence of carbonisation [7].

Different laser sources, optical fibres, modified tips and applicators are currently available. A nearly spherical volume of coagulative necrosis up to 20 mm in diameter can be obtained with a single optical fibre. A larger volume of necrosis may be induced firing multiple fibres, arrayed at 1.5 cm spacing throughout the target lesion [6, 7], or with the use of cooled-tip diffusers that deliver large amounts of energy over a wide area, thus preventing the occurrence of local charring [5–11].

The penetration of light is optimal in the near-infrared spectrum [7]. Hence, laser procedures are mostly performed with neodymium-doped yttrium aluminium garnet (Nd:YAG) or with diode lasers, operating with a wavelength of 800–980 nm. Current laser devices induce a predictable and reproducible area of tissue thermal ablation and, at the same time, minimally affect the tissue surrounding the targeted lesion [6, 12].

Laser treatment is performed on conscious patients after mild intravenous sedation and local anaesthesia with xylocaine (from the skin entry site down to the thyroid capsule) [6]. After preliminary information and reassurance, the patient is placed in the supine position and his/her neck is appropriately positioned (Fig. 6.1). Then, under ultrasound guidance, one or more spinal needles with diameter from 20 to 22 G are inserted into the target lesion [9, 11, 13]. Thereafter, the optical fibres are easily positioned through the sheath of the needles and 5–10 mm of their bare tip is placed in direct contact with the tissue. LA sessions may be performed either under US guidance or assistance, using an ultrasound (US) system equipped with a high-frequency linear probe (7.5–15 MHz) and a removable guiding device. During laser firing, US monitoring demonstrates in the area under treatment the appearance of hyperechoic spots due to gas microbubbles produced by tissue heating. The procedure is stopped after 400–600 s or when the zone of hyperechogenicity caused by the evaporation of the water content of the tissue is steady and complete [9, 14–20]. In order to increase the volume of ablation in large-size lesions, the energy may be delivered continuously while retracting the needles by 1–2 cm ("pull back technique") [11, 21]. Spinal needles and optical fibres are then withdrawn, the patient is given an analgesics injection and is observed for an hour before US control and discharge [16].

## 6.2 Experience

### 6.2.1 Cold Nodules

The feasibility of percutaneous laser thermal ablation was initially tested on animal models (New Zealand rabbits and laboratory pigs) [6]. After ex vivo studies on resected thyroid glands [6] that provided reproducible energy-damage curves, a

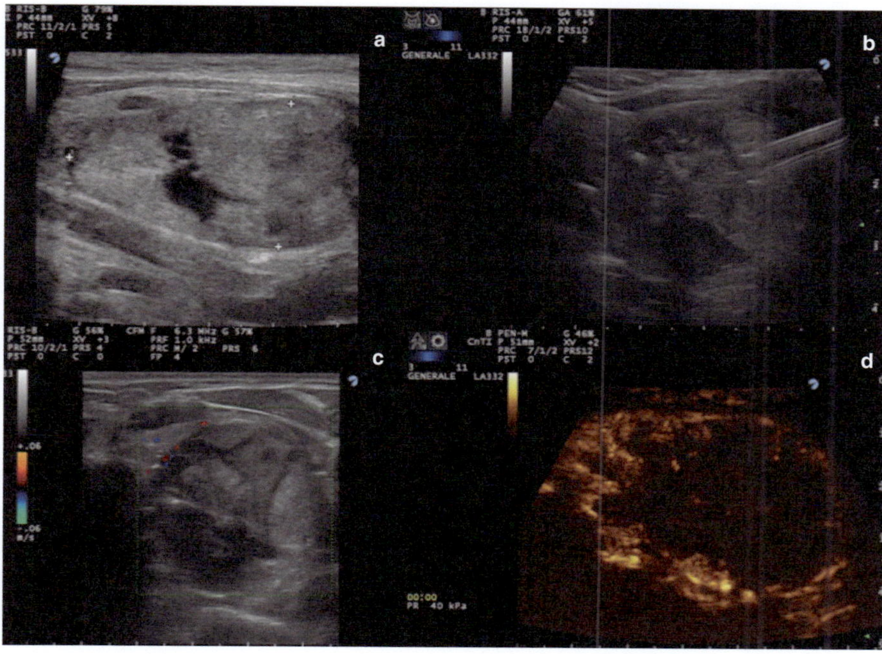

**Fig. 6.1** (**a**) Ultrasound scan of a large, prevalently solid, cold thyroid nodule (DM 4.6 × 2.3 × 3.7 cm vol 20.3 cc). (**b**) Under ultrasound monitoring, two optical fibres are inserted into the nodule and start laser firing. (**c**) After 600 s of energy delivery, colour-Doppler examination of the target lesions demonstrates a large area of thermal necrosis devoid of vascular signals. (**d**) Contrast-enhanced ultrasound, performed 24 h after treatment, clearly depicts a large area of tissue ablation with no evidence of blood supply

feasibility study was performed on two human volunteers with large thyroid nodules immediately before their surgical resection. Since then, several non-randomised [9–11, 22–26] trials showed consistent results for LAT treatment of thyroid lesions. Cytological and histological samples, obtained by fine-needle aspiration, core needle biopsy or surgical resection, demonstrated in the treated lesions the presence of an area of complete coagulative necrosis surrounded by degenerative changes and inflammatory reaction. No evidence of extrathyroidal damage or cervical fibrosis along the needle tract was observed [26]. Two single-centre randomised studies compared the clinical and US changes induced by LAT with those observed in patients under thyroxine suppressive therapy or plainly followed-up [15, 27, 28]. Even if the first trial was conducted with a Nd:YAG and the second one with a diode laser source, both studies confirmed that a single laser treatment results in a nodule volume decrease greater than 40 % versus baseline at the 6- and 12-month US controls. No significant volume change was found in the suppressive therapy or in the control group.

In a retrospective study, volume reduction remained stable up to 5 years after the initial treatment and the majority of patients described a sustained improvement of their local symptoms after LAT [19]. A recent Italian multicentre prospective randomised trial provided a conclusive evidence of the outcomes of LAT in clinical practice [16]. The study assessed the long-term clinical efficacy, tolerability and predictability of outcome of LAT in four different centres operating according to the same procedure. Two hundred and one euthyroid patients with a solid not hyperfunctioning nodule were randomly assigned to a single laser session or to follow-up. Three years after LAT, in the active treatment group, mean nodule volume reduction was about 58 %. Thermal ablation induced a nodule decrease >50 % in nearly 70 % of cases and no significant difference in the outcomes was reported by the various centres. Presence of local symptoms decreased from 31 % at baseline to 5 % of cases 36 months after LAT, and cosmetic signs from 74 to 12 % of cases. The procedure was fairly well tolerated by most patients and the only major complication was one case of vocal cord paresis that self-resolved in 2 weeks. No changes in thyroid function or autoimmunity were observed. Hence, a single LAT session of solid thyroid nodules, performed by experienced operators, results in the majority of cases in a significant and persistent volume reduction and in the improvement of local symptoms in absence of late thyroid function changes.

### 6.2.2 Autonomously Functioning Thyroid Nodules

Initial reports on small series of hyperfunctioning thyroid nodules treated with LAT showed normalisation of thyroid function and effacement of the hyperfunctioning area at the post-ablation radioisotope scan [10, 14, 29, 30]. Data from larger studies, however, demonstrated that multiple laser treatments are necessary to normalise serum TSH levels [11, 17, 31]. In a prospective trial on hyperfunctioning nodules with suppression of extranodular parenchyma, laser ablation and radioiodine (131-I) treatment resulted in similar nodule shrinkage. It is noteworthy, however, that LAT induced the return to detectable levels of serum TSH in only 50 % of patients, a successful control of hyperfunction that was definitely lower than after 131-I treatment [18]. As a whole, these trials demonstrate an acceptable efficacy of laser ablation when treating small-size and mildly hyperfunctioning nodules [22]. On the other hand, in large hyperfunctioning thyroid lesions, normalisation of thyroid function is obtained less consistently and requires repeated laser treatments [11, 31].

A recent prospective controlled trial on large toxic thyroid nodules evaluated the efficacy of the combined treatment with a single laser ablation followed by 131-I therapy with respect to the rapidity of control of local symptoms and hyperthyroidism [32]. The reduction of 131-I activity administered 1 month after laser LAT was assessed versus a matched control group treated with radioiodine alone. After 2 years, nodule volume decrease was significantly higher in the combined treatment than in the control group (71.3 % vs 47.4 %, $p<0.001$). Moreover, the use of a preliminary LAT allowed a >20 % decrease in the administered 131-I activity. The reduction of local symptoms was more rapid in the combined treatment group and, in three cases, no radioiodine therapy was needed after LAT. These data are of interest because in large hyperfunctioning thyroid lesions nodule shrinkage and the ease of pressure symptoms are rather slow after radioiodine treatment and the activities of 131-I required for treatment are usually elevated [32]. A combined treatment may be of use in large hyperfunctioning nodules because it allows a faster volume reduction and the disappearance of local symptoms, an earlier control of hyperthyroidism and permits the use of lower doses of 131-I in an outpatient treatment setting.

### 6.2.3 Cystic Lesions

Due to its high efficacy and safety and very low cost of percutaneous ethanol injection (PEIT) [17], few contributes are available on the use of LAT for cystic thyroid lesions.

In a recent trial, a series of cystic thyroid nodules were randomised to aspiration alone or to drainage followed by LAT [20]. After 6 months, a nearly complete disappearance of the cystic component was observed in 68 % of LAT patients as opposed to 18 % in the aspiration-alone group. Local symptoms improved significantly in the LAT patients as compared with the drainage-only group, and thyroid function remained unaffected in all cases. These results indicate a possible convenience of combined treatment with fluid aspiration followed by LAT in patients with large relapsing complex lesions with relevant solid component.

### 6.2.4 Cervical Recurrences of Thyroid Tumours

The majority of differentiated thyroid tumours are effectively treated by the initial surgical approach, with or without subsequent 131-I ablation of thyroid remnants. However, the recurrence rate during follow-up is up to 20 % in patients with differentiated thyroid tumours and is even higher in patients with medullary thyroid cancer [33]. In these last tumours and in some differentiated cancers, 131-I treatment is not effective in eradicating nodal metastases due to the absence of 131-I uptake. Part of the nonpalpable cervical metastases that are revealed by US examination of the neck, moreover, may be at difficult surgical reach. Some of these patients have already undergone repeat neck dissection and a further resection of nodal metastases may be technically difficult and at risk of surgical complications [33].

Due to the usually slow progression of the small-size cervical recurrences of differentiated thyroid carcinoma, MIT are currently under investigation for patients at elevated surgical risk [34].

LAT for thyroid malignancies was first tested in an elderly woman with undifferentiated thyroid carcinoma [6]. Repeated LAT sessions debulked large areas of the tumour, the patient underwent external beam radiation therapy and local symptoms improved for several months. A similar response to LAT was reported in a second inoperable anaplastic carcinoma, but in both cases the favourable course was transient and was followed by fatal outcome [35].

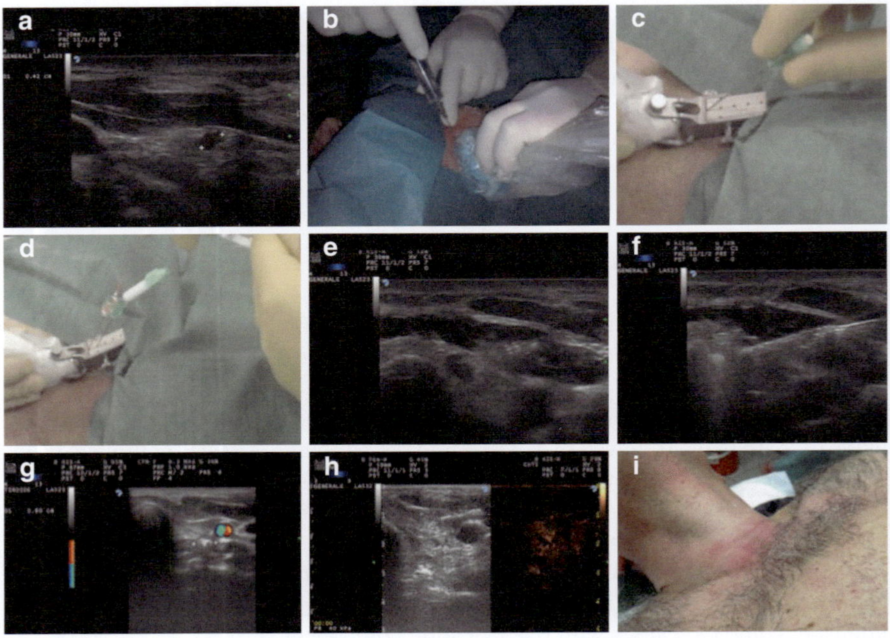


**Fig. 6.2** (**a**) Ultrasound scan of a small size (4×4×6 mm) nodal recurrence of papillary thyroid carcinoma (left laterocervical region, level IV); (**b**) ultrasound-guided local anaesthesia performed along the planned needle path; (**c–e**) insertion under ultrasound guidance of two spinal needles, progression of the optical fibres into the target lesion and subsequent laser firing; (**f**) complete effacement of the metastatic lymph node by the hyperechoic spots generated by gas microbubbles; (**g–h**) the metastatic lymph node is not revealed by post-treatment ultrasound controls; (**i**) absence of skin or subcutaneous damage after the end of the procedure

Favourable experiences with laser ablation have been reported small-size cervical recurrences of differentiated thyroid cancer [36]. A first series of eight cervical recurrences of papillary thyroid carcinoma in patients already submitted to cervical dissection was treated with a single session of Nd:YAG laser ablation with two optical fibres (Fig. 6.2). Twelve months after treatment, all the lymph node metastases showed a marked volume reduction (from 0.64±0.58 to 0.07±0.06 ml, $p=0.01$) and the mean thyroglobulin levels decreased significantly from 8.0±3.2 to 2.0±2.5 ng/ml. Laser ablation was a rapid and usually well-tolerated procedure and no major complications were registered. These results were confirmed in a subsequent study performed in a different centre with the same technique [37]. Twenty-four metastatic lymph nodes (mean size 1.1 cm) from papillary cancer of the thyroid gland that relapsed after thyroidectomy and cervical dissection were enrolled in the study. All recurrences showed absent uptake at 131-I whole body scan but revealed a marked uptake at 18-FDG PET/TC. In most cases, LAT induced a marked shrinkage or the disappearance of the treated lesions at US and colour-Doppler examination and loss of 18-FDG uptake at the post-treatment PET/CT control.

The issue concerning the opportunity to surgically treat papillary thyroid microcarcinomas (PTMC) incidentally revealed by imaging studies in fragile patients is still unsettled [38]. Due to their indolent course, indeed, a wait-and-see clinical management is frequently advocated for these cases. A feasibility study was performed on a solitary PTMC (8 mm in maximum diameter), with no US evidence of spreading outside the thyroid gland, in an elderly patient at high surgical risk because of liver and kidney failure. The small tumour was completely ablated with a single laser treatment without complications [39]. During a 2-year follow-up, US cervical examination and contrast-enhanced US scan demonstrated that the PTMC was completely replaced by a larger hypoechoic zone devoid of vascular supply. Both US-guided fine-needle aspiration biopsy and core-needle biopsy provided necrotic debris only with no viable neoplastic cells.

Despite the limited number of cases, LAT is a promising therapeutic tool for PTMC ablation in fragile patients at surgical risk and for isolated neck metastases from differentiated or medullary thyroid carcinoma in patients already treated with neck dissection. Laser ablation could be used for local recurrences that are not amenable to traditional surgical treatments for improving local symptoms or concern and for decreasing the bulk of tumour tissue prior to external radiation therapy or target therapy [34].

## 6.3 Tolerability and Safety

### 6.3.1 Tolerability

Mild to moderate cervical pain or low-grade fever (<38 °C) may occur after LAT. These symptoms usually last 24–48 h and are easily controlled by acetaminophen or ketoprophene by mouth. The occurrence of local bruising is infrequent [16, 17].

### 6.3.2 Complications

Subcapsular haematoma and dizziness may occur, even if infrequently [25, 40, 41]. Skin burn, cervical swelling, tracheal injury, transient hyperthyroidism and late hypothyroidism have been reported, but are definitely rare [25]. No pathological changes have been found in cervical tissues adjacent to the ablated area in patients who subsequently underwent surgery [6, 42].

The fairly good tolerability of LAT and the low risk of major complications (about 1 %) were recently confirmed in the large, externally monitored, series of the Italian multicentre trial [16].

## 6.4 Conclusions and Indications

- Minimally invasive procedures are thoroughly evaluated techniques and are available in specialised centres for selected patients.
- Relapsing thyroid cysts and complex nodules are best managed with US-guided aspiration followed by PEIT as first-line treatment.

- In solid nonfunctioning symptomatic thyroid nodules, LAT achieves, in a single session, a nearly 50 % volume decrease and the improvement of local pressure symptoms. These results are obtained in most patients and are stable during a period of at least 3 years.
- Hyperfunctioning thyroid nodules remain best treated with radioactive iodine, which provides an inexpensive and safe tool for long-term control of hyperthyroidism. In large-size toxic nodules, a pre-treatment with LAT may allow an earlier control of hyperthyroidism and a more rapid nodule volume reduction.
- LAT may be employed for local control of small size, non-radioiodine-avid, neck recurrences of PTC in patients who are not candidates for a repeat cervical lymph node dissection. LAT seems to be a potential alternative to the simple follow-up of cancer recurrences and may be used in larger or progressive cervical metastasis, as part of a multimodality therapeutic approach.
- LAT was proposed for the ablation of PTMC without evidence of multifocality or extrathyroidal spreading in patients at high surgical risk. This application should be considered as experimental and reserved to highly selected cases.
- Head-to-head prospective studies of LAT versus surgery comparing long-term efficacy, side effects, overall expense and impact on quality of life are needed to better define the role of MIT in everyday practice.

## References


1. Papini E, Petrucci L, Guglielmi R et al (1998) Long-term changes in nodular goiter. A 5-year prospective randomized trial of levothyroxine suppressive therapy for benign cold thyroid nodules. J Clin Endocrinol Metab 83:780–783
2. Tan GH, Gharib H (1997) Thyroid incidentalomas: management approaches to nonpalpable nodules discovered incidentally on thyroid imaging. Ann Intern Med 126:226–231
3. Bergenfelz A, Jansson S, Kristoffersson A, Martensson H, Reihner E, Wallin G, Lausen I (2008) Complications to thyroid surgery: results as reported in a database from a multicenter audit comprising 3,660 patients. Langenbecks Arch Surg 393:667–673
4. Hegedus L (2009) Therapy: a new nonsurgical therapy option for benign thyroid nodules? Nat Rev Endocrinol 5:476–478
5. Bown SG (1983) Phototherapy in tumors. World J Surg 7:700–709
6. Pacella CM, Bizzarri G, Guglielmi R, Anelli V, Bianchini A, Crescenzi A, Pacella S, Papini E (2000) Thyroid tissue: US-guided percutaneous interstitial laser ablation-a feasibility study. Radiology 217:673–677
7. Jacques SL (1992) Laser-tissue interactions. Photochemical, photothermal, and photomechanical. Surg Clin North Am 72:531–558
8. Bennedbaek FN, Hegedus L (1995) Alcohol sclerotherapy for benign solitary solid cold thyroid nodules. Lancet 346:1227
9. Dossing H, Bennedbaek FN, Karstrup S, Hegedus L (2002) Benign solitary solid cold thyroid nodules: US-guided interstitial laser photocoagulation–initial experience. Radiology 225:53–57
10. Spiezia S, Vitale G, Di Somma C, Pio Assanti A, Ciccarelli A, Lombardi G, Colao A (2003) Ultrasound-guided laser thermal ablation in the treatment of autonomous hyperfunctioning thyroid nodules and compressive nontoxic nodular goiter. Thyroid 13:941–947
11. Pacella CM, Bizzarri G, Spiezia S, Bianchini A, Guglielmi R, Crescenzi A, Pacella S, Toscano V, Papini E (2004) Thyroid tissue: US-guided percutaneous laser thermal ablation. Radiology 232:272–280

12. Prapavat V, Roggan A, Walter J, Beuthan J, Klingbeil U, Muller G (1996) In vitro studies and computer simulations to assess the use of a diode laser (850 nm) for laser-induced thermotherapy (LITT). Lasers Surg Med 18:22–33
13. Amabile G, Rotondi M, De Chiara G, Silvestri A, Di Filippo B, Bellastella A, Chiovato L (2006) Low-energy interstitial laser photocoagulation for treatment of nonfunctioning thyroid nodules: therapeutic outcome in relation to pretreatment and treatment parameters. Thyroid 16:749–755
14. Dossing H, Bennedbaek FN, Hegedus L (2003) Ultrasound-guided interstitial laser photocoagulation of an autonomous thyroid nodule: the introduction of a novel alternative. Thyroid 13:885–888
15. Dossing H, Bennedbaek FN, Hegedus L (2005) Effect of ultrasound-guided interstitial laser photocoagulation on benign solitary solid cold thyroid nodules – a randomised study. Eur J Endocrinol 152:341–345
16. Papini E, Rago T, Gambelunghe G et al (2014) Long-term efficacy of ultrasound-guided laser ablation for benign solid thyroid nodules. Results of a three-year multicenter prospective randomized trial. J Clin Endocrinol Metab 99(10):3653–3659
17. Gharib H, Hegedus L, Pacella CM, Baek JH, Papini E (2013) Clinical review: nonsurgical image-guided, minimally-invasive therapy for thyroid nodules. J Clin Endocrinol Metab 98:3947–3957
18. Dossing H, Bennedbaek FN, Bonnema SJ, Grupe P, Hegedus L (2007) Randomized prospective study comparing a single radioiodine dose and a single laser therapy session in autonomously functioning thyroid nodules. Eur J Endocrinol 157:95–100
19. Dossing H, Bennedbaek FN, Hegedus L (2011) Long-term outcome following interstitial laser photocoagulation of benign cold thyroid nodules. Eur J Endocrinol 165:123–128
20. Dossing H, Bennedbaek FN, Hegedus L (2013) Interstitial laser photocoagulation (ILP) of benign cystic thyroid nodules-a prospective randomized trial. J Clin Endocrinol Metab 98:E1213–E1217
21. Amabile G, Rotondi M, Pirali B, Dionisio R, Agozzino L, Lanza M, Buonanno L, Di Filippo B, Fonte R, Chiovato L (2011) Interstitial laser photocoagulation for benign thyroid nodules: time to treat large nodules. Lasers Surg Med 43:797–803
22. Valcavi R, Bertani A, Pesenti M, Al Jandali Rifa'Y LR, Frasoldati AFD, Pacella CM (2008) Laser and radiofrequency ablation procedures. In: Baskin BJ, Duick DS, Levine RA (eds) Thyroid ultrasound and ultrasound-guided FNA, 2nd edn. Springer, New York, pp 198–218
23. Valcavi R, Riganti F, Bertani A, Formisano D, Pacella CM (2010) Percutaneous laser ablation of cold benign thyroid nodules: a 3-year follow-up study in 122 patients. Thyroid 20:1253–1261
24. Papini E, Guglielmi R, Bizzarri G, Pacella CM (2004) Ultrasound-guided laser thermal ablation for treatment of benign thyroid nodules. Endocr Pract 10:276–283
25. Gambelunghe G, Fede R, Bini V, Monacelli M, Avenia N, D'Ajello M, Colella R, Nasini G, De Feo P (2013) Ultrasound-guided interstitial laser ablation for thyroid nodules is effective only at high total amounts of energy: results from a three-year pilot study. Surg Innov 20:345–350
26. Cakir B, Topaloglu O, Gul K, Agac T, Aydin C, Dirikoc A, Gumus M, Yazicioglu K, Ersoy RU, Ugras S (2006) Effects of percutaneous laser ablation treatment in benign solitary thyroid nodules on nodule volume, thyroglobulin and anti-thyroglobulin levels, and cytopathology of nodule in 1 yr follow-up. J Endocrinol Invest 29:876–884
27. Gambelunghe G, Fatone C, Ranchelli A, Fanelli C, Lucidi P, Cavaliere A, Avenia N, d'Ajello M, Santeusanio F, De Feo P (2006) A randomized controlled trial to evaluate the efficacy of ultrasound-guided laser photocoagulation for treatment of benign thyroid nodules. J Endocrinol Invest 29:RC23–RC26
28. Papini E, Guglielmi R, Bizzarri G, Graziano F, Bianchini A, Brufani C, Pacella S, Valle D, Pacella CM (2007) Treatment of benign cold thyroid nodules: a randomized clinical trial of percutaneous laser ablation versus levothyroxine therapy or follow-up. Thyroid 17:229–235
29. Rotondi M, Amabile G, Leporati P, Di Filippo B, Chiovato L (2009) Repeated laser thermal ablation of a large functioning thyroid nodule restores euthyroidism and ameliorates constrictive symptoms. J Clin Endocrinol Metab 94:382–383

30. Cakir B, Gul K, Ugras S, Ersoy R, Topaloglu O, Agac T, Aydin C, Dirikoc A, Gumus M, Korukluoglu B, Kusdemir A (2008) Percutaneous laser ablation of an autonomous thyroid nodule: effects on nodule size and histopathology of the nodule 2 years after the procedure. Thyroid 18:803–805
31. Barbaro D, Orsini P, Lapi P, Pasquini C, Tuco A, Righini A, Lemmi P (2007) Percutaneous laser ablation in the treatment of toxic and pretoxic nodular goiter. Endocr Pract 13:30–36
32. Chianelli M, Bizzarri G, Todino V, Misischi I, Bianchini A, Graziano F, Guglielmi R, Pacella CM, Gharib H, Papini E (2014) Laser ablation and 131-iodine: a 24-month pilot study of combined treatment for large toxic nodular goiter. J Clin Endocrinol Metab 99(7):E1283–E1286. Published online: 31 Mar 2014
33. Burman KD (2013) Treatment of recurrent or persistent cervical node metastases in differentiated thyroid cancer: deceptively simple options. J Clin Endocrinol Metab 97:8. Published online: 2 Jul 2013
34. Papini E, Bianchini A, Guglielmi R, Pacella CM, Misischi I, Papini L, Bizzarri G (2011) Image-guided mini-invasive ablation of thyroid tumors and distant metastases. In: Carpi A, Mechanick JI (eds) Thyroid cancer: from emergent biotechnologies to clinical practice guidelines. CRC Press, New York, pp 213–230
35. Cakir B, Topaloglu O, Gul K et al (2007) Ultrasound-guided percutaneous laser ablation treatment in inoperable aggressive course anaplastic thyroid carcinoma: the introduction of a novel alternative palliative therapy–second experience in the literature. J Endocrinol Invest 30:624–625
36. Papini E, Bizzarri G, Bianchini A, Valle D, Misischi I, Guglielmi R, Salvatori M, Solbiati L, Crescenzi A, Pacella CM, Gharib H (2013) Percutaneous ultrasound-guided laser ablation is effective for treating selected nodal metastases in papillary thyroid cancer. J Clin Endocrinol Metab 98(1):E92–E97
37. Mauri G, Cova L, Tondolo T, Ierace T, Baroli A, Di Mauro E, Pacella CM, Goldberg SN, Solbiati L (2013) Percutaneous laser ablation of metastatic lymph nodes in the neck from papillary thyroid carcinoma: preliminary results. J Clin Endocrinol Metab 98(7):E1203–E1207
38. Ito Y, Miyauchi A (2007) Appropriate treatment for asymptomatic papillary microcarcinoma of the thyroid. Expert Opin Pharmacother 8(18):3205–3215
39. Papini E, Guglielmi R, Gharib H, Misischi I, Graziano F, Chianelli M, Crescenzi A, Bianchini A, Valle D, Bizzarri G (2011) Ultrasound-guided laser ablation of incidental papillary thyroid microcarcinoma: a potential therapeutic approach in patients at surgical risk. Thyroid 21(8):917–920
40. Gambelunghe G, Bini V, Monacelli M, Avenia N, D'Ajello M, Colella R, De Feo P (2013) The administation of anesthetic in the thyroid pericapsular region increase the possibility of side effects during percutaneous laser ablation of thyroid nodules. Lasers Surg Med 45(1):34–37
41. Cakir B, Gul K, Ersoy R, Topaloglu O, Korukluoglu B (2008) Subcapsular hematoma complication during percutaneous laser ablation to a hypoactive benign solitary thyroid nodule. Thyroid 18:917–918
42. Cakir B, Ugras NS, Gul K, Ersoy R, Korukluoglu B (2009) Initial report of the results of percutaneous laser ablation of benign cold thyroid nodules: evaluation of histopathological changes after 2 years. Endocr Pathol 20:170–176

# Percutaneous Radiofrequency Ablation 7

Eun Ju Ha and Jung Hwan Baek

## 7.1 Introduction

Although most thyroid nodules are benign, some patients require treatment because of cosmetic problems or subjective symptoms. Surgery, radioiodine therapy, and thyroid hormone medication have been used to reduce the size of benign thyroid nodules; however, they have many drawbacks such as scarring, the need for general anesthesia, hospital admission, hypoparathyroidism, hypothyroidism, bleeding, infection, and voice change. Radiofrequency ablation (RFA) is a method of thermal ablation that could induce the necrosis of nodule tissue. It has been used to treat various benign and malignant tumors with good results. In the thyroid gland, RFA has been used to treat benign thyroid nodules and recurrent thyroid cancers [1–4]. In this chapter, we discuss four topics regarding RFA: (1) procedures, (2) indications, (3) clinical outcomes, and (4) complications.

E.J. Ha
Department of Radiology, Ajou University School of Medicine, Wonchon-Dong, Yeongtong-Gu, Suwon 443-380, Korea
e-mail: radhej@naver.com

J.H. Baek (✉)
Department of Radiology and Research Institute of Radiology, University of Ulsan College of Medicine, Asan Medical Center, 86 Asanbyeongwon-Gil, Songpa-Gu, Seoul 138-736, Korea
e-mail: radbaek@naver.com



C.P. Lombardi, R. Bellantone (eds.), *Minimally Invasive Therapies for Endocrine Neck Diseases*, DOI 10.1007/978-3-319-20065-1_7

## 7.2 Procedure

Regarding the application of RFA techniques, thyroid nodules are different from liver tumors. In contrast to the liver, the thyroid gland is a relatively superficial and small organ, whereas thyroid nodules are large and ellipsoidal in shape. Therefore, a new device and technique have been developed for thyroid RFA.

### 7.2.1 Devices

Before the development of thyroid-dedicated devices, straight internally cooled and multi-tined expandable electrodes have been used [5–11]. A multi-tined expandable electrode (14-gauge, 10 cm in length, with 4–9 hooks expandable to 3.5–4.0 cm) has been employed in Italy [9, 10], and a straight, internally cooled electrode (17-gauge, 15 cm in length, with a 1 cm active tip) has been used in Korea [5–8, 11]. In Korea, a modified, straight, internally cooled electrode has also been developed [8]. This modified electrode, which is used worldwide, is short (7 cm) for easy control and thin (18- or 19-gauge) to minimize injury to the normal thyroid gland; in addition, it can be used with active tips of various sizes (0.5–2.0 cm).

### 7.2.2 The Trans-isthmic Approach and Moving Shot Technique

Regarding the procedure, a patient is placed in the supine position with mild neck extension. Two grounding pads are firmly attached to both thighs. Local anesthesia is sufficient to control pain during the procedure [5, 7, 10–12]. After sterilization, the electrode is inserted through the isthmic portion of the thyroid (called the trans-isthmic approach), and ablation proceeds via a transverse ultrasound (US) view (Fig. 7.1). This method has several advantages: (1) during the procedure, the entire length of the electrode can be monitored on the transverse US view; (2) minimal exposure of the danger triangle (including the recurrent laryngeal nerve and/or esophagus) to heat is possible; and (3) the electrode passes through a sufficient amount of thyroid parenchyma, preventing a change in the position of the electrode tip during swallowing or talking, as well as leakage of ablated hot fluid outside the thyroid gland.

Baek et al. [7] proposed a moving shot technique for thyroid RFA [5–8, 12] (Fig. 7.1). In the fixed-electrode technique, which has been used to treat liver tumors [13–16], the electrode is fixed in position during ablation, resulting in a round ablation zone. A round ablation zone could be dangerous to the surrounding critical structures, because thyroid nodules are ellipsoidal in shape. To resolve this problem, the moving shot technique has been suggested: dividing thyroid nodules into multiple, small conceptual ablation units, and performing RFA unit-by-unit, by moving the electrode tip. The conceptual units are smaller at the margin of the nodules and larger in the central area of the nodules. Initially, the electrode tip is positioned in the deepest, most posterior portion of the nodule to enable the tip to be easily monitored in the absence of any

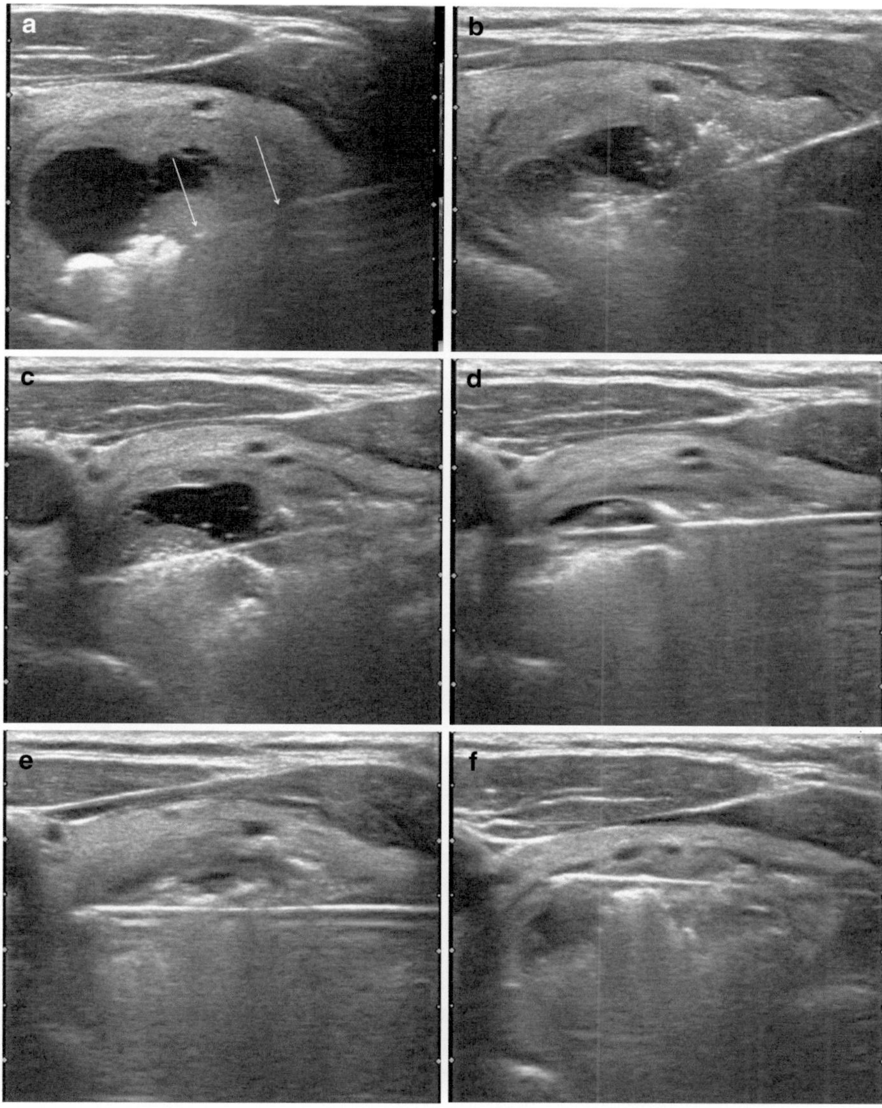


**Fig. 7.1** Sequential US images of the moving shot technique. (**a**, **b**) The electrode is initially positioned at the periphery of the deep and remote portions of the target nodule, and continuously moves backward (*arrows*) within the thyroid nodule. (**c**, **d**) Next, the electrode tip is relocated in the untreated superficial area, and the ablation is repeated until it covers the entire nodule. (**e**, **f**) The procedure is terminated when all of the conceptual units of the targeted nodule have become transient hyperechoic zones

disturbance caused by the transient hyperechoic zone. Ablation is commenced with 20 W (0.5 cm active tip), 30 W (0.7 cm active tip), and 50 W (1.0 cm active tip) of RF power. When a transient hyperechoic zone appears at the targeted unit, RF power starts to decrease, and the electrode tip is moved to an untreated area. The electrode moves continuously both backward and in the superficial direction within the thyroid nodule. The extent of the ablated area is determined by the echogenic area around the electrode. If a transient hyperechoic zone does not appear at the electrode tip within 5 s, RF power is increased in 10-W increments to a maximum of 100 W. If a patient cannot tolerate the pain, injection of a local anesthetic around the thyroid capsule is effective to reduce pain. To treat cystic or predominantly cystic nodules, the cystic fluid is first aspirated, and then RFA is performed. RFA is terminated when all of the conceptual units of the targeted nodule become transient hyperechoic zones (Fig. 7.1). However, certain regions of each thyroid nodule, including those close to critical structures such as the recurrent laryngeal nerve and esophagus, may remain undertreated. Operators must monitor any complications that might occur during and immediately after a procedure. The patient is observed for 1–2 h in the hospital with mild compression of the neck [5, 10].

## 7.3 Indications

According to the 2012 consensus statement and recommendations of the Korean Society of Thyroid Radiology, RFA can be used to treat both benign thyroid nodules and inoperable, recurrent thyroid cancers in the neck [5–12, 17–24]. The Korean Society of Thyroid Radiology does not recommend RFA for follicular neoplasms or primary thyroid cancers because there is no evidence of a benefit by RFA in these tumors [5, 25]. Caution should be taken regarding the use of thyroid RFA in pregnant women, patients with serious heart problems, and those with contralateral vocal cord palsy [26–30]. Patients with cystic thyroid nodules that regrow after simple aspiration should be treated first with ethanol ablation (EA) rather than RFA [6, 18, 31–33]. A retrospective study and a randomized clinical trial both suggested EA to be a first-line treatment for cystic thyroid nodules [18, 34].

Indications for RFA of benign thyroid nodules include patients with nodule-related clinical problems [5, 7, 8, 10, 11, 22]. The symptom score can be self-measured by patients using a 10-cm visual analog scale (grade 0–10) [6, 7, 31], and the cosmetic score [6, 7, 9, 10, 31] can be measured by a physician (score 1–4: 1, no palpable mass; 2, no cosmetic problem but a palpable mass; 3, a cosmetic problem on swallowing only; and 4, a readily detected cosmetic problem) [6, 7, 18]. Patients with autonomously functioning thyroid nodules (AFTNs) causing thyrotoxicosis are also indicated for RFA [8–10, 12, 35–39]. The nodules with a maximum diameter >2 cm that continue to grow may be considered for RFA.

Indications for RFA of recurrent thyroid cancers include patients at high surgical risk and patients who refuse to undergo repeated surgery [20, 21, 23, 24]. The recommendations suggest that tumor recurrence should be confirmed before treatment by US-guided fine-needle aspiration cytology and/or measurement of the washout thyroglobulin concentration [2, 40]. The treatment strategy of RFA for recurrent thyroid cancers is not well established; however, two strategies have been suggested: complete ablation of any recurrent thyroid cancers visible on US [23, 41] or conservative treatment to improve any symptomatic problems [21]. To achieve complete ablation, several studies have suggested that RFA should be restricted to patients with three or less recurrent tumors in the neck and no metastatic tumors beyond the neck at the time of treatment [2, 23, 41, 42]. Conservative treatment has been applied to treat large recurrent cancers that cause symptomatic problems, such as pain, dysphagia, hoarseness, and dyspnea [21].

## 7.4 Clinical Outcomes

The efficacy of RFA for benign thyroid nodules can be evaluated by the symptom score, cosmetic score, volume reduction ratio [5, 7, 8], and therapeutic success rate (volume reduction >50 %) [18]. US is recommended for routine follow-up at 1, 6, and 12 months, and every 6–12 months, and changes in size, echogenicity, and intranodular vascularity are evaluated by US. The reduction in volume is calculated using the following equation: volume reduction (%) = ([initial volume (mL) − final volume (mL)] × 100)/initial volume (mL) [5]. The echogenicity of a nodule would be lower than noted before ablation (Fig. 7.2), and intra-nodular vascularity should disappear in regions receiving complete ablation [5]. Additional ablation should be performed if a viable portion of the nodule (i.e., the region showing the same echogenicity as the initial nodule with intra-nodular vascularity) remains on follow-up

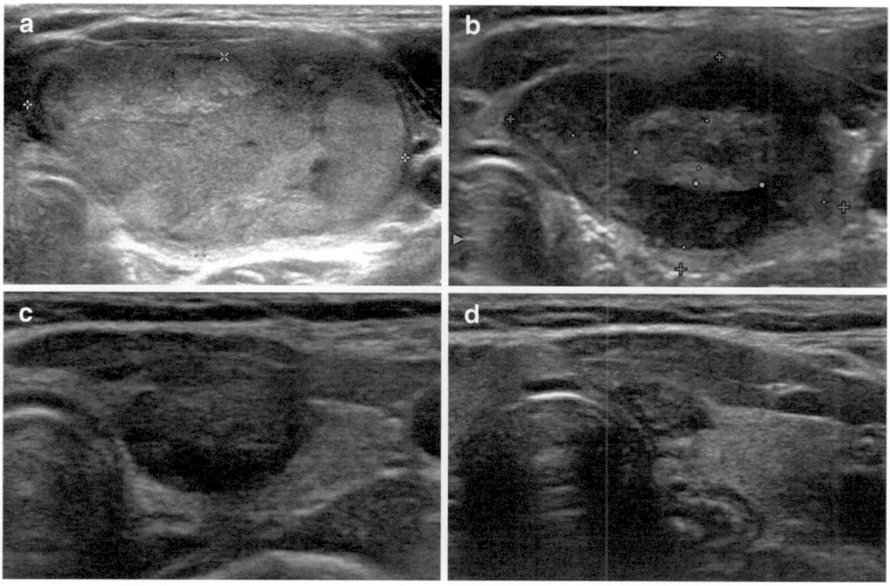

**Fig. 7.2** Transverse US images of a well-ablated thyroid nodule. Images obtained before (**a**), and 12 and 36 months after (**b**, **c**) RFA showing the reduced size and decreased echogenicity of the ablated nodule. Only a small scar-like lesion remained at the last follow-up of 56 months (**d**)

US, or if a patient complains of incompletely resolved clinical problems, including cosmetic and symptomatic concerns [5, 9]. Proper additional treatment interval is 1–3 months after initial treatment, because rapid volume reduction can be achieved the first 3 months after ablation. Although no guidelines are available to identify a time when follow-up US should cease, additional routine US is not considered necessary when a treated nodule disappears completely or remains as a small scar-like lesion (Fig. 7.2). For the evaluation of AFTNs, a thyroid scan and the measurement of serum thyroid hormone and thyrotropin levels are recommended [8–10]. The efficacy of RFA for recurrent thyroid cancers can be evaluated by the volume reduction ratio, serum thyroglobulin concentrations, and improvement of symptoms [20, 21, 23, 24].

RFA cannot remove thyroid nodules immediately; rather, it induces the necrosis and involution of thyroid nodules, resulting in volume reduction and improvement in clinical symptoms, with an efficacy similar to that of thyroid surgery [5, 10, 11]. Hyperthyroidism caused by AFTNs can be cured or improved by RFA [8–10]. Regarding benign, non-functioning thyroid nodules, the volume reduction after RFA has been found to range from 33 to 58 % at 1 month and from 51 to 92 % at 6 months [5–11, 43]. A long-term study reported that the volume reduction was 90 % at 1 year and 93 % at 4 years [44]. Prospective randomized studies have revealed that RFA is effective for solid thyroid nodules, with 76.5–79.7 % volume reduction at 6 months after RFA [7, 45]. Regarding benign AFTNs, one study [8] reported a volume reduction of 44–81.9 % at 6 months; normalization of thyroid function was 31–87 %. In that study, the volume reduction of treated nodules was slightly lower than that of cold thyroid nodules, possibly due to the autonomy of AFTNs. In addition, incomplete ablation of the nodule margins allowed marginal regrowth of treated nodules, particularly for patients with AFTNs.

Although the moving shot technique can successfully prevent marginal regrowth in many patients, undertreated portions adjacent to the critical structures, as well as large-sized nodules, remain vulnerable to marginal regrowth following RFA [1, 8, 9]. For example, a patient with a large thyroid nodule greater than 20 mL may require additional RFA due to incomplete treatment and unresolved clinical problems [19]. Recent review articles have suggested that RFA is a safe and effective treatment for symptomatic benign thyroid nodules [46–48]. These articles emphasized the proper selection of patients with benign nodules and subsequent monitoring.

RFA of recurrent thyroid cancers results in a mean volume reduction of 56–93 % [21, 23], with 42–58 % of nodules completely disappearing [20, 23, 24], 64 % of patients experiencing symptom improvement [21], and the serum thyroglobulin concentration decreasing [20, 21, 23, 24].

## 7.5 Complications

The reported complications are summarized in Table 7.1. Physicians who perform thyroid RFA should understand the broad spectrum of complications and proper prevention methods [3, 49]. In 2012, the Korean Society of Thyroid Radiology

**Table 7.1** Complications of RFA for benign thyroid nodules

| | Kim et al. | Jeong et al. | Deandrea et al. | Spiezia et al. | Baek et al. | Baek et al. | Lee et al. | Sung et al. | Huh et al. | Jang et al. | Faggiano et al. | Ha et al. | Sung et al. | Total |
|---|---|---|---|---|---|---|---|---|---|---|---|---|---|---|
| Year | 2006 | 2008 | 2008 | 2009 | 2009 | 2010 | 2010 | 2011 | 2012 | 2012 | 2012 | 2013 | 2013 | |
| No. of patients | 30 | 236 | 31 | 94 | 9 | 15 | 27 | 21 | 15 | 20 | 20 | 11 | 21 | 550 |
| Hematoma | 1 | 5 | – | – | – | – | 1 | – | – | – | – | – | – | 7 |
| Skin burn | 1 | – | – | – | – | – | – | – | – | – | – | – | – | 1 |
| Pain | 1 | 13 | Few | 13 | Few | Few | Few | Few | Few | Few | Few | Few | Few | 27+ |
| Transient hyperthyroidism | 3 | 3 | – | – | – | – | – | – | – | – | – | – | – | 6 |
| Hypothyroidism | – | – | – | – | 1 | – | – | – | – | – | – | – | – | 1 |
| Edema | – | – | 3 | – | – | – | – | – | – | – | – | – | – | 3 |
| Fever | – | – | – | 5 | – | – | – | – | – | – | – | – | – | 5 |
| Voice change | 1 | 3 | – | – | – | – | – | – | – | – | – | – | – | 4 |

**Table 7.2** Complications of RFA for recurrent thyroid cancers

| | Dupuy et al. | Monchik et al. | Baek et al. | Park et al. | Guenette et al. | Total |
|---|---|---|---|---|---|---|
| Year | 2001 | 2006 | 2011 | 2011 | 2013 | |
| No. of patients | 8 | 16 | 10 | 11 | 14 | 59 |
| Voice change | 1[a] | 1[a] | 1[a] | – | 1[b] | 4 (6.8 %) |
| Skin burn | 1 | 1 | – | 1 | – | 3 (5.1 %) |

Recurrent tumors in [a]central neck; [b]lateral neck

reported various complications for benign nonfunctioning thyroid nodules in a large population multicenter study [49]. The overall complication rate was 3.3 % (48/1459) and the major complication rate was 1.4 % (20/1459). The reported sequelae rate was 0.14 % (2/1459): hypothyroidism in one patient and abscess formation with nodule rupture in the other patient [49]. Regarding the complications related to RFA of recurrent thyroid cancers (Table 7.2), voice change due to recurrent laryngeal nerve injury, skin burn, and procedure-related pain have been reported. Although other nerve injuries have not been reported, any type of injury is possible according to the site of recurrent tumors. Therefore, the operator should monitor the relationship between the nerve and tumor during RFA.

Pain is the most common complaint in most patients during the procedure. Various degrees of pain in the neck and/or radiating to the head, ear, shoulders, chest, back, or teeth can be present; however, patients are usually tolerant of the pain, which decreases rapidly when the generator output is reduced or turned off [1, 5, 7, 49]. In addition, injection of local anesthetics around the thyroid capsule effectively reduces the pain. Painkillers could reduce post-procedural pain [1].

Voice change is a major complication of thyroid RFA that is caused by thermal damage to the recurrent laryngeal or vagus nerve [50, 51]. In most cases, voice change is detected during or immediately after ablation. Voice changes are usually transient, with most patients recovering within 3 months [1, 49]; however, some patients recover more slowly. To prevent voice change, both the trans-isthmic approach and moving shot technique can be helpful. Using these techniques, unit-by-unit ablation of conceptual ablation units and under-treatment of the danger triangle (i.e., the area of the thyroid nodule adjacent to the recurrent laryngeal nerve) may minimize recurrent laryngeal nerve injury [1, 3, 49]. The vagus nerve is located within the carotid sheath, usually posteriorly between the common carotid artery and internal jugular vein; however, a bulging large thyroid nodule may alter the location of the vagus nerve, making it closer to the thyroid nodule [50–53]. To avoid thermal injury to the vagus nerve, the operators should be aware of the location of the vagus nerve and its variations as viewed in US [50, 51]. If the electrode moves beyond the thyroid nodule (outside the thyroid gland), it may induce thermal injury to surrounding critical structures such as the vagus nerve or sympathetic ganglion. To avoid this complication, continuous US-guided tracing of the electrode tip is mandatory during the ablation.

Hematomas, resulting from electrode-induced vessel injury, can occur in the perithyroidal, subcapsular, and intranodular locations [49]. Hematomas can usually be controlled by compression of the neck for several minutes, with most hematomas disappearing within 1–2 weeks [1]. Because serious hematomas may compress the airways, close observation is recommended during and after the procedure [1].

Transient thyrotoxicosis may occur after RFA, although the patient is usually asymptomatic and normalizes within 1 month [5]. Hypothyroidism has been reported after treating nonfunctioning and hyperfunctioning thyroid nodules [8, 49]. Consequently, thyroid function tests are recommended during the follow-up period for patients with hyper- or hypothyroid symptoms [5, 8, 11, 49, 54]. To prevent an infection or abscess, the puncture site should be sterilized, and prophylactic antibiotics can be used; however, infection or abscess formation is a rare complication.

Thyroid nodule rupture after RFA may be suspected in patients with sudden neck bulging and pain at the treatment site [1, 49, 55]. Prior to nodule rupture, the ablated thyroid nodule gradually decreases in size. The rupture might occur due to volume expansion by a delayed hemorrhage or tumor wall tear. US usually shows a breakdown of the anterior thyroid capsule and formation of a new nodule in the anterior neck [1, 49, 55]. In cases of suspected nodule rupture, an initial conservative treatment (simple compression) without invasive procedures, such as needle aspiration is recommended. However, drainage or excision may be required if the symptoms of redness and pain progress [55].

Skin burns have been reported at the electrode puncture site [11, 21, 49]. Application of an ice bag during ablation or injection of fluid between the nodule and skin may prevent skin burns [56]. The risk of burns at the pad attachment site is relatively low because RF energy is lower in the thyroid [49]. Nausea and vasovagal reflection may be caused by severe tension, pain, or hypersensitivity to lidocaine [49]. Life-threatening complications, including trachea injury [57] and myocardial infarction [26, 27, 29, 30, 58], have been reported in patients undergoing RFA of tumors other than those of the thyroid gland. Although the RF current can cause esophageal or tracheal injury and heart problems, those complications have not been reported in thyroid. Thermal injury to critical structures in the neck such as the cervical sympathetic nerve and spinal accessory nerve have also not been reported, but the operator should be aware of the significance of such possible complications, particularly when a recurrent tumor is close to neck nerves. To prevent nerve injury, the moving shot technique, which uses a small active tip (<1 cm), and the hydrodissection technique are helpful [2]. When operators use the hydrodissection technique, continuous infusion of fluid is necessary because the injected fluid spreads gradually along the muscle plane of the neck [59]. Coughing can be induced by thermal propagation to the trachea and is managed by stopping the ablation [1, 49]. To prevent thermal injury to the esophagus, patients should be asked to swallow cold water during the ablation of a nodule adjacent to the esophagus [1, 26, 28, 49].

To prevent life-threatening complications, the operators should strictly trace the electrode tip during the procedure and should have knowledge of the neck's anatomy and experience with an image-guided intervention.

**Conclusion**

Thyroid RFA is an effective and safe treatment modality in patients with thyroid lesions. RFA may be as effective as surgery if it is performed by experienced physicians in optimally selected patients. RFA may also have an effective complementary role in the management of recurrent thyroid cancers.

## References


1. Baek JH, Lee JH, Valcavi R, Pacella CM, Rhim H, Na DG (2011) Thermal ablation for benign thyroid nodules: radiofrequency and laser. Korean J Radiol 12(5):525–540
2. Na DG, Lee JH, Jung SL et al (2012) Radiofrequency ablation of benign thyroid nodules and recurrent thyroid cancers: consensus statement and recommendations. Korean J Radiol 13(2):117–125
3. Ha EJ, Baek JH, Lee JH (2011) The efficacy and complications of radiofrequency ablation of thyroid nodules. Curr Opin Endocrinol Diabetes Obes 18(5):310–314
4. Shin JH, Baek JH, Ha EJ, Lee JH (2012) Radiofrequency ablation of thyroid nodules: basic principles and clinical application. Int J Endocrinol 2012:919650
5. Jeong W, Baek J, Rhim H et al (2008) Radiofrequency ablation of benign thyroid nodules: safety and imaging follow-up in 236 patients. Eur Radiol 18(6):1244–1250
6. Lee J, Kim Y, Lee D, Choi H, Yoo H, Baek J (2010) Radiofrequency ablation (RFA) of benign thyroid nodules in patients with incompletely resolved clinical problems after ethanol ablation (EA). World J Surg 34(7):1488–1493
7. Baek J, Kim Y, Lee D, Huh J, Lee J (2010) Benign predominantly solid thyroid nodules: prospective study of efficacy of sonographically guided radiofrequency ablation versus control condition. AJR Am J Roentgenol 194(4):1137–1142
8. Baek J, Moon W, Kim Y, Lee J, Lee D (2009) Radiofrequency ablation for the treatment of autonomously functioning thyroid nodules. World J Surg 33(9):1971–1977
9. Deandrea M, Limone P, Basso E et al (2008) US-guided percutaneous radiofrequency thermal ablation for the treatment of solid benign hyperfunctioning or compressive thyroid nodules. Ultrasound Med Biol 34(5):784–791
10. Spiezia S, Garberoglio R, Milone F et al (2009) Thyroid nodules and related symptoms are stably controlled two years after radiofrequency thermal ablation. Thyroid 19(3):219–225
11. Kim YS, Rhim H, Tae K, Park DW, Kim ST (2006) Radiofrequency ablation of benign cold thyroid nodules: initial clinical experience. Thyroid 16(4):361–367
12. Baek J, Jeong H, Kim Y, Kwak M, Lee D (2008) Radiofrequency ablation for an autonomously functioning thyroid nodule. Thyroid 18(6):675–676
13. Goldberg SN (2001) Radiofrequency tumor ablation: principles and techniques. Eur J Ultrasound 13(2):129–147
14. Kang TW, Rhim H, Kim EY et al (2009) Percutaneous radiofrequency ablation for the hepatocellular carcinoma abutting the diaphragm: assessment of safety and therapeutic efficacy. Korean J Radiol 10(1):34–42
15. Rhim H, Goldberg SN, Dodd GD 3rd et al (2001) Essential techniques for successful radiofrequency thermal ablation of malignant hepatic tumors. Radiographics 21 Spec No, S17–S35; discussion S36–19
16. Goldberg SN, Gazelle GS, Mueller PR (2000) Thermal ablation therapy for focal malignancy: a unified approach to underlying principles, techniques, and diagnostic imaging guidance. AJR Am J Roentgenol 174(2):323–331
17. Sung JY, Baek JH, Kim YS et al (2008) One-step ethanol ablation of viscous cystic thyroid nodules. AJR Am J Roentgenol 191(6):1730–1733
18. Sung JY, Kim YS, Choi H, Lee JH, Baek JH (2011) Optimum first-line treatment technique for benign cystic thyroid nodules: ethanol ablation or radiofrequency ablation? AJR Am J Roentgenol 196(2):W210–W214

19. Huh JY, Baek JH, Choi H, Kim JK, Lee JH (2012) Symptomatic benign thyroid nodules: efficacy of additional radiofrequency ablation treatment session–prospective randomized study. Radiology 263(3):909–916
20. Monchik J, Donatini G, Iannuccilli J, Dupuy D (2006) Radiofrequency ablation and percutaneous ethanol injection treatment for recurrent local and distant well-differentiated thyroid carcinoma. Ann Surg 244(2):296–304
21. Park KW, Shin JH, Han BK, Ko EY, Chung JH (2011) Inoperable symptomatic recurrent thyroid cancers: preliminary result of radiofrequency ablation. Ann Surg Oncol 18(9): 2564–2568
22. Spiezia S, Garberoglio R, Di Somma C et al (2007) Efficacy and safety of radiofrequency thermal ablation in the treatment of thyroid nodules with pressure symptoms in elderly patients. J Am Geriatr Soc 55(9):1478–1479
23. Baek JH, Kim YS, Sung JY, Choi H, Lee JH (2011) Locoregional control of metastatic well-differentiated thyroid cancer by ultrasound-guided radiofrequency ablation. AJR Am J Roentgenol 197(2):W331–W336
24. Dupuy D, Monchik J, Decrea C, Pisharodi L (2001) Radiofrequency ablation of regional recurrence from well-differentiated thyroid malignancy. Surgery 130(6):971–977
25. Papini E, Guglielmi R, Hosseim G et al (2011) Ultrasound-guided laser ablation of incidental papillary thyroid microcarcinoma: a potential therapeutic approach in patients at surgical risk. Thyroid 21(8):917–920
26. Livraghi T, Solbiati L, Meloni MF, Gazelle GS, Halpern EF, Goldberg SN (2003) Treatment of focal liver tumors with percutaneous radio-frequency ablation: complications encountered in a multicenter study. Radiology 226(2):441–451
27. Rhim H, Dodd GD, Chintapalli KN et al (2004) Radiofrequency thermal ablation of abdominal tumors: lessons learned from complications. Radiographics 24(1):41–52
28. Rhim H, Yoon KH, Lee JM et al (2003) Major complications after radio-frequency thermal ablation of hepatic tumors: spectrum of imaging findings. Radiographics 23(1):123–134; discussion 134–126
29. Tong NY, Ru HJ, Ling HY, Cheung YC, Meng LW, Chung PC (2004) Extracardiac radiofrequency ablation interferes with pacemaker function but does not damage the device. Anesthesiology 100(4):1041
30. Nemcek AA (2006) Complications of radiofrequency ablation of neoplasms. Semin Intervent Radiol 23(2):177–187
31. Jang SW, Baek JH, Kim JK et al (2012) How to manage the patients with unsatisfactory results after ethanol ablation for thyroid nodules: role of radiofrequency ablation. Eur J Radiol 81(5):905–910
32. Bennedbaek FN, Hegedus L (2003) Treatment of recurrent thyroid cysts with ethanol: a randomized double-blind controlled trial. J Clin Endocrinol Metab 88(12):5773–5777
33. Kim DW, Rho MH, Kim HJ, Kwon JS, Sung YS, Lee SW (2005) Percutaneous ethanol injection for benign cystic thyroid nodules: is aspiration of ethanol-mixed fluid advantageous? AJNR Am J Neuroradiol 26(8):2122–2127
34. Sung JY, Baek JH, Kim KS et al (2013) Single-session treatment of benign cystic thyroid nodules with ethanol versus radiofrequency ablation: a prospective randomized study. Radiology 269(1):293–300
35. Gharib H, Papini E, Paschke R et al (2010) American Association of Clinical Endocrinologists, Associazione Medici Endocrinologi, and European Thyroid Association Medical guidelines for clinical practice for the diagnosis and management of thyroid nodules. Endocr Pract 16(Suppl 1):1–43
36. Dossing H, Bennedbaek FN, Hegedus L (2003) Ultrasound-guided interstitial laser photocoagulation of an autonomous thyroid nodule: the introduction of a novel alternative. Thyroid 13(9):885–888
37. Fassi J, Lambertini R, Farias P et al (2005) Treatment of uremic hyperparathyroidism with percutaneous ethanol injection. Nephron Clin Pract 101(2):c53–c57
38. Guglielmi R, Pacella CM, Bianchini A et al (2004) Percutaneous ethanol injection treatment in benign thyroid lesions: role and efficacy. Thyroid 14(2):125–131

39. Cooper DS, Doherty GM, Haugen BR et al (2009) Revised American Thyroid Association management guidelines for patients with thyroid nodules and differentiated thyroid cancer. Thyroid 19(11):1167–1214
40. Jeon SJ, Kim E, Park JS et al (2009) Diagnostic benefit of thyroglobulin measurement in fine-needle aspiration for diagnosing metastatic cervical lymph nodes from papillary thyroid cancer: correlations with US features. Korean J Radiol 10(2):106–111
41. Heilo A, Sigstad E, Fagerlid KH et al (2011) Efficacy of ultrasound-guided percutaneous ethanol injection treatment in patients with a limited number of metastatic cervical lymph nodes from papillary thyroid carcinoma. J Clin Endocrinol Metab 96(9):2750–2755
42. Kim BM, Kim MJ, Kim EK, Park SI, Park CS, Chung WY (2008) Controlling recurrent papillary thyroid carcinoma in the neck by ultrasonography-guided percutaneous ethanol injection. Eur Radiol 18(4):835–842
43. Wallace LB, Berber E (2011) Percutaneous and video-assisted ablation of endocrine tumors: liver, adrenal, and thyroid. Surg Laparosc Endosc Percutan Tech 21(4):255–259
44. Lim HK, Lee JH, Ha EJ, Sung JY, Kim JK, Baek JH (2013) Radiofrequency ablation of benign non-functioning thyroid nodules: 4-year follow-up results for 111 patients. Eur Radiol 23(4):1044–1049
45. Faggiano A, Ramundo V, Assanti AP et al (2012) Thyroid nodules treated with percutaneous radiofrequency thermal ablation: a comparative study. J Clin Endocrinol Metab 97(12): 4439–4445
46. Fuller CW, Nguyen SA, Lohia S, Gillespie MB (2014) Radiofrequency ablation for treatment of benign thyroid nodules: systematic review. Laryngoscope 124(1):346–353
47. Wong KP, Lang BH (2013) Use of radiofrequency ablation in benign thyroid nodules: a literature review and updates. Int J Endocrinol 2013:428363
48. Gharib H, Hegedus L, Pacella CM, Baek JH, Papini E (2013) Nonsurgical, image-guided, minimally invasive therapy for thyroid nodules. J Clin Endocrinol Metab 98(10):3949–3957
49. Baek JH, Lee JH, Sung JY et al (2012) Complications encountered in the treatment of benign thyroid nodules with US-guided radiofrequency ablation: a multicenter study. Radiology 262(1):335–342
50. Park JK, Jeong SY, Lee JH, Lim GC, Chang JW (2011) Variations in the course of the cervical vagus nerve on thyroid ultrasonography. AJNR Am J Neuroradiol 32(7):1178–1181
51. Ha EJ, Baek JH, Lee JH, Kim JK, Shong YK (2011) Clinical significance of vagus nerve variation in radiofrequency ablation of thyroid nodules. Eur Radiol 21(10):2151–2157
52. Gibson A (1915) Bilateral abnormal relationship of the vagus nerve in its cervical portion. J Anat Physiol 49(Pt 4):389–392
53. Giovagnorio F, Martinoli C (2001) Sonography of the cervical vagus nerve: normal appearance and abnormal findings. AJR Am J Roentgenol 176(3):745–749
54. Valcavi R, Riganti F, Bertani A, Formisano D, Pacella CM (2010) Percutaneous laser ablation of cold benign thyroid nodules: a 3-year follow-up study in 122 patients. Thyroid 20(11): 1253–1261
55. Shin JH, Jung SL, Baek JH, Kim JH (2011) Rupture of benign thyroid tumors after radiofrequency ablation. AJNR Am J Neuroradiol 32(11):2165–2169
56. Koo JH, Shin JH, Oh YL, Ko EY, Han BK (2012) Sonographically guided radiofrequency ablation with and without a superficial saline injection to prevent skin burns in a rabbit model. J Ultrasound Med 31(6):873–878
57. Choi JW, Kwak S-H, Yoo SM et al (2005) Ultrasound-guided radiofrequency ablation of thyroid gland: a preliminary study in dogs. J Korean Radiol Soc 52:333–341
58. Mulier S, Mulier P, Ni Y et al (2002) Complications of radiofrequency coagulation of liver tumours. Br J Surg 89(10):1206–1222
59. Shin JE, Baek JH, Lee JH (2013) Radiofrequency and ethanol ablation for the treatment of recurrent thyroid cancers: current status and challenges. Curr Opin Oncol 25(1):14–19

# High-Intensity Focused Ultrasound Ablation (HI-FU) in Endocrine Neck Diseases

8

Fabrice Menegaux, Laurence Leenhardt, and Olivier Esnault

Thyroid nodules and primary hyperparathyroidism (HPT) are highly prevalent endocrine disorders. Fortunately, almost 100 % of parathyroid tumors and more than 95 % of thyroid nodules are benign. Some patients with thyroid nodules will need surgery for diagnostic purpose despite the improved accuracy of noninvasive procedures, and others for HPT. Complications of thyroid and parathyroid surgery such as recurrent laryngeal nerve (RLN) injury, superior laryngeal nerve injury, hypocalcaemia after total thyroid resection, and hemorrhage are not so rare and permanent complications can occur, respectively, at 2.1 % and 2.7 % RLN palsy, and hypoparathyroidism rates have been reported in a prospective multicenter study including departments specialized in endocrine surgery [1].

Moreover, some patients in poor medical condition are contraindicated for a surgical neck exploration for a local recurrence of thyroid carcinoma or for a parathyroid adenoma because of a high risk of surgery and/or general anesthesia.

This is why minimally invasive or noninvasive methods have been developed to ablate thyroid nodules and parathyroid glands without surgery: percutaneous ethanol injection therapy, percutaneous thermal procedures (radiofrequency ablation, laser coagulation), microwave ablation, and high-intensity focused ultrasound (HIFU) [2].

F. Menegaux, MD, PhD (✉)
Department of General Surgery, Hopital de la Pitié, Paris 6 University, 83 boulevard de l'hopital, Paris F-75013, France
e-mail: fabrice.menegaux@psl.aphp.fr

L. Leenhardt
Department of Nuclear Medicine, Hopital de la Pitié, Paris 6 University, Paris F-75013, France

O. Esnault
ENT, 6 Rue Puvis de Chavannes, Paris F-75017, France



C.P. Lombardi, R. Bellantone (eds.), *Minimally Invasive Therapies for Endocrine Neck Diseases*, DOI 10.1007/978-3-319-20065-1_8

HIFU has been studied for 50 years, with recent technological developments allowing its use for tumors of various sites. This technique was initially employed to treat localized prostate cancer [3] and is currently widely used in clinical practice in this indication. A recent review showed that localized prostate cancer could be eradicated by HIFU with a reduction of associated side effects of radical treatment, although long-term follow-up studies are still needed to evaluate cancer-specific and overall survival [4]. In the field of prostate cancer, HIFU has also been described among salvage local therapies after failure of radiotherapy [5].

For other tumor locations, clinical applications are still to be established [6]. With the exception of prostate cancer, literature is relatively poor. However, recent technological developments allow its use for tumors of the liver to treat unresectable advanced stages of hepatocellular carcinoma and liver metastases [7].

Concerning HIFU ablation of thyroid nodules or parathyroid glands, there is no randomized cohort studies. The only reported experience is limited to studies from two teams using this procedure to treat thyroid nodules [8] or HPT [9].

The first experience of HIFU for localized thyroid tissue ablation in an animal was published only 10 years ago by Esnault O. et al. [8]. This preliminary study confirmed the possibility of using HIFU for ablation of a defined area in thyroid tissue in an experimental model performed in ewes with a device not fully suitable for this purpose (it was a device for prostate cancer treatment). An additional study was performed on ewes to evaluate the reproducibility of a HIFU prototype designed specifically for human use [10]. First human feasibility studies are very recent since HIFU ablation of thyroid nodules was published only in 2011 for 25 patients included from 2003 to 2006 [11], and HIFU ablation of parathyroid adenoma was only reported in 2010 (4 patients, date of inclusion unknown) [9].

## 8.1 Technique

The originality of HIFU ablation is that this procedure induces thermal destruction without any skin penetration. It delivers a large amount of heat energy to a restricted space, where ultrasound (US) produces necrosis with a minimum effect on surrounding structures. Energy deposit caused by the interaction between high-intensity US and the tissue will raise the temperature locally in the target area [6].

Ultrasound guidance is used to position the device accurately over the right or the left lobe of the thyroid: an extracorporeal probe (3 MHz frequency) can locate the zone to be treated during the session and trachea, esophagus, and other parts potentially at risk such as the carotid are carefully avoided.

Two parameters must be defined: acoustic intensity and focus of the US beam. Acoustic intensity is usually set at around 100 W/cm$^2$. The focus of US beam is activated by using multiple, convergent, and specific transducers, creating a concentration of energy at a focal point and producing the ablative effect. Focus within the tissue is highly collimated and allows an energy concentration that is followed by an increased temperature within the focal volume, resulting in tissue coagulative necrosis. Multiple impulses are needed to induce an ablation volume of clinical significance. An effective treatment area of 2 mm in diameter by 5 to 8 mm in depth is obtained for each sequence of US impulses, which generally lasts about 5 s. For each treatment cycle, around 100 J of energy are delivered, heating up the focal point, the objective being to exceed 70–75 °C locally in order to destroy the target cells. This method is extremely accurate since energy drops sharply outside the focal zone: tissue 0.3 mm away from the point focal remains unchanged [12].

The procedure is usually performed under conscious sedation, can be employed in an ambulatory setting, and requires from 1 h to a few hours to achieve an effective volume ablation [11]. Local anesthesia is administered on the skin, and in some cases, inside the nodule itself. Not every thyroid nodule can be treated all at once, but experience in prostate disease shows that a 40 g prostate can be entirely treated in one session [13]. For thyroid nodules, HIFU can be repeated if the first treatment was incomplete: it was the case for 2 patients (out of 25 in the clinical study) who had a second HIFU session on day 8 for no significant reduction in vascularization in the treated nodule by Doppler ultrasonography [11].

## 8.2 Indications

Clinical experience is limited and no study was performed to compare HIFU ablation with other noninvasive or minimally invasive alternative treatments such as ethanol injection therapy, radiofrequency ablation, or laser coagulation [14].

As with diagnostic US, sound waves do not pass through air or solid structures, like bone. This prevents the treatment of tumors behind the sternum (substernal goiter and mediastinal parathyroid adenoma).

### 8.2.1 Thyroid Disease

#### 8.2.1.1 Euthyroid Nodular Goiters

HIFU ablation could be used to treat benign or malignant lesions of the thyroid without having to resort to surgery and without disrupting any subsequent treatment. However, the only clinical data on HIFU ablation for the thyroid gland nodules come from a single research center [11, 14, 15]. In an open feasibility study, 25 patients were treated with HIFU two weeks before surgery for nodular goiter [11]. Treatment was disrupted in 3 patients. Among the remaining 22 patients, macroscopic and histological examinations showed that all lesions were confined to the targeted nodule without affecting adjacent structures. Although 17 out of the 22 treated patients showed no US change in nodule size at 15 days, an extent of nodule destruction (ranged from 2 to 80 %) was observed on pathology in every patient, including 5 patients who had over 20 % pathological lesions unmistakably attributed to HIFU: Typical lesions were coagulative necrosis, multiple fibrotic scars, thrombosis, surrounding a cystic area; less specific lesions associated with ultrasound changes were noncoagulative necrosis, hemorrhage, nodule detachment, cavitations, and cysts). The last three patients ablated at a highest energy level showed a significant ultrasound change and complete coagulative necrosis in 80 %, 78 %, and 58 % of the targeted area, respectively.

#### 8.2.1.2 Nodular Hyperthyroidism

A pilot study of HIFU ablation of a single 8 mm toxic nodule was also recently reported [15]: 2 weeks after treatment, the nodule had become cystic with a nonvascularized hypoechoic scar of 1.4 × 1.6 mm at 12 and 18 months. Biologic euthyroidism was achieved at 3 months with a TSH = 1.91 μU/mL and was maintained at 6, 12, and 18 months. Thyroid scintigraphy performed 18 months after treatment showed a recovery of the thyroid iodine uptake.

#### 8.2.1.3 Not Estimated Indications

HIFU ablation has not been studied in thyroid carcinoma as an alternative treatment to surgery. However, in the only field largely studied in the literature for impact of HIFU ablation on survival of a solid organ cancer, prostate carcinoma, HIFU seems to result in short- to medium-term localized cancer control, although long-term follow-up studies are needed to evaluate cancer-specific and overall survival [4]. If the promising results on HIFU for definitive treatment of prostate cancer were confirmed in future prospective trials, this procedure could be studied in the management of localized thyroid carcinoma.

HIFU ablation could also be interesting in patients with a neck recurrence after total thyroid resection for carcinoma with no possible surgery for local or general reasons. This procedure could theoretically reduce nonresectable tumors but experimental and clinical studies are to be set up since there is actually no reported experience on HIFU ablation of neck recurrences.

### 8.2.2 Parathyroid Neck Disease

Clinical data on the parathyroid gland are also limited. Only one team from Bulgaria reported clinical experience of HIFU ablation on hyperparathyroidism.

A feasibility study was performed in 4 patients [9] followed by a clinical study that was conducted in patients with a secondary HPT [16]: Five chronic hemodialysis patients with severe HPT underwent one to three HIFU treatments. They had at least one enlarged parathyroid gland. This first experience illustrated the procedure potential benefits with a marked decrease of serum parathyroid hormone (PTH) achieved in three patients, but also its limitations, since in the long run, HIFU treatment was successful in only two patients. Authors concluded that the presence of diffuse major parathyroid hyperplasia in three or more glands clearly was a limitation for the success of the HIFU method, as well as the accessibility of the targeted gland.

In a more recent study, the same team studied in patients with primary hyperparathyroidism (PHPT) [17]: 13 patients PHPT were eligible for HIFU treatment, performed in 1 or 2 sessions. A significant parathyroid volume reduction was observed after the final HIFU treatment. Similarly, PTH decreased significantly 1 month after HIFU therapy and the value remained lower during the following months. However,

6 months after the final HIFU session, PTH decreased from 5.7 to 75.3 % (mean 48±28 %) in ten patients, while in three others an increase of PTH was observed. Permanent cure was obtained in 3 patients (23 %, all after 2 HIFU sessions), and good control of the disease was achieved in 9 patients (69 %, including 7 patients after only 1 HIFU session and 2 after 2 sessions); the procedure was unsuccessful in 1 patient (8 %) only. Number of sessions was significantly related to treatment success ($p<0.05$). Authors concluded that HIFU was a promising noninvasive technique for PHPT treatment, which could serve as therapeutic alternative for selected patients.

## 8.3 Experience and Complications

Although clinical experience is limited, first pilot studies were useful in evaluating specific risks of HIFU ablation of thyroid nodules or parathyroid glands but morbidity needs to be assessed on a larger scale.

In the preliminary animal study [8], some injuries to neighboring organs, such as skin, trachea, esophagus, and recurrent nerves, were observed; however, the device that was used in this study was not fully suited for this purpose.

In clinical studies, no long-term side effects are described, especially those affecting the recurrent nerves (permanent recurrent laryngeal nerve palsy) or the trachea.

Pain and skin damage are the most common HIFU-related adverse events.

In the clinical trial of HIFU ablation of thyroid nodules, three patients among 25 (12 %) discontinued treatment due to pain or the appearance of skin microblister [11]. Skin blisters appeared with increasing energy levels. In this study, adaptation of treatment parameters allowed to reduce the focal point and thus cutaneous problems. Local subcutaneous edema was also quite frequent (23 %) but was mild and transient, disappearing in a few days [16].

Patient discomfort and pain increase proportionally with increases in delivered energy, and pain ceases between pulses. Transient cough is also a frequent complication with an 8 % rate [11].

Vocal cord palsy is the most feared complication. However, first reported experiences show that vocal cord mobility impairment were always transient, although their rates varied a lot since they ranged from 0 % [11] to 23 % (3/13 patients) [17] and even 40 % (2/5 patients) [16]. It is related to the depth of the thyroid nodule or the parathyroid adenoma since they require higher pulse acoustic energies to overcome the absorption by tissues between the skin and the nodule. On the other hand, location of the thyroid nodule or the parathyroid gland (superior or inferior) and the applied energy do not seem to be risk factors [17].

## 8.4 Management of Complications

It is necessary to adapt the analgesia to the degree of energy delivered. Conscious intravenous analgesia is delivered in all cases and an additional injection of the nodule with 1 % lidocaine under sonographic guidance can be done to prevent pain.

However, injection into the nodule could cause dissipation of thermal energy due to the locally induced edema, and conversely, local vasoconstriction may decrease the energy required for ablation [11].

Risks of recurrent nerve palsy and skin damages can be reduced with the improvement of the technique, including patient selection, preoperative localization of the nodule, treatment targeting assessments of the volume treated, and a better understanding of the factors that influence HIFU-induced tissue destruction.

**Conclusion**

HIFU appears as the potentially less invasive procedure due to the absence of skin penetration. Currently, advantages of this technique can be established: Age of the patient and numerous concomitant diseases do not represent limitation for treatment; HIFU can be performed as an outpatient procedure.

However, the high cost of the specific equipment, its limited availability, treatment duration, and very limited data do not allow a large use in current clinical practice. Moreover, we should be very careful for patients with HPT: The high risk of recurrent laryngeal nerve injury in patients treated with HIFU should limit this procedure to a very few selected patients. Larger studies are needed to establish the optimal treatment protocol and to better define the selection of patients.

## References


1. Duclos A, Peix JL, Colin C, Kraimps JL, Menegaux F, Pattou F, Sebag F, Touzet S, Bourdy S, Voirin N, Lifante JC, for the CATHY Study Group (2012) Influence of experience on performance of individual surgeons: observational multicentre study in thyroid surgery. BMJ 344:d8041. doi:10.1136/bmj.d8041.
2. Gharib H, Hegedüs L, Pacella CM, Baek JH, Papini E (2013) Clinical review: nonsurgical, image-guided, minimally invasive therapy for thyroid nodules. J Clin Endocrinol Metab 98:3949–3957
3. Madersbacher S, Kratzik C, Susani M, Marberger M (1994) Tissue ablation in benign prostatic hyperplasia with high intensity focused ultrasound. J Urol 152:1956–1960
4. Cordeiro ER, Cathelineau X, Thüroff S, Marberger M, Crouzet S, de la Rosette JJ (2012) High-intensity focused ultrasound (HIFU) for definitive treatment of prostate cancer. BJU Int 110:1228–1242
5. Parekh A, Graham PL, Nguyen PL (2013) Cancer control and complications of salvage local therapy after failure of radiotherapy for prostate cancer: a systematic review. Semin Radiat Oncol 23:222–234
6. Kennedy JE, Ter Haar GR, Cranston D (2003) High intensity focused ultrasound: surgery of the future? Br J Radiol 76:590–599
7. Mearini L (2013) High intensity focused ultrasound, liver disease and bridging therapy. World J Gastroenterol 19:7494–7499
8. Esnault O, Franc B, Monteil JP, Chapelon JY (2004) High-intensity focused ultrasound for localized thyroid-tissue ablation: preliminary experimental animal study. Thyroid 14:1072–1076
9. Kovatcheva RD, Vlahov JD, Shinkov AD, Borissova AM, Hwang JH, Arnaud F, Hegedüs L (2010) High-intensity focused ultrasound to treat primary hyperparathyroidism: a feasibility study in four patients. AJR Am J Roentgenol 195:830–835
10. Esnault O, Franc B, Chapelon JY (2009) Localized ablation of thyroid tissue by high-intensity focused ultrasound: improvement of noninvasive tissue necrosis methods. Thyroid 19:1085–1091

11. Esnault O, Franc B, Menegaux F, Rouxel A, De Kerviler E, Bourrier P, Lacoste F, Chapelon JY, Leenhardt L (2011) High-intensity focused ultrasound ablation of thyroid nodules: first human feasibility study. Thyroid 21:965–973
12. Leenhardt L, Borson-Chazot F, Calzada M, Carnaille B, Charrié A, Cochand-Priollet B, Cao CD, Leboulleux S, Le Clech G, Mansour G, Menegaux F, Monpeyssen H, Orgiazzi J, Rouxel A, Sadoul JL, Schlumberger M, Tramalloni J, Tranquart F, Wemeau JL, French Society of Endocrinology (SFE) and of the Thyroid Study Group (GRT) (2011) Good practice guide for cervical ultrasound scan and echo-guided techniques in treating differentiated thyroid cancer of vesicular origin. Ann Endocrinol (Paris) 72:173–197
13. Mearini L, Porena M (2010) Transrectal high-intensity focused ultrasound for the treatment of prostate cancer: past, present, and future. Indian J Urol 26:4–11
14. Bandeira-Echtler E, Bergerhoff K, Richter B (2014) Levothyroxine or minimally invasive therapies for benign thyroid nodules. Cochrane Database Syst Rev 6:CD004098
15. Esnault O, Rouxel A, Le Nestour E, Gheron G, Leenhardt L (2010) Minimally invasive ablation of a toxic thyroid nodule by high-intensity focused ultrasound. AJNR Am J Neuroradiol 31:1967–1968
16. Kovatcheva RD, Vlahov JD, Stoinov JI, Kirilov GG, Krivoshiev SG, Arnaud F, Ortuno C, Drüeke TB (2012) High-intensity focussed ultrasound (HIFU) treatment in uraemic secondary hyperparathyroidism. Nephrol Dial Transplant 27:76–80
17. Kovatcheva R, Vlahov J, Stoinov J, Lacoste F, Ortuno C, Zaletel K (2014) US-guided high-intensity focused ultrasound as a promising non-invasive method for treatment of primary hyperparathyroidism. Eur Radiol 24:2052–2058

# Mini-Invasive Techniques for the Treatment of Thyroid Nodules: Critical Issues

9

Paolo Piero Limone, Alberto Mormile, Maurilio Deandrea, Francesca Garino, Elena Gamarra, and Federico Ragazzoni

In the last few decades, the introduction of US-guided mini-invasive techniques such as percutaneous ethanol injection (PEI), laser thermal ablation (LTA), and radiofrequency thermal ablation (RFA) has dramatically changed the approach to benign thyroid nodules, for which surgical excision had previously been the sole definitive treatment option [1, 2]. Quite recently, high-intensity focused ultrasound (HIFU) [3] and microwave (MW) [4] have been preliminarily reported as potential tools for thermal ablation.

The advantages of mini-invasive techniques are that they are less expensive and have fewer complications [5] than surgery, they do not require a general anesthesia, they are fast, and the patients can generally be discharged soon after the procedure. Therefore many patients at high surgical or anesthesiological risk can be safely treated this way. Another important advantage is that they do not affect thyroid function [6] and do not leave skin scars.

Despite these evident advantages, and the increasing diffusion of mini-invasive techniques, some critical issues still remain, regarding both technical and clinical aspects; we therefore review these issues, with the aim of focusing on the implications for clinical practice.

## 9.1 PEI

PEI has been proven as a fast and cheap tool for treating both cystic and solid nodules, as well as lymph nodal metastasis of differentiated thyroid cancer.

P.P. Limone (✉) • A. Mormile • M. Deandrea • F. Garino • E. Gamarra • F. Ragazzoni
Division of Endocrinology, Diabetes and Metabolism, "Centre for Thyroid Diseases", A.O. Ordine Mauriziano di Torino, Via Magellano 1, Torino 10128, Italy
e-mail: plimone@mauriziano.it; amormile@mauriziano.it



C.P. Lombardi, R. Bellantone (eds.), *Minimally Invasive Therapies for Endocrine Neck Diseases*, DOI 10.1007/978-3-319-20065-1_9

**Solid Cold Nodules** Bennedbaek et al. in a randomized study aiming to compare a single PEI session with L-thyroxine reported a volume reduction of around 50 % 12 months after PEI, whereas medical therapy was almost ineffective [7]. Further treatment sessions were able to induce only small additive effects, which were also confirmed by another report [8]. The most relevant drawback of this method is the possibility of leakage of alcohol into the surrounding neck tissue, causing immediate pain and long-term development of fibrotic scars, which could create difficulties in tissue dissection in case of subsequent surgical intervention [9]. Moreover, rare, laryngeal nerve damage can occur. The factors that could predict the outcome were specifically assessed by Kim et al., who reported a significant association of nodule vascularity and degree of intranodular echo-staining just after ethanol injection with a successful outcome, while such association was not observed with regard to nodule size, ratio of cystic component, amount of infused ethanol, and the number of treatment sessions [10].

**Solid Hot Nodules** Some studies have been carried out in autonomous nodules, but none was prospective and randomized. Multiple sessions were required to obtain normalization of TSH levels, which was obtained in all pretoxic adenomas, but in only 71 % of nodules causing overt hyperthyroidism [11–14]. Regrowth of the nodules associated with recurrence of hyperfunction is not uncommon in the long-term follow-up [14]. The side effects are the same as those seen in cold nodules.

**Cystic nodules** Many studies have shown the efficacy of PEI in cystic nodules, both pure cystic and hemorrhagic, as well as in those with a minor solid component [15, 16]. Bennedbaek et al. showed a greater efficacy of PEI vs. saline in cystic nodules (82 % of success rate vs. 18 %) [17]. The shrinkage has been shown to last for a long time [16]. (For comparison of PEI with LTA and RFA, see below in the paragraph concerning thermoablative techniques.) The outcome was inversely related to baseline volume and to the number of previous aspirations; moreover it has been suggested that internal bleeding could reduce the efficacy of PEI [18].

**Recurrent Cervical Cancer** Sixty-three patients with 109 neck lymph node metastases treated by PEI underwent follow-up for a mean time of 38.4 months. 84 % of the lymph nodes completely responded to PEI, and 9 % responded incompletely. In the follow-up, a cancer recurrence was seen in two nodes. The treatment was well tolerated in all patients [19]. In a long-term follow-up of an average of 5.4 years, 25 patients with neck nodal metastasis showed a decrease in size in 95 % of the treated nodes, and blood flow was undetectable at Doppler evaluation. 46 % of the nodes disappeared on US [20].

*To summarize, according to clinical experience and to the suggestions of the current available guidelines, PEI is the treatment of choice for cystic or mainly cystic nodules which recur after aspiration* [21, 22]. *Concerning the solid nodules, both cold and autonomous, the risk of alcohol diffusion outside the nodule, and the need for multiple sessions* (*in particular in order to obtain function normalization in hot nodules*), *the use of PEI is limited to a few selected patients and has nearly been abandoned in most centers, where it has been replaced by thermoablative techniques* (*see below*). *In centers with extensive experience, PEI could be considered to selectively treat neck nodal metastasis of well-differentiated cancer in patients who had previously undergone surgical dissection or are at high surgical risk* [23].

## 9.2 Laser and Radiofrequency Thermal Ablation

**Laser Disposals** Laser (*l*ight *a*mplification by *s*timulated *e*mission of *r*adiation) is able to induce necrosis coagulation of the tissues by heat generated by the interaction of photons transmitted by the tip of an optical fiber within the tissue. From a technical point of view, one of the main advantages of laser technology is that the area of tissue damage is predictable with high precision: indeed a single fiber induces coagulative necrosis with a spherical volume of about 20 mm in diameter [24]. Larger areas of necrosis may be obtained by inserting multiple fibers (two to four) 15–18 mm apart.

**Radiofrequency Disposals** Radiofrequency can be carried out using various devices. In our country, we [25] and others [26] at first used a rather large 14 G needle, with nine tips inside, which were expanded after the needle was inserted inside the nodule, to spread heating. Thereafter, two new devices became available, one with four expandable tips and the other, slightly thinner, with a single tip. At the same time, in Korea, a new thinner 18 G internally cooled needle (and more recently 19 G) was made available, with an active tip of 5–15 mm in length. Using this device, JH Baek proposed a new technique for treatment, called moving shot [27]. The main advantage of the moving-shot technique is that it allows us to treat almost the whole nodule; besides, the trans-isthmic approach makes it possible for the operator to spare the inner area of the nodule, the so-called danger triangle, which is close to the laryngeal nerve. At present the "moving-shot" technique is the best choice for RFA, due to its relative handiness, the cost of the device, and its efficacy.

**Learning Curve** It is generally believed that the learning curve is rather short. In our practice, the experience in this technique has enabled us to progressively deliver more energy and to treat the nodules more extensively, thus achieving better results. We have also realized that a large number of sessions are required to acquire confidence with these techniques and that extensive experience is required to minimize the complications of thermal ablation. We can argue that at least 30–40 cases are required to achieve a solid skill.

### 9.2.1 Are There US or Clinical Features or Physical Parameters Which Can Predict the Extent of Volume Reduction? Or That Can Predict Poor Response?

**Radiofrequency** In the experimental animal, Holmer et al. showed a dose–response relationship for RFA of thyroid tissue [28], but this was not confirmed in humans, probably because other influencing parameters intervene, such as vascularity of the nodules, the presence of fibrosis, and so on. Indeed, the human studies which addressed this topic provided conflicting results, due to different methodological approaches (number of treatment sessions, time of follow-up, differences in nodule volume, etc). In most reports an inverse relationship was found between basal volume and solidity and the extent of shrinkage [25, 26, 29–31], while other reports failed to show a similar relationship. In our first report we were unable to find a relationship between volume reduction of nodules treated by large electrode with nine tips and the amount of delivered energy [25]. Working together with Baek's group, we recently found, using moving-shot technique, that the energy delivered per mL of tissue volume was the only factor related to volume reduction observed at 6 months, while the time of effective treatment and the total energy were not critical [32].

**Laser** A significant correlation was reported in 2004 by Pacella et al. between energy delivered and volume of coagulation achieved and between energy delivered and reduction in nodule size [32], but this observation was not confirmed by other authors [34–36]. Furthermore, the initial nodule volume [32, 35, 37] and the echostructure [32, 36, 37] of the nodules did not seem to influence the response to treatment, whereas Valcavi et al. reported that the spongiform aspect was the only US feature which was predictive of good shrinkage; furthermore, smaller nodules showed a trend toward greater shrinkage [38].

*To summarize, data in literature (which is in agreement with our experience in about 400 cases) point to the spongiform aspect as the only US feature that predicts a good shrinkage; moreover, as a general rule, the larger initial volume is predictive of less response, as well as the nodule conglomerate.*

As to factors predictive of poor response, extensive fibrosis and coarse calcifications could limit the efficacy of the treatment by impairing the heat diffusion within the nodular tissue. What is more, some observations suggest that an increase of intranodular blood flow could reduce the extent of ablation through perfusion-mediated tissue cooling [39], but this is in contrast with other findings that hyperfunctioning nodules, which in general have an increased internal blood flow, had a volume reduction similar to cold nodules [25, 40].

Another factor that we should consider is the temperature reached during treatment; indeed, when we aim to destroy tissue by heat, whatever the adopted technique, the best results are obtained when the temperature ranges between 50 and 100 °C; this is when irreversible damage and coagulation necrosis occur, while at higher temperatures carbonization takes place, which impairs the diffusion of heat to the surrounding tissue. Therefore it is essential that the operator maintains an adequate temperature during treatment (this could be obtained infusing saline solution inside the nodule during the procedure in order to prevent overheating the tissue).

### 9.2.2 What Is the Best Nodule Volume for Treatment?

One of the most intriguing issues, and one which is closely related to the above considerations, is what is the optimal nodule size in order to obtain the best results. In other words, do we have to wait for the nodule to grow or do we treat it when it is still rather small? By intuition, an early treatment could be advantageous, but small nodules are generally asymptomatic, so an interventional procedure (though quite safe) could be unjustified, bearing in mind that there are no criteria to predict the growth of a nodule. On the other hand, very large nodules could show a less

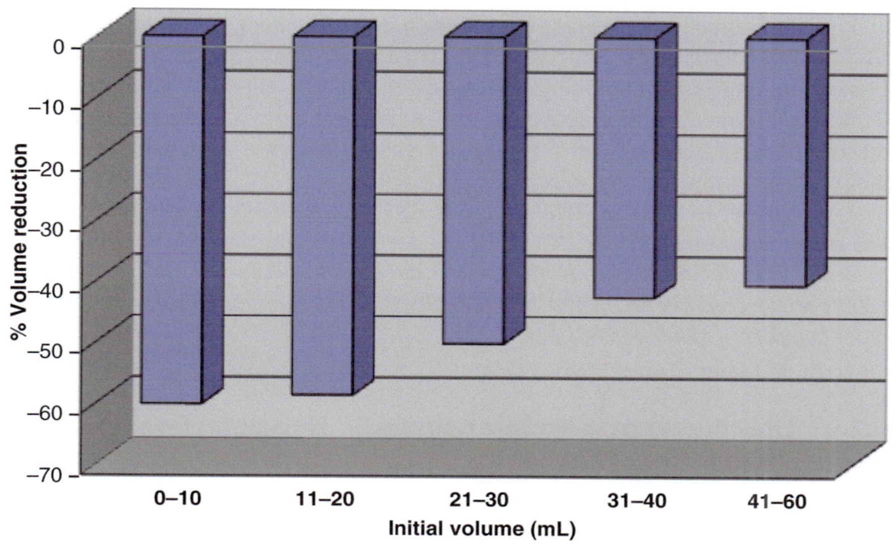


**Fig. 9.1** Volume reduction at 6-month follow-up after a single RFA session performed by moving-shot technique, according initial nodule volume

satisfactory shrinkage. Indeed Baek et al. reported that RFA is less effective in nodules more than 4 cm in size [39].

In our experience of using RFA by moving-shot technique, the best volume reduction was obtained in nodules less than 15–20 mL in volume, which showed a shrinkage greater than 60 %, while in larger nodules (up to 25–30 mL), the reduction was less than 40 % (unpublished data, Fig. 9.1).

*To summarize, in our opinion the optimal volume for submitting patients to thermal ablation is less than 20 mL (provided the nodules are responsible for compressive or aesthetic discomfort). Larger nodules can be effectively treated, bearing in mind that volume reduction could only be partial, but that it could be enough to relieve compressive symptoms, which, in most cases, is the primary objective of thermal ablation, and that more treatment sessions could be performed in order to obtain further reduction in size.*

### 9.2.3 Is Thermal Ablation Better Than PEI in Cystic Nodules? Is There a Limit in the Solid/Colloid Ratio for Selecting Nodules to Submit to Mini-Invasive Procedures?

Sung initially reported a superiority of PEI vs. RFA in cystic nodules, but in their first experience, internal fluid was not aspirated before RFA [41]. In a more recent prospective trial of the same authors, at six-month follow-up volume reduction was 96.9 % in the PEI group and 93.3 % in the RFA group [42].

PEI is less effective for treating thyroid nodules with a larger solid component [18], so further thermal ablation could be required to achieve significant shrinkage [43, 44].
**Laser** Dossing et al. randomized 44 cystic nodules to single aspiration with or without subsequent LTA. A reduction to a volume $\leq$ 1 ml was reported in 18 % in the aspiration group and in 68 % of the LTA group (thanks to a greater reduction of the solid part of the nodules induced by LTA) [45].

*In summary, no clear superiority of a technique over the other in cystic nodules has been demonstrated, but PEI is by far less expensive than thermal ablation; therefore it is definitely preferable. Only large mixed nodules with a considerable solid portion could be sequentially treated by PEI and thermal ablation to obtain a more complete volume reduction.*

### 9.2.4 How Frequent Is Nodule Regrowth? How Long Does Volume Reduction Last?

**Radiofrequency** Lim et al. followed 111 patients for up to 4 years; a regrowth (defined as a > 50 % increase in the volume compared to initial volume) was recorded in 5.6 % of the patients. The regrowth generally affected the peripheral areas of the nodule, which had been undertreated [29].
**Laser** Valcavi et al. in a retrospective 3 year follow-up reported a regrowth (defined as an increase to a volume larger than that before treatment) in 9 % of the subjects [38]; 5 % of 101 nodules treated by Papini et al. showed a regrowth (defined as a >20 % increase vs. the one-year posttreatment volume) 36 months after a single LTA session [37].

*In summary, the effects of thermal ablation generally last over time, and a regrowth of the treated nodules occurs in only 5–10 % of cases. The regrowing nodules can be further treated by thermal ablation or surgically; in few of our patients who were operated on because of a poor response to RFA, no scars were found in the extranodular tissue which could impair the outcome of the surgery. This clinical observation is in agreement with the findings of Holmer et al. who in experimental animals showed a clear demarcation between areas of radiofrequency induced necrosis and the surrounding vital tissue* [28].

### 9.2.5 Is a Single Treatment Session Enough? How Many Repeated Treatment Sessions Are Required to Significantly Increase the Nodule Volume Reduction? How Long After the First Procedure Can a Second Treatment Be Planned?

**Radiofrequency** In 58 out of 111 patients reported by Lim et al., more than one treatment session (mean 2.2 ± 1.4) was required to achieve an adequate shrinkage of the nodule, and the need of multiple treatments was related to the initial volume of the nodule [29].

Hu HY enrolled 30 patients with a nodule volume of about 13 mL, randomly assigned to receive one or two treatments; at six months volume reduction was 70.2 +/– 13.2 % in the group assigned to one treatment, while in the patients who received two treatment sessions one month apart, the volume reduction was 78.3 %. Thus, a second treatment produced a slight but not significant further benefit [46]. We can speculate that the second session was performed too early after the first treatment.

**Laser** Dossing et al. showed that the volume reduction induced by three monthly LTA sessions was slightly but significantly greater than that induced by a single session (58 % vs. 45 %, $p=0.03$) [47].

In a series of 77 patients with very large nodules (mean volume about 55 ml) treated by two or three LTA cycles (each consisting of three sessions 1 month apart), volume reduction was 43 % after one cycle, 72 % after two cycles, and 81 % after three cycles [48].

*In summary, a second or third procedure is able to obtain a further volume reduction of 15–20 %, which could lead to a global reduction of about 80 % or more; in our opinion more treatment sessions should be considered for larger nodules, when a significant portion of untreated tissue remains after the first procedure and/or when the patient complains of incomplete resolution of the symptoms. However, in these cases, a careful analysis of the cost-effectiveness should be performed, taking into account the cost of the many devices required, the clinical condition of the patients, and the aim of the treatment.*

*As regards the timing of a second treatment, up until now no studies have specifically investigated this issue, but, as the maximum volume reduction is obtained between 6 and 12 months after the first thermal ablation, it would be reasonable to plan it after this period of follow-up.*

### 9.2.6 Are the Hyperfunctioning Nodules Suitable for Thermal Ablation?

**Laser** As far as hyperfunctioning nodules are concerned, complete normalization of thyroid function was observed in 100 % of patients with small lesions treated by Spiezia et al. three months after a single LTA session [49], but in only 31 % of patients treated by Pacella et al. with a mean of 2.7 LTA sessions, despite good volume reduction [33]; moreover, LTA was shown to be inferior to 131I in normalizing serum TSH [50]. Interestingly, the combination of LTA and 131I in very large hyperfunctioning nodules obtained a more rapid reduction of the nodule volume and of compressive symptoms than 131I alone; furthermore, the patients treated by laser required lower 131I activity [51].

Amabile et al. treated large (>40 mL) hyperfunctioning nodules by 1 to 3 cycles of LTA (each cycle consisted of three sessions performed at an interval of 1 month); normal serum TSH was obtained in 87 % of the patients after three cycles of LTA [48].

**Radiofrequency** A complete recovery of hyperthyroidism was seen in 22–40 % of patients with toxic nodules treated by different radiofrequency techniques, whereas an improvement in thyroid function, allowing a reduction of the methimazole dose, occurred in 40–78 % of cases [25, 40, 52].

Some evidence suggests that the efficacy of RFA in hot nodules depends on the extent of hyperfunction, pretoxic nodules showing a normalization of their function more frequently than toxic nodules [26].

*In summary, thermal ablation should not be the first choice for the treatment of hyperfunctioning thyroid nodules, due to the difficulty of obtaining complete ablation of the whole nodular tissue, so the peripheral untreated areas could maintain hyperactivity* [53]. *On the other hand, radioiodine treatment is more effective in nodules < 4 cm and is by far less expensive, while surgery is the best choice for very large nodules following a course of antithyroid drugs to normalize thyroid function, providing there are no serious contraindications to surgery. We argue that thermoablation may be considered in two opposite conditions, the first being small autonomous nodules in young patients who refuse surgery or radioiodine (though, this is not a frequent condition), because a complete ablation can be achieved, and the second being very large nodules in patients at high surgical risk, in combination with radioiodine.*

### 9.2.7 Is There a Risk of Not Detecting Malignancy in Nodules Undergoing Thermal Ablation?

In the series with the longest follow-up, no malignancies are reported [29, 37, 38, 54, 57]; in our experience no cases of malignancy were found, and in those few patients who underwent subsequent surgery due to poor response to thermal ablation, the histological examination confirmed the benignancy.

If we examine this problem from the opposite point of view, we cannot ignore that in patients undergoing surgery for benign thyroid nodules, microcarcinomas are occasionally found on histological examination. This aspect is highlighted in the study of Bernardi et al., who compared RFA and surgery; in their series of 74 patients operated on, 8 microcarcinomas were found on histology [55]. However, this percentage seems quite elevated; we believe that there is a strong bias related to the retrospective analysis.

*In summary, the risk of malignancies is almost inexistent, providing that an accurate cytological evaluation has been carried out before treatment, possibly by performing two FNABs. Furthermore, we can speculate that small foci of cancer which are occasionally present inside the nodule could be ablated by heat.*

### 9.2.8 Is There a Precocious Thyroid Hormone Release After Treatment Causing Risk of Transient Thyrotoxicosis?

Both our group and Baek et al. did not report any case of hyperthyroidism in patients with nodules treated by RFA, neither cold nor autonomous [25, 27, 52].

A transient TSH decrease and fT4 increase were seen by Valcavi et al. at day 1 and week 1, respectively, after LTA; they returned to baseline levels within one month. Serum fT3 did not change. Two patients developed overt hyperthyroidism one month after the procedure, associated with a transient TRAb peak, and were treated with methimazole and 131I, respectively [38]. No changes in thyroid function or antithyroid antibodies were reported in the recent trial of Papini et al. [37].

*These observations give evidence that the risk of symptomatic thyrotoxicosis after thermal ablation is negligible.*

### 9.2.9 Is Thermal Ablation Cost-Effective?

This issue has been accurately and extensively addressed by Bernardi et al., who demonstrated that a single RFA session is cheaper than hemithyroidectomy (1,661.50 euros vs. 4,556.30) [55]. According to the analysis performed by the aforementioned authors, RFA could still be advantageous in patients with very large nodules who require further treatment sessions; indeed, we have to note that such patients are generally poor candidates for surgery due to their age or clinical conditions. Therefore, we should also take into account this aspect in the overall evaluation of the cost/benefit ratio in these cases.

The same considerations could be applied to the LTA, bearing in mind that the cost of the latter procedure is dependent on the number of fibers which are used in any single session (about 300–400 euros/fiber). We can argue that the cost of LTA is inferior not only to that of the surgery but even to that of radiofrequency when small nodules are treated by one or two fibers, while it could be similar to or greater than that of RFA when three or four fibers are required to treat large nodules. These aspects should be taken into consideration in the choice of the technique to be used for individual patients in centers, such as our institution, where both laser and radiofrequency are adopted.

### 9.2.10 Is Thermal Ablation Suitable for Treating Thyroid Cancer?

#### 9.2.10.1 Local Recurrent Thyroid Cancer

**Radiofrequency** Dupuy et al. first reported significant disappearance of vascular flow, coupled with necrosis of the regional recurrencies of papillary and follicular carcinomas in eight patients treated by RFA [56]. The same group treated twelve other patients, undergoing a mean follow-up at 41 months: no regrowth occurred in over 80 % of the subjects [57]. However, a case of vocal cord paralysis was reported in each series.

Park et al. treated 16 patients with cervical nodal metastasis responsible for local symptoms using one RFA session and reported complete ablation in six cases at 6-month follow-up, while in the other patients ablation was incomplete, mainly due to early interruption of the procedure due to severe local pain or the proximity of the node to vessels [58]. Ten patients in one of the Baek et al. series showed a significant volume reduction and 6 lesions completely disappeared. One patient complained of vocal cord paralysis [59].

We treated few cases of recurrent thyroid cancer by RFA: in a patient with a large cervical metastasis with ulcerated skin, an important shrinkage, followed by skin healing, was seen (unpublished observation). In another case RFA induced a substantial volume reduction of metastatic cervical lymph nodes.

**Laser** Some reports pointed to a significant volume decrease (and in most cases complete disappearance) of cervical nodal metastasis of papillary cancer after LTA and a parallel reduction of serum thyroglobulin. There were no cases of regrowth [60, 61].

#### 9.2.10.2 Primary Tumor

**Laser** Pacella et al. first treated an anaplastic cancer by LTA, followed by external beam irradiation. The combined treatment obtained a volume reduction and an improvement in compressive symptoms lasting 4 months [33].

Another patient with aggressive anaplastic carcinoma reported no significant improvement after LTA, and the disease rapidly progressed; this observation is in agreement with our experience in a case of a rapidly progressive anaplastic cancer undergoing RFA [62].

Papini et al. successfully treated an 8 mm papillary microcarcinoma in an elderly patient at high surgical risk, with complete ablation, which persisted at 24-month follow-up [63].

More recently, Valcavi et al. carried out LTA in 3 patients with papillary microcarcinoma (8 to 10 mm in diameter), who were candidates for surgery. Histological examination of the gland surgically excised immediately after LTA showed destructured and carbonized tissue, and lack of vitality was confirmed by loss of TTF1 and antimitochondria antibody expression in the ablated area. In 2 cases microfoci of papillary cancer were detected in extranodal tissue, and lymph node metastasis was present in one patient [64].

*In summary, thermal ablation (by both laser and radiofrequency) could be a useful tool for palliative treatment of patients with recurrent cervical differentiated thyroid cancer, not amenable to surgical excision or radiometabolic treatment. With regard to primary tumors, the response of few anaplastic carcinomas was very poor, so thermal ablation is almost useless in such cases. The preliminary reported cases of intrathyroidal papillary microcarcinomas treated by LTA seem to point to an efficacy of this technique in inducing complete destruction of the lesions, though we have some concerns regarding this modality of treatment, due to the not infrequent multifocality of papillary cancer. Therefore, considering the very low morbidity of surgery and the impossibility of identifying tumor microfoci with currently available imaging techniques, at present we cannot advise thermal ablation as primary treatment choice, with the exception of those very few patients at high surgical risk. However, considering the current trend toward a less aggressive treatment of intrathyroidal papillary cancer, this topic could be addressed by future trials.*

### 9.2.11 Is a Technique (Laser or Radiofrequency) More Effective Than the Other?

LTA is reported to be able to induce a reduction of the volume of benign thyroid nodules ranging between 36 and 60 %, depending on baseline volume, number of treatment sessions, and the morphology of the nodules [33–37, 65].

As well as LTA, the volume reduction obtained by RFA varies depending on the devices used, the baseline volume, and the other characteristics of the nodule. The reported reduction ranges between 50 and 84 % [25, 27, 30, 31, 40] and thyroid function is not compromised, even in patients who had previously undergone lobectomy [6].

Up until now, only one study was made on porcine thyroid gland to compare LTA and RFA, showing that both these techniques are suitable for singular thyroid nodules and induce reproducible clinically relevant lesions; moreover, the maximum inducible lesion volumes by LTA were significantly larger than by RFA [66]. However, it is not easy to translate these results to human nodular thyroid disease, due to different devices and experimental/clinical conditions. Furthermore, it is difficult to attempt to compare the various clinical trials performed by radiofrequency or laser, due to differences in clinical and technical settings; the only two studies in which patients with nodules with similar volume (10–20 mL) were enrolled, were that of Papini et al., who treated patients with a single LTA session [37], and that of our group together with Baek who treated patients with a single RFA session [32]. In the former, at six-month follow-up the volume reduction was about 50 %, whereas in the latter it was about 66 %. However, in the long-term follow-up, the LTA-treated group showed a further reduction which attained a mean of 57 %; in our study the follow-up is at present shorter, so a long-term comparison is impossible. Therefore, while at a glance the RFA ablation could appear more effective in the short term, this is only a speculative remark, and no conclusions can be drawn, because the above studies were not designed to compare the two techniques. Only specifically addressed trials in standardized conditions could help us to clarify this issue.

## 9.3 HIFU

HIFU was initially used for treating prostate cancer. More recently, HIFU has been used for ablating thyroid nodules or parathyroid adenomas in only two centers [3, 67]. The HIFU ablation has the advantage of being a noninvasive procedure, since it delivers heat energy without penetrating the skin. The nodule can be treated selectively in this way, avoiding damage to the surrounding thyroid tissue. The HIFU ablation is usually carried out under conscious sedation, can be performed as an outpatient procedure, and requires up to a few hours of treatment to achieve effective volume ablation [3].

Regarding side effects, local pain or skin microblisters requiring interruption of the treatment were recorded in 12 % of the patients; however the most serious complication is transient vocal cord paralysis, which was reported in a percentage ranging from 0 to 40 %, in particular, in patients treated for parathyroid adenoma [67].

However, due to high cost of the specific equipment, limited availability, treatment duration, very limited data, and the rather high risk of recurrent nerve damage, HIFU is limited to a very few selected patients in centers with experience in this technique. Larger studies should be undertaken to define the possibility of its use in clinical practice.

## 9.4 Microwave

Microwave ablation (MWA) has been used to treat benign and malignant tumors of various organs, and it has recently been adopted in few centers for the treatment of benign thyroid nodules. Compared to other thermoablative techniques, MWA seems able to induce a larger area of necrosis.

Feng et al. first carried out a preliminary study in 11 patients (9 with nodular goiter and 2 with Hashimoto's thyroiditis), undergoing unconscious anesthesia to allow the insertion of a 16 G microwave antenna inside the nodule (2 antennae were used in two patients). Baseline volume was 5.3 +/– mL; at 12-month follow-up, the mean volume reduction was 45.99 +/– 29.9 %. All patients complained of heat sensation and of a slight pain after the procedure; one patient showed vocal cord paralysis, which recovered within two months after steroids and vocal exercises [4].

MWA has also recently been used in 21 patients to treat papillary microcarcinoma without apparent lymph node metastasis; complete ablation was obtained in all patients. Complete necrosis of the tumor was confirmed in three subjects operated on shortly after MWA, as well as on five patients undergoing biopsy. In the other patients US showed absence of vascularization of the treated lesions. No recurrence was recorded during the follow-up (mean 11 months). Four patients had transient vocal cord paralysis which spontaneously resolved a few months later [68].

No randomized studies are currently available. Considering the small number of patients treated up until now, the need for unconscious anesthesia, and the reported complications, at present MWA cannot be recommended in clinical practice and should still be considered an experimental procedure.

## References

1. Gharib H, Hegedüs L, Pacella CM et al (2013) Clinical review: nonsurgical, image-guided, minimally invasive therapy for thyroid nodules. J Clin Endocrinol Metab 98:3949–3957
2. Papini E, Pacella CM, Hegedus L (2014) Thyroid ultrasound (US) and US-assisted procedures: from the shadows into an array of applications. Eur J Endocrinol 170:R133–R146
3. Esnault O, Franc B, Menegaux F et al (2011) High-intensity focused ultrasound ablation of thyroid nodules: first human feasibility study. Thyroid 21:965–973
4. Feng B, Liang P, Cheng Z et al (2012) Ultrasound-guided percutaneous microwave ablation of benign thyroid nodules: experimental and clinical studies. Eur J Endocrinol 166:1031–1037
5. Baek JH, Lee JH, Sung JY et al (2012) Korean society of thyroid radiology complications encountered in the treatment of benign thyroid nodules with US-guided radiofrequency ablation: a multicenter study. Radiology 262:335–342
6. Ha EJ, Baek JH, Lee JH et al (2013) Radiofrequency ablation of benign thyroid nodules does not affect thyroid function in patients with previous lobectomy. Thyroid 23:289–293
7. Bennedbaek FN, Nielsen LK, Hegedüs L (1998) Effect of percutaneous ethanol injection versus suppressive doses of L-thyroxine on benign solitary solid cold thyroid nodules: a randomized trial. J Clin Endocrinol Metab 83:830–835
8. Bennedbaek FN, Hegedüs L (1999) Percutaneous ethanol injection therapy in benign solitary solid cold thyroid nodules: a randomized trial comparing one with three injections". Thyroid 9:225–233
9. Monzani F, Caraccio N, Basolo F et al (2000) Surgical and pathological changes after percutaneous ethanol injection therapy of thyroid nodules. Thyroid 10:1087–1092

10. Kim DW, Rho MH, Park HJ et al (2012) Ultrasonography-guided ethanol ablation of predominantly solid thyroid nodules: a preliminary study for factors that predict the outcome. Br J Radiol 85:930–936
11. Livraghi T, Paracchi A, Ferrari C et al (1990) Treatment of autonomous thyroid nodules with percutaneous ethanol injection: preliminary results. Work in progress. Radiology 175: 827–829
12. Lippi F, Ferrari C, Manetti L et al (1996) Treatment of solitary autonomous thyroid nodules by percutaneous ethanol injection: results of an Italian multicenter study. The Multicenter Study Group. J Clin Endocrinol Metab 81:3261–3264
13. Tarantino L, Francica G, Sordelli I et al (2008) Percutaneous ethanol injection of hyperfunctioning thyroid nodules: long-term follow-up in 125 patients. Am J Roentgenol 190: 800–808
14. Yano Y, Sugino K, Akaishi J et al (2011) Treatment of autonomously functioning thyroid nodules at a single institution: radioiodine therapy, surgery and ethanol injection therapy. Ann Nucl Med 25:749–754
15. Verde G, Papini E, Pacella CM (1994) Ultrasound guided percutaneous ethanol injection in the treatment of cystic thyroid nodules. Clin Endocrinol 41:719–724
16. Zingrillo M, Torlontano M, Chiarella R et al (1999) Percutaneous ethanol injection may be a definitive treatment for symptomatic thyroid cystic nodules not treatable by surgery: five-year follow-up study. Thyroid 9:763–767
17. Bennedbaek FN, Hegedüs L (2003) Treatment of recurrent thyroid cysts with ethanol: a randomized double-blind controlled trial. J Clin Endocrinol Metab 88:5773–5777
18. Kim YJ, Baek JH, Ha EJ et al (2012) Cystic versus predominantly cystic thyroid nodules: efficacy of ethanol ablation and analysis of related factors. Eur Radiol 22:1573–1578
19. Heilo A, Sigstad E, Fagerlid KH et al (2011) Efficacy of ultrasound-guided percutaneous ethanol injection treatment in patients with a limited number of metastatic cervical lymph nodes from papillary thyroid carcinoma. J Clin Endocrinol Metab 96:2750–2755
20. Hay ID, Lee RA, Davidge-Pitts C, Reading CC et al (2013) Long-term outcome of ultrasound-guided percutaneous ethanol ablation of selected "recurrent" neck nodal metastases in 25 patients with TNM stages III or IVA papillary thyroid carcinoma previously treated by surgery and 131I therapy. Surgery 154:1448–1454
21. Gharib H, Papini E, Pashke R et al (2010) American Association of Clinical Endocrinologists, Associazione Medici Endocrinologi, and European Thyroid Association medical guidelines for clinical practice for the diagnosis and management of thyroid nodules. Endocr Pract 16(suppl 1):1–43
22. Cooper DS, Doherty GM, Haugen BE et al (2009) Revised American Thyroid Association management guidelines for patients with thyroid nodules and differentiated thyroid cancer. Thyroid 19:1167–1214
23. Shin JE, Baek JH, Lee JH (2013) Radiofrequency and ethanol ablation for the treatment of recurrent thyroid cancers: current status and challenges. Curr Opin Oncol 25:14–19
24. Pacella CM, Bizzarri G, Guglielmi R et al (2000) Thyroid tissue: US-guided percutaneous interstitial laser ablation-a feasibility study. Radiology 217:673–677
25. Deandrea M, Limone P, Basso E et al (2008) US-guided percutaneous radiofrequency thermal ablation for the treatment of solid benign hyperfunctioning or compressive thyroid nodules. Ultrasound Med Biol 34:784–791
26. Spiezia S, Garberoglio R, Milone F et al (2009) Thyroid nodules and related symptoms are stably controlled two years after radiofrequency thermal ablation. Thyroid 19:219–225
27. Baek JH, Kim YS, Lee D et al (2010) Benign predominantly solid thyroid nodules: prospective study of efficacy of sonographically guided radiofrequency ablation versus control condition. Am J Roentgenol 194:1137–1142
28. Holmer C, Lehmann KS, Knappe V et al (2011) Bipolar radiofrequency ablation for nodular thyroid disease–ex vivo and in vivo evaluation of a dose–response relationship. J Surg Res 169:234–240
29. Lim HK, Lee JH, Ha EJ et al (2013) Radiofrequency ablation of benign non-functioning thyroid nodules: 4-year follow-up results for 111 patients. Eur Radiol 23:1044–1049

30. Kim YS, Rhim H, Tae K et al (2006) Radiofrequency ablation of benign cold thyroid nodules: initial clinical experience. Thyroid 16:361–367
31. Jeong WK, Baek JH, Rhim H et al (2008) Radiofrequency ablation of benign thyroid nodules: safety and imaging follow-up in 236 patients. Eur Radiol 18:1244–1250
32. Deandrea M, Kee Shong Y, Sung JY et al (2013) Radiofrequency ablation using moving-shot technique is a reproducible, effective technique for treating benign thyroid nodules. Preliminary results of an international randomized controlled study. 37th annual meeting of the European thyroid association, Leiden, 7–11 Sept
33. Pacella CM, Bizzarri G, Spiezia S et al (2004) Thyroid tissue: US-guided percutaneous laser thermal ablation. Radiology 232:272–280
34. Døssing H, Bennedbaek FN, Karstrup S et al (2002) Benign solitary solid cold thyroid nodules: US-guided interstitial laser photocoagulation–initial experience. Radiology 225:53–57
35. Døssing H, Bennedbaek FN, Hegedüs L (2005) Effect of ultrasound-guided interstitial laser photocoagulation on benign solitary solid cold thyroid nodules – a randomised study. Eur J Endocrinol 152:341–345
36. Amabile G, Rotondi M, De Chiara G et al (2006) Low-energy interstitial laser photocoagulation for treatment of nonfunctioning thyroid nodules: therapeutic outcome in relation to pretreatment and treatment parameters. Thyroid 16:749–755
37. Papini E, Rago T, Gambelunghe G et al (2014) Long-term efficacy of ultrasound-guided laser ablation for benign solid thyroid nodules. Results of a three-year multicenter prospective randomized trial. J Clin Endocrinol Metab 99:3653–3659
38. Valcavi R, Riganti F, Bertani A et al (2010) Percutaneous laser ablation of cold benign thyroid nodules: a 3-year follow-up study in 122 patients. Thyroid 20:1253–1261
39. Baek JH, Lee JH, Valcavi R et al (2011) Thermal ablation for benign thyroid nodules: radiofrequency and laser. Korean J Radiol 12:525–540
40. Faggiano A, Ramundo V, Assanti AP et al (2012) Thyroid nodules treated with percutaneous radiofrequency thermal ablation: a comparative study. J Clin Endocrinol Metab 97:4439–4445
41. Sung JY, Kim YS, Choi H et al (2011) Optimum first-line treatment technique for benign cystic thyroid nodules: ethanol ablation or radiofrequency ablation? Am J Roentgenol 196:210–214
42. Sung JY, Baek JH, Kim KS et al (2013) Single-session treatment of benign cystic thyroid nodules with ethanol versus radiofrequency ablation: a prospective randomized study. Radiology 269:293–300
43. Jang SW, Baek JH, Kim JK et al (2012) How to manage the patients with unsatisfactory results after ethanol ablation for thyroid nodules: role of radiofrequency ablation. Eur J Radiol 81:905–910
44. Lee JH, Kim YS, Lee D et al (2010) Radiofrequency ablation (RFA) of benign thyroid nodules in patients with incompletely resolved clinical problems after ethanol ablation (EA). World J Surg 34:1488–1493
45. Døssing H, Bennedbæk FN, Hegedüs L (2013) Interstitial laser photocoagulation (ILP) of benign cystic thyroid nodules–a prospective randomized trial. J Clin Endocrinol Metab 98:1213–1217
46. Huh JY, Baek JH, Choi H et al (2012) Symptomatic benign thyroid nodules: efficacy of additional radiofrequency ablation treatment session–prospective randomized study. Radiology 263:909–916
47. Døssing H, Bennedbaek FN, Hegedüs L (2006) Effect of ultrasound-guided interstitial laser photocoagulation on benign solitary solid cold thyroid nodules: one versus three treatments. Thyroid 16:763–768
48. Amabile G, Rotondi M, Pirali B et al (2011) Interstitial laser photocoagulation for benign thyroid nodules: time to treat large nodules. Lasers Surg Med 43:797–803
49. Spiezia S, Vitale G, Di Somma C et al (2003) Ultrasound-guided laser thermal ablation in the treatment of autonomous hyperfunctioning thyroid nodules and compressive nontoxic nodular goiter. Thyroid 13:941–947
50. Døssing H, Bennedbaek FN, Bonnema SJ et al (2007) Randomized prospective study comparing a single radioiodine dose and a single laser therapy session in autonomously functioning thyroid nodules. Eur J Endocrinol 157:95–100

51. Chianelli M, Bizzarri G, Todino V et al (2014) Laser ablation and 131-iodine: a 24-month pilot study of combined treatment for large toxic nodular goiter. J Clin Endocrinol Metab 99: 1283–1286
52. Baek JH, Moon WJ, Kim YS et al (2009) Radiofrequency ablation for the treatment of autonomously functioning thyroid nodules. World J Surg 33:1971–1977
53. Shin JH, Baek JH, Ha EJ et al (2012) Radiofrequency ablation of thyroid nodules: basic principles and clinical application. Int J Endocrinol 2012:919650
54. Døssing H, Bennedbæk FN, Hegedüs L (2011) Long-term outcome following interstitial laser photocoagulation of benign cold thyroid nodules. Eur J Endocrinol 165:123–128
55. Bernardi S, Dobrinja C, Fabris B et al (2014) Radiofrequency ablation compared to surgery for the treatment of benign thyroid nodules. Int J Endocrinol 2014:934595
56. Dupuy DE, Monchik JM, Decrea C et al (2001) Radiofrequency ablation of regional recurrence from well-differentiated thyroid malignancy. Surgery 130:971–977
57. Monchik JM, Donatini G, Iannuccilli J et al (2006) Radiofrequency ablation and percutaneous ethanol injection treatment for recurrent local and distant well-differentiated thyroid carcinoma. Ann Surg 244:296–304
58. Park KW, Shin JH, Han BK et al (2011) Inoperable symptomatic recurrent thyroid cancers: preliminary results of radiofrequency ablation. Ann Surg Oncol 18:2564–2568
59. Baek JH, Kim YS, Sung JY et al (2011) Locoregional control of metastatic well-differentiated thyroid cancer by ultrasound-guided radiofrequency ablation. Am J Roentgenol 197:331–336
60. Papini E, Bizzarri G, Bianchini A et al (2013) Percutaneous ultrasound-guided laser ablation is effective for treating selected nodal metastases in papillary thyroid cancer. J Clin Endocrinol Metab 98:92–97
61. Solbiati L, Cova L, Ierace T et al (2011) Percutaneous US-guided interstitial laser ablation of new metastatic lymph nodes in the neck from papillary thyroid carcinoma following thyroidectomy and lymphadenectomy (abstract) In: Radiological Society of North America scientific assembly and annual meeting. Radiological Society of North America, Oak Brook
62. Pacella CM, Papini E (2013) Image-guided percutaneous therapies for local recurrences of thyroid tumors. J Endocrinol Invest 36:61–70
63. Papini E, Guglielmi R, Gharib H et al (2011) Ultrasound-guided laser ablation of incidentally papillary thyroid carcinoma: a potential therapeutic approach in patients at high surgical risk. Thyroid 21:917–920
64. Valcavi R, Piana S, Bortolan GS et al (2013) Ultrasound-guided percutaneous laser ablation of papillary thyroid microcarcinoma: a feasibility study on three cases with pathological and immunohistochemical evaluation. Thyroid 23:1578–1582
65. Papini E, Guglielmi R, Bizzarri G et al (2007) Treatment of benign cold thyroid nodules: a randomized clinical trial of percutaneous laser ablation versus levothyroxine therapy or follow-up. Thyroid 17:229–235
66. Ritz JP, Lehmann KS, Schumann T et al (2011) Effectiveness of various thermal ablation techniques for the treatment of nodular thyroid disease: comparison of laser-induced thermotherapy and bipolar radiofrequency ablation. Lasers Med Sci 26:545–552
67. Kovatcheva R, Vlahov JD, Stoinov J et al (2014) US-guided High-intensity focused ultrasound as a promising non-invasive method for treatment of primary hyperparathyroidism. Eur Radiol 24:2052–2058
68. Yue W, Wang S, Yu S et al (2014) Ultrasound-guided percutaneous microwave ablation of solitary T1N0M0 papillary thyroid microcarcinoma: initial experience. Int J Hyperthermia 30:150–157

# Part III

# Minimally Invasive Surgical Techniques

# Minimally Invasive Video-Assisted Thyroidectomy (MIVAT)

# 10

Annamaria D'Amore, Carmela De Crea, Marco Raffaelli, Celestino Pio Lombardi, and Rocco Bellantone

## 10.1 Introduction

The traditional Kocher operation is characterized by a 10–12 cm long skin incision which results in a visible large scar in the neck. The main objective that led to the introduction of minimally invasive techniques to perform thyroidectomy was just the reduction of the cosmetic damage since the main part of patients who undergo thyroid surgery is represented by nearly young women, particularly careful to the cosmetic outcome in a very visible region like the neck. [1].

In recent years, since the first reported case of endoscopic parathyroidectomy by M. Gagner in 1996 [2], several minimally invasive techniques for thyroidectomy have been developed. [3–16].

Some techniques which require the use of endoscope [3–14] and others which do not need its use [14–17] have been proposed.

Procedures that imply the use of the endoscope (purely endoscopic and video-assisted techniques) take advantages not only of the reduction of the incision length, as well as the minimally invasive operations, but also of the endoscopic magnification. It consents to perform the same intervention through a very minimal access, with theoretical lower risk of complications, because of the optimal visualization of the neck structures (recurrent laryngeal nerve and parathyroid glands).

A. D'Amore (✉)
Unità Operativa di Chirurgia Endocrina CIC, Università Cattolica del Sacro Cuore, Roma, Largo Agostino Gemelli, 8, Rome 00168, Italy
e-mail: annadamore@alice.it

C. De Crea • M. Raffaelli • C.P. Lombardi • R. Bellantone
Unità Operativa di Chirurgia Endocrina E Metabolica, Università Cattolica del Sacro Cuore, Roma, Largo Agostino Gemelli, 8, Rome 00168, Italy
e-mail: carmela.decrea@rm.unicatt.it; marcoraffaelli@rm.unicatt.it; cp.lombardi@rm.unicatt.it; rbellantone@rm.unicatt.it



C.P. Lombardi, R. Bellantone (eds.), *Minimally Invasive Therapies for Endocrine Neck Diseases*, DOI 10.1007/978-3-319-20065-1_10

The different techniques implying the use of the endoscope can be classified in purely endoscopic [3–10] and video-assisted [11–14] procedures. In the totally endoscopic techniques, surgical dissection is completely carried out under endoscopic vision. This requires a continuous $CO_2$ insufflation [3–6, 9, 10] or the use of external devices (retractors) to maintain the operative space for dissection and trocars positioning [7, 8].

Among the totally endoscopic techniques, we find both the procedures with cervical access (firstly described by Gagner and subsequently utilized, even if modified, by some authors) [2–6] and the procedures with extra-cervical accesses, mainly supported by Asian authors who proposed approaches from the chest wall, the breast and the axilla, in order to avoid any visible scar in the neck and maximize the cosmetic outcome [9, 10].

The totally endoscopic approaches have as major limit the more difficult dissection in comparison with conventional techniques, above all in case of extra-cervical accesses. They are difficult to be reproduced in different settings, especially by not skilled endoscopic surgeons, and they are technically demanding. Moreover, the totally endoscopic techniques with extra-cervical accesses, in order to maximally improve the cosmetic outcome, require an extensive and difficult dissection to reach the operation site from the far access, increasing the risk of complications and the invasiveness of the procedure.

The long operative time reported represents another major limit for the diffusion of these approaches. Moreover, the risks related to $CO_2$ absorption (hypercarbia, subcutaneous emphysema, metabolic acidosis) are not completely eliminated.

Probably, for all these reasons, the totally endoscopic procedures encountered only limited diffusion and are usually performed only by the proponents.

On the contrary MIVAT, short after its first description in 1999 [11], gained a quite large worldwide diffusion, maybe because it combines the advantages related to the endoscopic magnification with those due to its close similarity with the conventional surgery that make it quite easy to be reproduced in different surgical settings. Actually, it is a completely gasless procedure that reproduces in all the steps the conventional operation. The endoscope represents only a tool that allows to perform the same intervention through a very minimal skin incision [11–13, 18, 19].

This makes a huge difference, in particular for surgeons not skilled in laparoscopic surgery, in comparison with the other endoscopic techniques which have an access completely different from conventional surgery. Moreover, the excellent visualization of the neck structures due to the two- to threefold endoscopic magnification permits an easy and prompt identification of the laryngeal nerve and parathyroid glands, reducing the risk of nerve palsy and postoperative hypoparathyroidism.

The minimal access guarantees for an optimal cosmetic result. Moreover, the absence of neck hyperextension and extensive dissections results in less postoperative pain. Several comparative studies have indeed demonstrated the advantages of MIVAT in terms of reduced postoperative pain, better cosmetic result and higher patient satisfaction over conventional thyroidectomy [20–26].

Moreover, data from multicentre studies on large series of patients showed that MIVAT is a safe and quite easy to be reproduced technique. Obviously for obtaining the best results, with similar or even less complication rate than conventional intervention, surgeons should be well trained in both endocrine and endoscopic surgery [27–29].

Its low invasiveness and the similarity with the conventional procedure render this approach feasible also under loco-regional anaesthesia (cervical block) [30], at least in selected patients, with the benefits to avoid the major side effects of general anaesthesia.

By the time, some criticisms concerning MIVAT were demonstrated baseless. In fact, in a published prospective randomized study [31], we demonstrated that thyroid gland manipulation is not substantially different between MIVAT and conventional thyroidectomy and that there is no additional risk of thyroid capsule rupture and thyroid cells seeding in patients who undergo MIVAT if the procedure is correctly conducted.

Moreover, we as well as other authors [32–34] demonstrated the possibility and the feasibility to treat thyroid malignancy by a video-assisted approach. After an adequate period of development, we showed the validation and standardization of the technique, so that MIVAT can be proposed also for the surgical treatment of small "low risk" papillary thyroid carcinoma (PTC).

We recently published the results of MIVAT in a large series of patients with PTC [35].

Though the study is retrospective, the very large sample size and the medium follow-up period allow us to conclude that the completeness of the resection achieved with MIVAT and the short-to-medium term recurrence seems comparable with that reported for conventional surgery. The excellent oncological results led some authors to a progressive increase in the treatment of differentiated thyroid carcinomas (DTCs) by MIVAT, starting from the so-called low-risk tumours to the "intermediate-risk" ones that have been recently demonstrated to be another optimal target for this minimally invasive operation [35, 36].

Some studies to compare the results in terms of adequacy of resection between MIVAT and conventional thyroidectomy have been conducted [34, 37, 38]. The results show that MIVAT is safe and effective for the treatment of small PTC and has similar oncological effectiveness of traditional thyroidectomy.

Nonetheless, a longer follow-up is necessary to draw definitive conclusions in terms of late recurrence and survival rate.

Instead the possibility to perform a concomitant lymphadenectomy during a video-assisted thyroidectomy for PTC is still debated.

Although the lymph-node involvement has been widely demonstrated, often microscopic, of the central compartment in case of PTC [39, 40], to date the prophylactic VI level lymphadenectomy is not considered mandatory yet [40, 41].

The only one worldwide recognized indication to perform a radical VI level lymphadenectomy is the preoperative or intraoperative evidence of macroscopic lymph-node involvement [41]. Nonetheless, it is quite frequent during a thyroidectomy for cancer to face a lymph-node enlargement not discovered by the preoperative neck ultrasonography. In such a case, it is mandatory to carry on a concomitant VI level lymphadenectomy.

A macroscopic preoperatively identified lymph-node involvement in case of PTC has been always considered an absolute contraindication for a video-assisted approach.

Anyway in our experience the incidental intraoperative evidence of lymph-node enlargement during MIVAT for PTC happened with a certain frequency.

Once familiarity with the technique was acquired, supported by the previous optimal results in terms of safety and completeness of the surgical resection, we decided to perform a video-assisted lymph node dissection (VALD) of the central compartment in case of incidental discovery of lymph-node enlargement during MIVAT for PTC or for suspicious nodules [42]. More recently, we as well other authors [43] have applied the technique to carry out a prophylactic thyroidectomy and central compartment lymphadenectomy in some cases of patients carrying the RET oncogene mutation for familial medullary thyroid carcinoma.

Despite the results of this approach are enthusiastic further controlled studies are necessary to evaluate the long-term results.

Finally, we evaluated the feasibility of minimally invasive video-assisted functional lateral neck dissection (VALNED) in patients with PTC with encouraging results [44]. Nonetheless for definitive conclusions, larger series and comparative studies are necessary.

## 10.2 Indications

An accurate patients' selection play a relevant role to ensure the success of MIVAT, especially at the beginning of the experience.

The early studies on MIVAT used limited indications. Initial contraindications included large nodules (>25–30 mm), thyroiditis, an abnormal thyroid gland volume (>20 $cm^3$), prior neck surgery, preoperative evidence of central compartment neck metastases and large malignant tumours with extra-thyroidal extension [45].

With increasing experience, selection criteria for MIVAT have been quite refined and widened. It is now possible to carry out this technique with expanded indications [46, 47].

Basing on the surgeons experience, in selected cases, patients with previous contralateral video-assisted neck surgery or thyroiditis can be selected for MIVAT. For example, in our experience also patients underwent video-assisted thyroid lobectomy needing a completion of thyroidectomy or patients with Basedow disease were treated by a video-assisted approach. Some authors demonstrated by prospective nonrandomized comparative studies that in selected patients with Graves' disease, MIVAT is feasible and can be performed safely with results comparable with open surgery [48–50].

In our experience, it has been possible to perform MIVAT also in case of nodule bigger than 35 mm in diameter. In these cases, the main limit is the nodule shape because it is possible to remove from a 15–20 mm of skin incision only nodules with a transverse diameter similar to the skin access.

The more and more frequent use of fine needle aspiration biopsy in the clinical practice has increased the diagnosis of asymptomatic little thyroid nodules with indeterminate or suspicious cytology. Regarding the preoperative diagnosis ideal candidates for MIVAT are just patients with little nodules with a certain degree of suspicious, for example follicular nodules or follicular nodules with atypia or polymorphism. Also small size hot nodules represent the best indication for this kind of surgery. As above reported also the results of MIVAT in case of little "low risk" papillary carcinoma are encouraging. Therefore we think that selected patients with PTC could be eligible for MIVAT. On the contrary despite we have successfully performed a large series of VALD in PTC cases with intraoperative evidence of lymph-node enlargement we still believe that a preoperatively diagnosed lymph-node involvement represents a contraindication for MIVAT.

Moreover from a purely theoretical point of view patients carrying RET oncogene mutation for familial forms of medullary thyroid carcinoma (FMTC, MEN IIA and MEN IIB), but not even expressing the disease (absence of detectable nodules and basal/stimulated calcitonin in the normal range) are excellent candidates for MIVAT, Indeed they are young patients with normal thyroid who need thyroidectomy as prophylactic treatment [51].

## 10.3 Instruments

Most part of endoscopic tools (endoscope, video, light source, camera, etc.) necessary for MIVAT is usually available in almost all operating rooms and so it cannot be considered a source of additional costs comparing with conventional surgery. The only instruments not commonly used for a conventional thyroidectomy are small dedicated tools (2–3 mm in diameter) necessary for dissection (ad hoc designed spatulas) which however are reusable so that their cost can be amortized with use.

Harmonic scalpel showed to be very useful in this kind of operation in reducing the operative time [52].

## 10.4 Surgical Technique

The operative technique has been previously described in detail [45].

### 10.4.1 Anaesthesia

At the beginning of the experience, MIVAT was described as procedure requiring general anaesthesia with orotracheal intubation. More recently and with increasing experience, the feasibility of MIVAT under loco-regional anaesthesia (MIVAT-LA) with superficial modified or deep cervical block has been demonstrated [30].

The indications are the same of MIVAT though, for this approach, smaller nodules ($\leq$2 cm) are preferable. In our experience, MIVAT-LA showed best results in patients with relative contraindications for general anaesthesia such as pregnant patients with PTC because the strong patient's motivation plays a relevant role in the feasibility of the procedure.

### 10.4.2 Patient Position

The patient, under general or loco-regional anaesthesia with cervical block, is positioned supine with the neck in slight extension, less than in conventional surgery. This may contribute to the lower postoperative pain complained by patients who have undergone MIVAT when compared to those undergone conventional thyroidectomy.

### 10.4.3 Surgical Equipment

The surgical team is represented by the surgeons and two assistants, one of whom handles the endoscope.

The need for at least three surgeons involved in the procedure has been considered one of the main limitations for the diffusion of this approach.

The monitor is positioned at the head of the patient in front of the surgeons, who is positioned on the right side of the patient. A second monitor is usually positioned in front of the assistants who are on the left side of the patient. The endoscope is held with two hands by the assistant. Even if the procedure is quite difficult to be accomplished, the absence of any external support allows modulating and changing the position of the endoscope in relationship to the particular exigencies of dissection. This represents an important advantage of the video-assisted procedure over purely endoscopic techniques. The tip of the endoscope is usually oriented towards the head of the patient, but it can be changed in order to expose and explore the upper mediastinum when, for example, a concomitant central compartment lymphadenectomy is required.

### 10.4.4 Surgical Steps

A small (1.5–2 cm) skin incision is performed between the cricoid cartilage and the sternal notch, in the midline. The skin incision is usually higher than in conventional cervicotomy and can also be modulated according to the neck conformation and the thyroid position. However, the skin incision is usually performed just below (1 cm) the cricoid cartilage in order to obtain a good exposure and a safe control of the superior vessels peduncle. The possibility to perform the skin incision nearby a skin line would optimize the cosmetic outcome. After cutting platysma muscle and preparing the upper and the lower flaps, the cervical *linea alba* is opened as far as possible. At the beginning of the experience, the procedure implied a short $CO_2$ insufflation to facilitate dissection of the thyroid lobe from the strap muscles. After this initial experience, the procedure became completely gasless. The thyroid lobe is separated from the strap muscles by means of small conventional retractors (Farabeuf retractors), which are also used to maintain the operative space. With this purpose, the thyroid lobe is medially retracted while the strap muscles, first on the most affected side, are retracted laterally, using two little Farabeuf. At this point, the

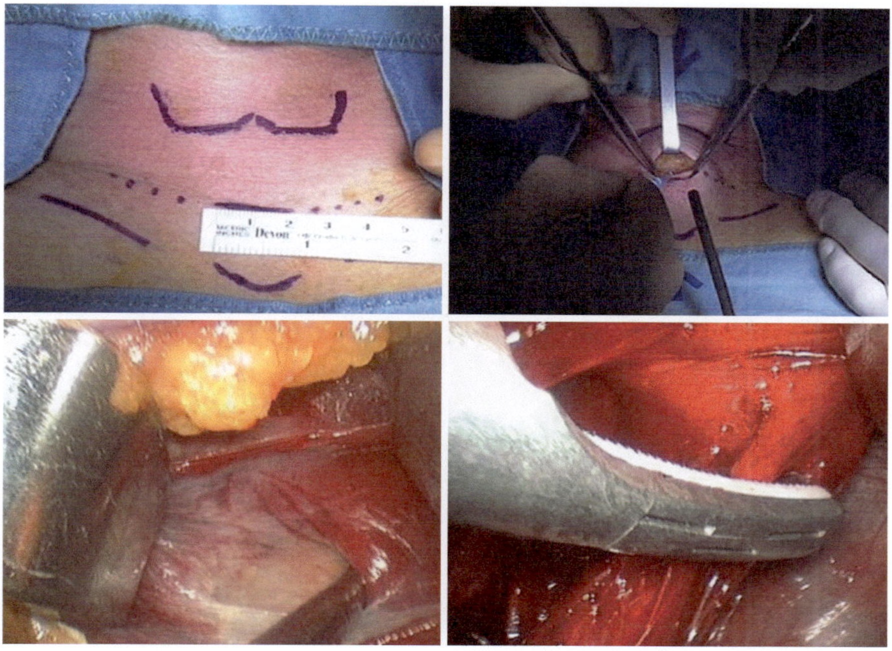

**Fig. 10.1** Skin incision; thyroid lobe is medially retracted while the strap muscles are retracted laterally, using two little Farabeuf; endoscope (5 mm – 30°) and the dedicated small surgical instruments are introduced through the single skin incision without any trocar utilization; the dissection is carried out by a blunt technique using two dedicated instruments called spatulas

endoscope (5 mm – 30°) and the dedicated small surgical instruments (2 mm in diameter) are introduced through the single skin incision without any trocar positioning. The first step of the procedure consists in complete freeing of the thyroid gland from the strap muscles, in order to have a good exposure of the pre-vertebral fascia that represents the posterior edge of the dissection. The lateral edge of the dissection is represented by the medial aspect of common carotid artery while the medial edge is represented by the trachea-oesophageal groove. The dissection is carried out by a blunt technique using two dedicated instruments called spatulas, one of them connected to an aspiration system. After its complete separation from the muscles, the thyroid lobe is downwards retracted in order to expose the superior peduncle vessels that are dissected using the spatula and the spatula-shaped aspirator and then selectively clipped and cut, or directly cut using an ultrasound knife system (Ultracision) (Fig. 10.1). It is very important to accurately control the tip of the instrument to avoid any pharynx or larynx thermal injury. During this phase, it is usually possible, thanks to the magnification of the endoscope, to identify the external branch of the superior laryngeal nerve. After cutting the superior thyroid vessels, the thyroid lobe is medially and slightly upwards retracted in order to identify the inferior laryngeal nerve and the parathyroid glands. The magnification

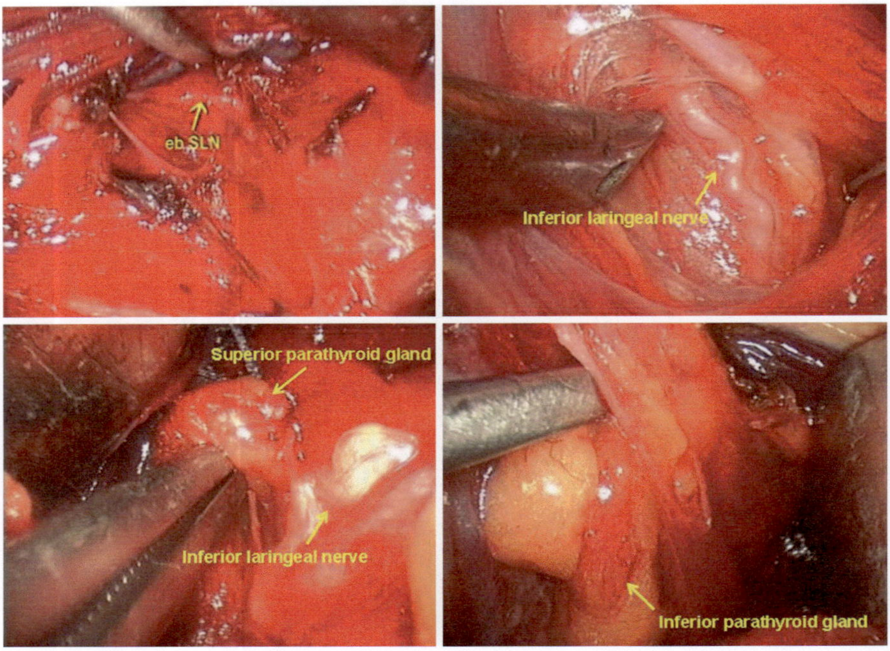


**Fig. 10.2** Visualization of external branch of the superior laryngeal nerve, inferior laryngeal nerve and parathyroid glands

(two- to threefold) of the endoscope permits a quite easy identification of these structures if the principles of blunt and bloodless dissection are respected. The traction on both the thyroid lobe (medially) and the strap muscles (laterally) allows to tense the trachea-oesophageal groove and the inferior thyroid artery in order to expose the nerve usually where it crosses the inferior thyroid artery. Once identified, the inferior laryngeal nerve is prepared and bluntly dissected, under endoscopic vision, from the thyroid gland till its entrance in the larynx. The parathyroid glands are usually easy identified and preserved thanks to the endoscopic magnification (Fig. 10.2). It is however very important to carry out a completely bloodless dissection that is facilitated by the use of the spatula-shaped aspirator. At this point, the thyroid lobe is extracted from the little skin incision and the procedure is carried on under both endoscopic and direct vision. Performing this manoeuvre, it is very important not to strongly pull the thyroid lobe because it is not yet completely freed and an excessive traction may determine some strain injury of the nerve. The separation of the thyroid from the trachea is usually carried out using Ultracision but close to the nerve and the parathyroid glands to cut the vessels after putting titanium clips or conventional ligature is preferable in order to avoid any thermal injury. If the planned intervention consists in a thyroid lobectomy, the thyroid lobe and the isthmus, once freed from the tracheal surface, are cut from the residual thyroid gland using Ultracision. Instead, if a total thyroidectomy was planned, the same steps are performed in the contralateral side.

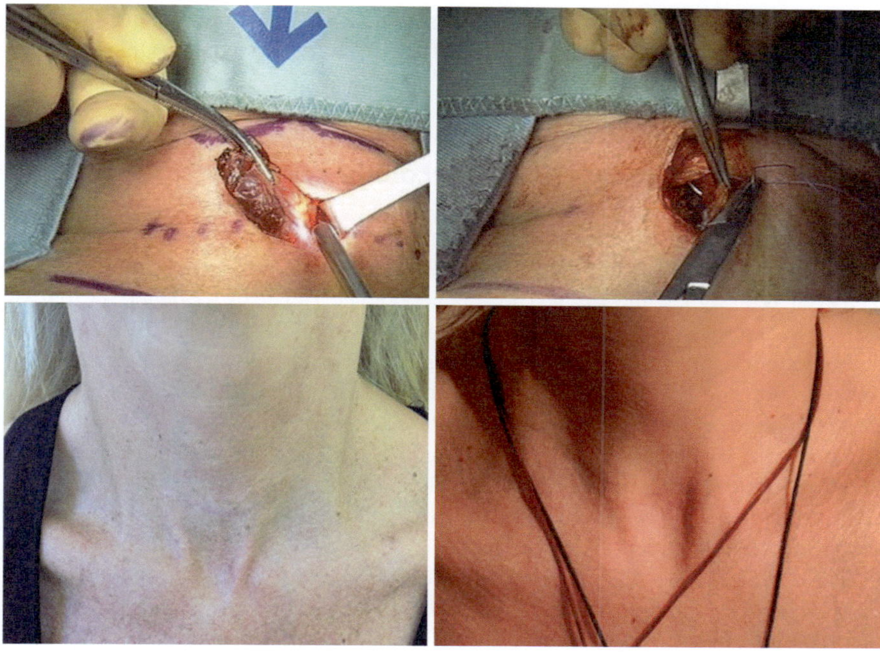

**Fig. 10.3** Thyroid lobe extraction; closure; aesthetics results

After checking the haemostasis, the strap muscles are sutured along the midline as well as the platysma. The skin is closed by means of a not re-absorbable subcuticular running suture or by a skin sealant. Usually, no drainage is left inside (Fig. 10.3).

## 10.5 Personal Series

We published a review of our experience [53] to evaluate the results obtained in a series of patients selected for MIVAT over a 10-year period. All patients who underwent MIVAT from June 1998 to June 2009 were considered. The eligibility criteria for video-assisted thyroidectomy were thyroid nodules < or = 35 mm; estimated thyroid volume < 30 ml; no previous conventional neck surgery and/or radiation therapy; small, low-risk papillary thyroid carcinoma. A total of 1363 video-assisted thyroidectomies were attempted in the time period considered. Conversion to the conventional procedure was necessary in 7 cases. Thyroid lobectomy was successfully performed in 157 cases, total thyroidectomy in 1175, and completion thyroidectomy in 24. In 126 patients, the central neck nodes were removed through the same access. Simultaneous video-assisted parathyroidectomy, for a parathyroid adenoma, was performed in 42 patients. Pathological studies showed benign disease in 986 cases, papillary thyroid carcinoma in 368 cases, C-cells hyperplasia in 1 case, and medullary microcarcinoma in 1 patient with RET germline mutation.

Postoperative complications included 27 transient and 1 definitive recurrent laryngeal nerve palsy, 230 transient hypocalcaemia, 10 definitive hypoparathyroidism, 4 postoperative haematoma, and 5 wound infection.

## 10.6 MIVAT: Evidence-Based Recommendations

Level of evidence in evidence-based medicine is frequently used for the recommendation of specific treatments [54, 55]. A well-conducted large prospective randomized trial is assigned the highest level of evidence (level of evidence 1) that by definition determines a high grade of recommendation (grade A) [56, 57].

Immediately after the first described case of minimally invasive thyroidectomy, several reports consisting in technical description of the feasibility of different techniques, without any grade of recommendation, were published [4–19].

Moreover, at least two multicentre studies [27, 58] demonstrated the feasibility of the technique. Their results did not reach a high level of evidence because of the retrospective model. Some other large retrospective studies had the same scarce power in terms of evidence [53, 59–63].

Gal et al. [23] and El Labban [24] reached by two well-designed randomized trials (level II B) the same conclusions. The studies show that the complication rate is comparable between the two approaches and that even if conventional thyroidectomy involves less operative time MIVAT offers distinct advantages in terms of less scarring and more satisfactory cosmetic results and reduced postoperative distress.

Searching for the same end points, Hegazy et al. [25] compared MIVAT to minimally invasive open thyroidectomy using the Sofferman technique (strap muscle transection). Also this prospective randomized study (level II B) demonstrated that MIVAT offers a significant better postoperative course and smaller incisions with the same cosmetic outcome but at the cost of a longer operative time.

In order to demonstrate that MIVAT improves postoperative pain compared with standard thyroidectomy, Miccoli et al. [26] recently published a prospective, randomized study that confirmed the most favourable postoperative outcome of MIVAT through the dosage of different biochemical pain mediators, before and after surgery.

In 2008, to stress other advantages of MIVAT over conventional thyroidectomy, we published a prospective randomized study [64] comparing MIVAT and conventional thyroidectomy for what concerns the voice and swallowing symptoms frequently reported after thyroidectomy even in absence of objective voice alterations. The study demonstrated with a level II B of evidence that the incidence and the severity of early voice and swallowing post-thyroidectomy symptoms are significantly reduced in patients who undergo MIVAT compared with conventional surgery.

Concerns regarding adequacy of resection of MIVAT in the treatment of malignancies were addressed by different studies with high level of recommendation (level II B) [31, 34].

Further data supporting the thesis of oncological safety of MIVAT in the treatment of PTC derive from two more recent comparative but retrospective studies on this topic [37, 38]. In conclusion, they contribute, though with a less power, to the growing body of evidence showing that MIVAT is safe and effective for the treatment of small papillary thyroid carcinomas and show similar oncological effectiveness of traditional thyroidectomy also at 5 years follow-up.

In addition to the more traditional advantages of MIVAT, the initial criticism concerning the costs seems evolving. Actually a very recent retrospective cost analysis shows that the cost of MIVAT appears to be equal to that of open thyroidectomy [65].

## References


1. Duh QY (2003) Presidential address: minimally invasive endocrine surgery – standard treatment of treatment or hype? Surgery 134:849–857
2. Gagner M (1996) Endoscopic subtotal parathyroidectomy in patients with primary hyperparathyroidism. Br J Surg 83:875
3. Gagner M, Inabnet WB (2001) Endoscopic thyroidectomy for solitary thyroid nodules. Thyroid 11:161–163
4. Huscher CS, Chiodini S, Napolitano C, Recher A (1997) Endoscopic right thyroid lobectomy. Surg Endosc 11:877
5. Inabnet WB III, Jacob BP, Gagner M (2003) Minimally invasive endoscopic thyroidectomy by a cervical approach. Surg Endosc 17:1808–1811
6. Yeung GH (1998) Endoscopic surgery of the neck: a new frontier. Surg Laparosc Endosc 8:227–232
7. Shimizu K, Akira S, Jasmi AY, Kitamura Y, Jasmi AY, Kitamura Y et al (1999) Video-assisted neck surgery: endoscopic resection of thyroid tumors with a very minimal neck wound. J Am Coll Surg 188:697–703
8. Yeh TS, Jan YY, Hsu BR, Chen KW, Chen MF (2000) Video-assisted endoscopic thyroidectomy. Am J Surg 180:82–85
9. Ikeda Y, Takami H, Tajima G, Sasaki Y, Takayama J, Kurihara H et al (2002) Total endoscopic thyroidectomy: axillary or anterior chest approach. Biomed Pharmacother 56(1 Suppl):72s–78s
10. Ohgami M, Ishii S, Arisawa Y, Ohmori T, Noga K, Furukawa T et al (2000) Scarless endoscopic thyroidectomy: breast approach for better cosmesis. Surg Laparosc Endosc Percutan Tech 10:1–4
11. Bellantone R, Lombardi CP, Raffaelli M, Rubino F, Boscherini M, Perilli W (1999) Minimally invasive, totally gasless video-assisted thyroid lobectomy. Am J Surg 177:342–343
12. Miccoli P, Berti P, Bendinelli C, Conte M, Fasolini F, Martino E (2000) Minimally invasive video-assisted surgery of the thyroid: a preliminary report. Langenbecks Arch Surg 385:261–264
13. Mourad M, Saab N, Malaise J, Ngongang C, Fournier B, Daumerie C et al (2001) Minimally invasive video-assisted approach for partial and total thyroidectomy: initial experience. Surg Endosc 15:1108–1111
14. Yamashita H, Watanabe S, Koike E, Ohshima A, Uchino S, Kuroki S et al (2002) Video-assisted thyroid lobectomy through a small wound in the submandibular area. Am J Surg 183:286–289
15. Ferzli GS, Sayad P, Abdo Z, Cacchione R (2001) Minimally invasive, nonendoscopic thyroid surgery. J Am Coll Surg 192:665–668
16. Sackett WR, Barraclough BH, Sidhu S, Reeve TS, Delbridge LW (2002) Minimal access thyroid surgery: is it feasible, is it appropriate? ANZ J Surg 72:777–780
17. Brunaud L, Zarnegar R, Wada N, Ituarte P, Clark OH, Duh QY (2003) Incision length for standard thyroidectomy and parathyroidectomy. When is it minimally invasive? Arch Surg 138:1140–1143

18. Bellantone R, Lombardi CP, Raffaelli M, Boscherini M, De Crea C, Traini E (2002) Video-assisted thyroidectomy. J Am Coll Surg 194:610–614
19. Miccoli P, Berti P, Raffaelli M, Conte M, Materazzi G, Galleri D (2000) Minimally invasive video-assisted thyroidectomy. Am J Surg 181:567–570
20. Miccoli P, Berti P, Raffaelli M, Materazzi G, Baldacci S, Rossi G (2001) Comparison between minimally invasive video-assisted thyroidectomy and conventional thyroidectomy: a prospective randomised study. Surgery 130:1039–1043
21. Bellantone R, Lombardi CP, Bossola M, Boscherini M, De Crea C, Alesina PF et al (2002) Video-assisted vs conventional thyroid lobectomy – A randomized trial. Arch Surg 137: 301–304
22. Chao TC, Lin JD, Chen MF (2004) Video-assisted open thyroid lobectomy through a small incision. Surg Laparosc Endosc Percutan Tech 14:15–19
23. Gal I, Solymosi T, Szabo Z, Balint A, Bolgar G (2008) Minimally invasive video-assisted thyroidectomy and conventional thyroidectomy: a prospective randomized study. Surg Endosc 22:2445–2449
24. El-Labban GM (2009) Minimally invasive video-assisted thyroidectomy versus conventional thyroidectomy: a single-blinded, randomized controlled clinical trial. J Minim Access Surg 5:97–102
25. Hegazy MA, Khater AA, Setit AE et al (2007) Minimally invasive video-assisted thyroidectomy for small follicular thyroid nodules. World J Surg 31:1743–1750
26. Miccoli P, Rago R, Massi M, Panicucci E, Metelli MR, Berti P, Minuto MN (2010) Standard versus video-assisted thyroidectomy: objective postoperative pain evaluation. Surg Endosc 24:2415–2417
27. Miccoli P, Bellantone R, Mourad M, Walz M, Raffaelli M, Berti P (2002) Minimally invasive video-assisted thyroidectomy: multiinstitutional experience. World J Surg 26:972–975
28. Papavramidis TS, Michalopoulos N, Pliakos J, Triantafillopoulou K, Sapalidis K, Deligiannidis N, Kesisoglou I, Ntokmetzioglou I, Papavramidis ST (2010) Minimally invasive video-assisted total thyroidectomy: an easy to learn technique for skillful surgeons. Head Neck 32: 1370–1376
29. Del Rio P, Sommaruga L, Cataldo S, Robuschi G, Arcuri MF, Sianesi M (2008) Minimally invasive video-assisted thyroidectomy: the learning curve. Eur Surg Res 41:33–36
30. Lombardi CP, Raffaelli M, Modesti C, Boscherini M, Bellantone R (2004) Video-assisted thyroidectomy under local anaesthesia. Am J Surg 187:515–518
31. Lombardi CP, Raffaelli M, Princi P, Lulli P, Rossi ED, Fadda G et al (2005) Safety of video-assisted thyroidectomy versus conventional surgery. Head Neck 27:58–64
32. Bellantone R, Lombardi CP, Raffaelli M, Alesina PF, De Crea C, Traini E et al (2003) Video-assisted thyroidectomy for papillary thyroid carcinoma. Surg Endosc 17:1604–1608
33. Lombardi CP, Raffaelli M, de Crea C, Princi P, Castaldi P, Spaventa A, Salvatori M, Bellantone R (2007) Report on 8 years of experience with video-assisted thyroidectomy for papillary thyroid carcinoma. Surgery 142:944–951
34. Miccoli P, Elisei R, Materazzi G, Capezzone M, Galleri D, Pacini F et al (2002) Minimally invasive video-assisted thyroidectomy for papillary carcinoma: a prospective study of its completeness. Surgery 132:1070–1074
35. Lombardi CP, Raffaelli M, De Crea C, D'Amore A, Oragano L, Salvatori M, Bellantone R (2010) Video-assisted thyroidectomy for papillary thyroid carcinoma. J Oncol. pii: 148542. doi: 10.1155/2010/148542
36. Miccoli P, Pinchera A, Materazzi G, Biagini A, Berti P, Faviana P, Molinaro E, Viola D, Elisei R (2009) Surgical treatment of low- and intermediate-risk papillary thyroid cancer with minimally invasive video-assisted thyroidectomy. J Clin Endocrinol Metab 94:1618–1622
37. Wu CT, Yang LH, Kuo SJ (2010) Comparison of video-assisted thyroidectomy and traditional thyroidectomy for the treatment of papillary thyroid carcinoma. Surg Endosc 24:1658–1662
38. DI JZ, Zhang HW, Han XD, Zhang P, Zheng Q, Wang Y (2011) Minimally invasive video-assisted thyroidectomy for accidental papillary thyroid microcarcinoma: comparison with conventional open thyroidectomy with 5 years follow-up. Chin Med J (Engl) 124:3293–3296

39. Kebebew E, Clark OH (2000) Differentiated thyroid cancer: "complete" rational approach. World J Surg 24:942–951
40. Mirallié E, Visset J, Sagan C, Hamy A, Le Bodic MF, Paineau J (1999) Localization of cervical node metastasis of papillary thyroid carcinoma. World J Surg 23:970–974
41. Bellantone R, Lombardi CP, Boscherini M, Ferrante A, Raffaelli M, Rubino F et al (1998) Prognostic factors in differentiated thyroid carcinoma: a multivariate analysis of 234 consecutive patients. J Surg Oncol 68:237–241
42. Bellantone R, Lombardi CP, Raffaelli M, Boscherini M, Alesina PF, Princi P (2002) Central neck lymph node removal during minimally invasive video-assisted thyroidectomy for thyroid carcinoma: a feasible and safe procedure. J Laparoendosc Adv Surg Tech A 12:181–185
43. Miccoli P, Elisei R, Donatini G et al (2007) Video-assisted central compartment lymphadenectomy in a patient with a positive RET oncogene: initial experience. Surg Endosc 21:120–123
44. Lombardi CP, Raffaelli M, Princi P, De Crea C, Bellantone R (2007) Minimally invasive video-assisted functional lateral neck dissection for metastatic papillary thyroid carcinoma. Am J Surg 193:114–118
45. Bellantone R, Lombardi CP, Raffaelli M. Tiroidectomia video-assistita. Trattato di Tecniche Chirurgiche, Chirurgia Generale, 46. EMC – Elsevier, Paris
46. Lai SY, Walvekar RR, Ferris RL (2008) Minimally invasive video-assisted thyroidectomy: expanded indications and oncologic completeness. Head Neck 30:1403–1407
47. Kim AJ, Liu JC, Ganly I, Kraus DH (2011) Minimally invasive video-assisted thyroidectomy 2.0: expanded indications in a tertiary care cancer center. Head Neck 33:1557–1560
48. Berti P, Materazzi G, Galleri D et al (2004) Video-assisted thyroidectomy for Graves' disease: report of a preliminary experience. Surg Endosc 18:1208–1210
49. Maeda S, Uga T, Hayashida N et al (2006) Video-assisted subtotal or near-total thyroidectomy for Graves' disease. Br J Surg 93:61–66
50. Alesina PF, Singaporewalla RM, Eckstein A, Lahner H, Walz MK (2011) Is minimally invasive, video-assisted thyroidectomy feasible in Graves' disease? Surgery 149:556–560
51. Dralle H, Gimm O, Simon D, Frank-Raue K, Gortz G, Niederle B et al (1998) Prophylactic thyroidectomy in 75 children and adolescents with hereditary medullary thyroid carcinoma: German and Austrian experience. World J Surg 22:744–751
52. Miccoli P, Berti P, Raffaelli M, Materazzi G, Conte M, Galleri D (2002) Impact of harmonic scalpel on operative time during video-assisted thyroidectomy. Surg Endosc 16:663–666
53. Lombardi CP, Raffaelli M, De Crea C, D'Amore A, Bellantone R (2009) Video-assisted thyroidectomy: lessons learned after more than one decade. Acta Otorhinolaryngol Ital 29:317–320
54. Agency for Health Care Policy and Research (1992) Acute pain management: operative or medical procedures and trauma, Clinical practice guideline number 1. AHPCR, Rockville
55. Agency for Health Care Policy and Research (1994) Management of cancer pain: adults, Clinical practice guideline number 9. AHPCR, Rockville
56. Sackett DL (1989) Rules of evidence and clinical recommendation on the use of antithrombotic agents. Chest 95(Suppl):2–4
57. Heinrich S, Schafer M, Rousson V et al (2006) Evidence –based treatment of acute pancreatitis : a look at estabilished paradigms. Ann Surg 243:154–168
58. Terris DJ, Angelos P, Steward DL, Simental AA (2008) Minimally invasive video-assisted thyroidectomy: a multi-institutional North American experience. Arch Otolaryngol Head Neck Surg 134:81–84
59. Miccoli P, Berti P, Frustaci GL et al (2006) Video-assisted thyroidectomy: indications and results. Langenbecks Arch Surg 391:68–71
60. Lombardi CP, Raffaelli M, Princi P et al (2006) Video-assisted thyroidectomy: report of a 7-year experience in Rome. Langenbecks Arch Surg 391:174–177
61. Lombardi CP, Raffaelli M, Princi P et al (2006) Video-assisted thyroidectomy: report on the experience of a single center in more than four hundred cases. World J Surg 30:794–800
62. Minuto MN, Berti P, Miccoli M, Ugolini C, Matteucci V, Moretti M, Basolo F, Miccoli P (2011) Minimally invasive video-assisted thyroidectomy: an analysis of results and a revision of indications. Surg Endosc 26(3):818–822

63. Radford PD, Ferguson MS, Magill JC, Karthikesalingham AP, Alusi G (2011) Meta-analysis of minimally invasive video-assisted thyroidectomy. Laryngoscope 21:1675–1681
64. Lombardi CP, Raffaelli M, D'Alatri L, De Crea C, Marchese MR, Maccora D, Paludetti G, Bellantone R (2008) Video-assisted thyroidectomy significantly reduces the risk of early post-thyroidectomy voice and swallowing symptoms. World J Surg 32:693–700
65. Byrd JK, Nguyen SA, Ketcham A, Hornig J, Gillespie MB, Lentsch E (2010) Minimally invasive video-assisted thyroidectomy versus conventional thyroidectomy: a cost-effective analysis. Otolaryngol Head Neck Surg 143:789–794

# Locoregional Anesthesia in Thyroid and Parathyroid Surgery

# 11

James Y. Lim and William B. Inabnet III

## 11.1 Introduction

The description of thyroid goiter dates back to centuries ago, one of the earliest descriptions appearing in Chinese literature in 2700 BC. Thyroid goiter also make appearances throughout historic artwork, even Leonardo Da Vinci sketched an anatomically correct thyroid gland in 1500 AD. It was not long until thyroid surgery was undertaken and in its early days, the procedure was highly morbid. Antiseptic technique had yet to be described by Joseph Lister and surgeons such as Samuel Gross and Theodor Bilroth considered operating on the thyroid only in emergent situations. The advent of general anesthesia and antiseptic technique ushered in an era of safer thyroid surgery, with Nikolai Pirogoff first using ether in 1849 to remove a large goiter causing tracheal compression in a 17-year-old girl [1]. Local anesthesia techniques soon followed, led by TP Dunhill and Emil Kocher in the early 1900s [2]. General anesthesia techniques continued to be refined and became the standard used during thyroidectomy surgery up until recently. Similarly, although the first parathyroidectomy was performed under local anesthesia by Felix Mandel in 1925, general anesthesia became the popularized technique as multigland disease and bilateral explorations became more common [1].

In the last couple of decades, there has been a renewed interest in performing both thyroid and parathyroid operations under locoregional anesthesia. As preoperative studies have enabled better localization of disease in both parathyroids and thyroid disorders, minimally invasive techniques have become popularized and the ability to

J.Y. Lim
Department of Surgery, The Mount Sinai Hospital, 5 E 98th St, New York, NY 10029, USA
e-mail: James.lim@mountsinai.org

W.B. Inabnet III (✉)
Department of Surgery, Mount Sinai Beth Israel, First Ave at 16th St, Baird Hall, Suite 16BH20, New York, NY 10003, USA
e-mail: william.inabnet@mountsinai.org



C.P. Lombardi, R. Bellantone (eds.), *Minimally Invasive Therapies for Endocrine Neck Diseases*, DOI 10.1007/978-3-319-20065-1_11

perform these procedures under locoregional anesthesia has improved. While the vast majority of parathyroid and thyroid operations are still performed under general anesthesia, locoregional anesthesia has been shown to be a safe and effective alternative that can potentially allow for a shorter recovery period, fewer costs, and obviate the potential risks that are inherent with general anesthesia [3–7].

## 11.2 Benefits of Locoregional Anesthesia

Although there are no absolute indications for the use of locoregional anesthesia in thyroid and parathyroid surgery, patients who may benefit the most are those for whom general anesthesia is considered high risk, such as in the case of amiodarone-induced thyrotoxicosis [8]. In addition, because endotracheal intubation is avoided, the potential for vocal cord trauma is removed making this technique particularly appealing for people who rely on their voice professionally. Similarly, since the patient is lightly sedated during the operation, the surgeon can assess voice integrity during thyroid gland dissection. Some critics have expressed concern that the potential for more frequent recurrent laryngeal nerve injury because the patient may move around more during the operation, but studies have shown no difference in nerve injury when comparing anesthetic techniques [9]. Studies have also shown that patients have less postoperative pain [10–14]. The reduction in pain can be attributed to the long action of the local anesthetic as well as the absence of postoperative nausea and vomiting that often accompanies general anesthesia. Locoregional anesthesia also allows for shorter operating room times and shorter postoperative recovery which can translate to shorter a hospital stay and lower overall costs [15, 16].

## 11.3 Contraindications to Locoregional Anesthesia

Although there are benefits to the use of locoregional anesthesia, certain groups of patients benefit from the use of general anesthesia. These patients include those with known adverse reactions to local anesthetics. Local anesthesia should be avoided in patients with seizure disorders, as the administration of local anesthesia can lower the seizure threshold. Since patients will be alert to a certain extent, if they are unable to follow directions such as staying still during the operation, general anesthesia would be more appropriate. Similarly, if the patient is claustrophobic, has significant anxiety, or is unable to physically maintain the position during surgery, locoregional anesthesia is contraindicated. If there are any airway concerns, such as in patients with morbid obesity, obstructive sleep apnea, chronic obstructive pulmonary disorder, or a "difficult airway," general anesthesia may be more appropriate. In addition, locoregional anesthesia may not be appropriate for patients for whom there are communication barriers such as deafness or foreign languages. Finally, anatomic features such as a substernal goiter or disease characteristics likely necessitating a longer surgery or extensive dissection are best managed with general anesthesia. One group identified the limits of patient tolerance with locoregional anesthesia to be approximately 2 h, after which patient cooperation and ability to maintain positioning proved difficult [2]. Ultimately, patients who undergo thyroidectomy or parathyroidectomy under locoregional anesthesia should be prepped in such a way as to facilitate the use of general anesthesia if intraoperative events favor conversion.

## 11.4 Relevant Anatomy

Sensory and motor innervation to the neck and posterior scalp is supplied by the cervical plexus which originates from the anterior rami of the first four cervical nerves (C1-C4) (figure would be nice). C1 is generally recognized as consisting of purely motor fibers. The cervical nerves pass laterally through the corresponding vertebrae and travel between the anterior and posterior tubercles of the transverse processes. The anterior and middle scalene muscles form a fascial compartment through which the cervical nerves traverse and within which the cervical plexus is formed. The cervical plexus is unique in that its sensory and motor components branch off into the superficial and deep branches early in its course. The deep branches supply the motor innervation to the neck muscles that insert onto the first four cervical vertebrae. The superficial branches course behind the anterior scalene muscle and emerge from the mid-posterior border of the sternocleidomastoid and provide sensory innervation to the anterior neck. Because of this division, selective blockade to the sensory component is able to be performed. The superficial branches form the lesser occipital (C2), greater auricular (C2, C3), transverse cervical (C2, C3), and supraclavicular (C3, C4) nerves (Fig. 11.1). The main sensory innervation to

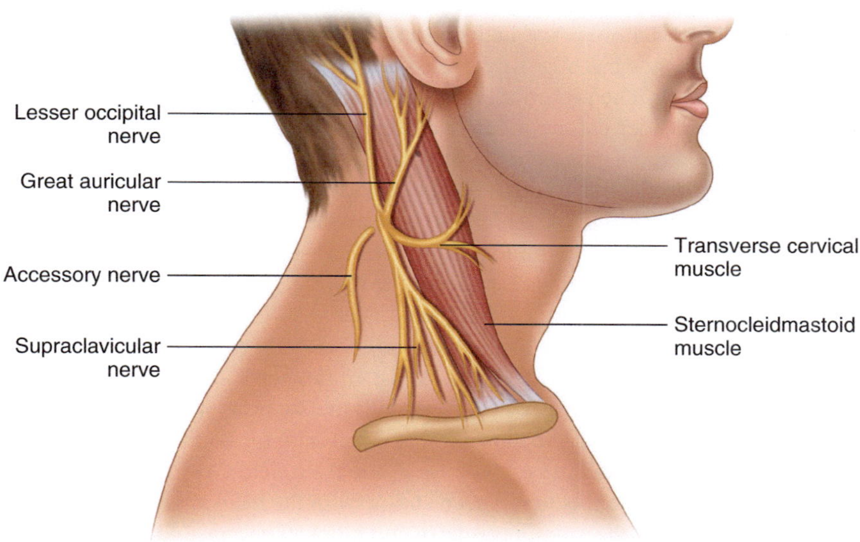


**Fig. 11.1** Diagram of superficial cervical plexus

the platysma, strap muscles, thyroid gland, and surrounding tissues relevant for thyroid or parathyroid surgery is the transverse cervical branch of the superficial cervical plexus. Close to the midline of the anterior neck, the contralateral cervical plexus contributes to sensation as many of the nerve endings of the transverse cervical nerve cross to the other side and so a bilateral block may provide for more complete analgesia. In addition, the roots from C3, C4, and C5 give rise to the phrenic nerve. The cranial nerves X, XI, and XII also communicate with the cervical plexus and this communication partially explain some of the complications seen with a cervical plexus block.

## 11.5 Types of Locoregional Block

There are three types of locoregional blocks that can be used for thyroid and parathyroid surgery: the anterior neck field block, the superficial cervical block, and the deep cervical block [17].

The anterior neck field block consists of infiltration of local anesthesia in the region of the anticipated incision. This block can be used alone, or in conjunction with any of the other two locoregional blocks. Just prior to incision, a small gauge needle is used to create a wide field block by passing the needle in multiple directions in the location of the incision. Isolated anterior neck field blocks are appropriate for central thyroid resections, although surgeons have used this block successfully in the past to perform total thyroidectomy and parathyroidectomy with the addition of intravenous sedation [9]. Cervical plexus blocks, though, allow for deeper dissection with less need for supplemental administration of local anesthesia throughout the case.

The superficial cervical plexus block provides the same sensory anesthesia as the deep cervical block but does not include the motor component. The patient is first placed supine with the head slightly elevated and turned toward the side opposite the opposite of the block. The posterior border of the sternocleidomastoid is then identified. The muscle border can be accentuated by asking the patient to lift his or her head against gentle resistance from the surgeon's hand. In addition, the external jugular vein can also be identified with a Valsalva maneuver or by placing the table in a slight Trendelburg position. The midpoint of the posterior border of the sternocleidomastoid muscle can then be identified and marked. This point usually corresponds to where the external jugular vein crosses over the muscle. Once identified, local anesthesia can be administered via a small gauge needle several inches superiorly and inferiorly into the subfascial plane along the posterior border of the muscle.

The deep cervical plexus block may assist in deeper surgical dissection as it anesthetizes not only the sensory nerves as with the superficial cervical block, but also the motor innervation to the muscles that insert onto the cervical vertebrae. The muscles will lose their tone and provide for optimal surgical conditions deep within the neck. Again, the patient is first placed supine with the head slightly elevated and turned slightly toward the side opposite of the block. The mastoid process is first identified. The transverse processes are then palpated and that of C6, the most prominent and easily palpable, is identified. The transverse process of C6 is also known as Chassaignac's tubercle and should be identified at the level of the cricoid cartilage. A line from the mastoid process to the transverse process of C6 should be marked out. The transverse processes of the C2, C3, and C4 can now be palpated approximately 0.5–1 cm posterior to the line drawn between the mastoid process and C6. If difficult to palpate, centimeter approximations can be used. As C1 does not have a transverse process, the first transverse process should be that of C2 and is located approximately 1.5 cm below the mastoid process. Each subsequent transverse process should be an additional 1.5 cm lower. The C4 transverse process should be at the level of the inferior most border of the mandible. These processes are then marked out. The area should be prepped in a sterile fashion and skin wheals can be raised at each transverse process. A small gauge needle can then be inserted perpendicularly and advanced until bone is contacted. Contact with the transverse process can be confirmed by walking the needle caudally. The needle will slip off the bone if it is on the transverse process as opposed to continuing to contact the bone if it is on the vertebral body. The needle is then walked laterally until the most superficial point of the process is identified. This is where the cervical nerves exit the vertebral body. The needle should be pulled back approximately 1 cm so it is within the interscalene groove and local anesthetic is injected.

The deep cervical plexus block can also be performed with a single injection at the level of the C3 or C4 transverse process. As the paravertebral space communicates freely within the cervical region, the local anesthetic can spread easily between levels. Placing pressure just caudad to the injection site can prevent caudal infiltration within the interscalene groove and prevents brachial plexus involvement.

## 11.6 Types of Local Anesthesia

Choice of local anesthetic is dependent on the preference of the surgeon or anesthesiologist and anticipated duration of the surgery. If the surgeon performs the block, it is essential to communicate the type of block and choice and dose of local anesthetic agent with the anesthesia team prior to performing the block. Recommended local anesthetics for use in cervical plexus blocks include lidocaine, bupivacaine, ropivicaine, and mepivicaine (Table 11.1). Few studies have compared the efficacy between these agents and there are few significant differences between them. Bupivacaine has the longest duration of action while mepivicaine had shortest time of analgesia based on studies looking at when the first request of postoperative analgesia occurred. The side effect profile of each anesthetic must be taken into consideration before use as well. Bupivacaine, for example, is markedly cardiotoxic and has been associated with irreversible asystolic arrest. Care must be taken to calculate the total dose that a patient can receive preoperatively in order to prevent systemic toxicity (what is the formula for this calculation?). This is particularly relevant when mixing local anesthetics together in order to obtain the short onset of action of lidocaine with long duration of bupivacaine, for example. If a bilateral block is being placed, the total calculated dose should be divided evenly between the two sides.

**Table 11.1** Characteristics of local anesthetics

| Local anesthetic | Typical concentration (%) | Onset of action (min) | Duration of action (min) | Duration of action with Epi (min) | Maximum total dose (mg) | Maximum total dose with Epi (mg) |
|---|---|---|---|---|---|---|
| Lidocaine | 1–2 | 2–5 | 50–120 | 60–180 | 300 | 500 |
| Bupivacaine | 0.25–0.5 | 5–10 | 240–480 | 240–480 | 175 | 225 |
| Ropivicaine | 0.5 | 10–30 | 300–480 | 300–480 | 300 | – |
| Mepivicaine | 1–2 | 2–5 | 50–120 | 60–180 | 300 | 500 |

Epinephrine can be added to prolong the duration of the local anesthetics at dilution factors varying between 1:100,000 and 1:300,000. A 15 % increase in heart rate is noted with the addition of epinephrine at concentrations as low as 1:200,000. The use of epinephrine with subsequent increase in heart rate must be balanced with the patient's comorbidities. Other studies have shown that there is a 7 % increase in systolic blood pressure after a cervical block, regardless of if epinephrine was used [18].

## 11.7 Monitored Anesthesia Care

While the block is being performed, light conscious intravenous sedation should be provided by the anesthesiologist with a combination of benzodiazepines, propofol, and/or opioids. During the surgical procedure, the goal is to maintain the patient's comfort while not oversedating the patient. Oversedation leading to respiratory depression requiring maneuvers to improve airway patency can be difficult to perform while maintaining a sterile field. The anesthesiologist must be diligent throughout the operation in order to balance the needs of both the patient and surgeon. Again, patients who undergo thyroidectomy or parathyroidectomy under locoregional anesthesia should be prepped in such a way as to facilitate the use of general anesthesia if intraoperative events favor conversion. A flexible ether screen is one such item that permits rapid, easy access to the airway without compromising the sterility of the surgical field (Fig. 11.2).

## 11.8 Patient Selection

Careful patient selection is paramount. Prior to the operation, the patients must be chosen carefully and have a knowledgeable understanding of the locoregional anesthesia technique. They must be able to communicate with the surgeon. The surgeon should prepare the patient by describing the positioning as well as sensations the patient will feel throughout the surgery. During the operation, the surgical drapes should be placed as a tent around the head and not directly on the face. Pressure points should be padded during the patient positioning process. In addition, patients should empty their bladder just prior to surgery and intravenous fluids should be carefully managed to prevent a distended and uncomfortable bladder during the operation.

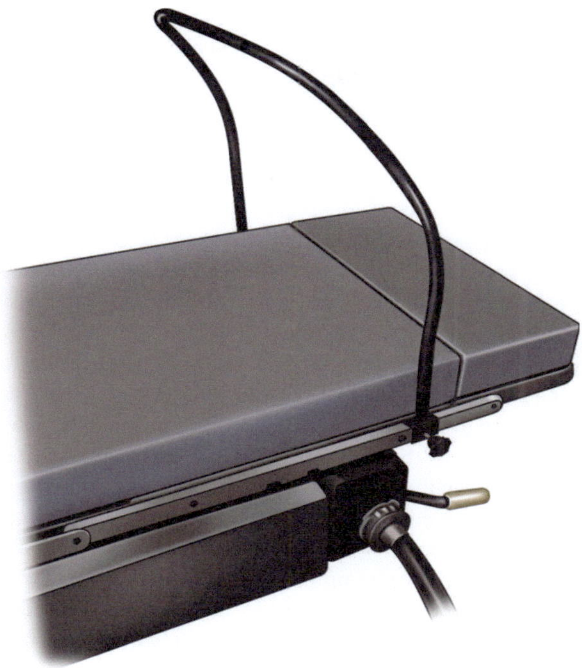

**Fig. 11.2** Example of flexible ether screen

## 11.9 Complications Specific to Locoregional Anesthesia

Cervical plexus blocks are safe in experienced hands and the type of complication varies depending on whether a superficial or deep cervical plexus block is performed. One meta-analysis reviewing over 2500 cases of cervical plexus blocks found that deep cervical plexus blocks were associated with serious life-threatening complications in 0.25 % of patients whereas not a single instance was identified with the superficial cervical plexus block [18].

The more serious complications are associated with intravascular injection of the local anesthesia and so it is of paramount importance to always aspirate prior to injection. Depending on the location, intravascular injections can occur into the vertebral and carotid arteries as well as the internal and external jugular veins. Accidental administration of volumes as small as 0.5 mL of local anesthetic into the vertebral or carotid artery can lead to immediate transient loss of consciousness or convulsions [19]. Intraspinal injections and subsequent injuries to the spinal cord can also occur with the deep cervical blocks in particular. Aspiration should also be performed to ensure there is no return of cerebrospinal fluid. Inadvertent subarachnoid space injection can lead to total brainstem anesthesia, whereas epidural injection at the cervical level can lead to anesthesia of the bilateral upper limbs and bilateral diaphragmatic paralysis. Administration of intravascular lipids has been shown to be an effective treatment for asystole that may occur with the inadvertent intravascular administration of local anesthetic. A 20 % lipid emulsion is initially bolused (1.5 mL/kg) and then followed by a continuous infusion (0.25–0.5 mL/kg/min) until vital signs are recovered. Early recognition and the bolus injection are the keys to rapid improvement [20].

Phrenic nerve block can also occur, more frequently with the deep cervical block. Some studies have shown that phrenic nerve anesthesia occurs in up to 60 % of patients who receive deep cervical blocks [21]. The consequence of ipsilateral diaphragm paralysis is usually not significant unless the patient has severe lung disease, such as chronic obstructive pulmonary disorder, at baseline. In addition, this diaphragm paralysis is temporary and usually resolves after several hours. Similarly, anesthesia of the vagus nerve and the recurrent laryngeal nerve can occur with the deep cervical blocks. Incidence of this complication ranges from 3 to 55 % in studies [21]. Involvement of the recurrent laryngeal nerve usually leads to hoarseness from vocal cord dysfunction and when combined with an increase in heart rate, usually means that the vagus nerve is involved. Again, the effect is usually transient and clears as the block dissipates. Because of these two potentially serious complications, bilateral deep cervical blocks must be performed judiciously (i.e., only for total thyroidectomy or planned bilateral neck exploration) to avoid potentially severe respiratory complications.

Many other adverse effects have been reported with cervical plexus blocks. Injection into the thyroid gland can cause localized hematomas. Dysphagia is reported to occur in up to 50 % of cases, likely secondary to involvement of cranial nerves IX and X, although this usually resolves in the post anesthesia care unit [21]. Horner's syndrome can occur when anesthesia is injected anterior to the transverse process and middle cervical sympathetic ganglion is blocked. Due to the potential of all these complications, knowledge of the relevant anatomy, cognizance of needle depth and direction, as well as routine aspiration are imperative in order to ensure safe administration of a cervical plexus block.

The conversion rate to general anesthesia was higher in patients who underwent deep cervical blocks. The deep cervical blocks were associated with a higher rate of conversion as compared to superficial cervical blocks, 2.1 % vs. 0.4 % ($P<0.0001$) [18]. Ultimately, patients who undergo thyroidectomy or parathyroidectomy under locoregional anesthesia should be prepped in such a way as to facilitate the use of general anesthesia if intraoperative events favor conversion.

## Conclusion

Locoregional anesthesia for parathyroid and thyroid surgery offers can offer several advantages over traditional general anesthesia and should have a place in the surgeon's armamentarium. Recent studies have shown that postoperative analgesia requirements and nausea is improved with locoregional anesthesia as compared to general anesthesia. In addition, locoregional anesthesia can be more cost efficient given the potential for decreased overall hospitalization times for patients. Finally, studies have shown that in appropriate patient populations, local anesthesia can be used safely during parathyroid and thyroid surgery.

## References

1. Rogers-Stevane J, Kauffman GL Jr (2008) A historical perspective on surgery of the thyroid and parathyroid glands. Otolaryngol Clin North Am 41(6):1059–1067. doi:10.1016/j.otc.2008.08.003, vii
2. Arora N, Dhar P, Fahey TJ 3rd (2006) Seminars: local and regional anesthesia for thyroid surgery. J Surg Oncol 94(8):708–713. doi:10.1002/jso.20694
3. Saxe AW, Brown E, Hamburger SW (1988) Thyroid and parathyroid surgery performed with patient under regional anesthesia. Surgery 103(4):415–420
4. Chen H, Sokoll LJ, Udelsman R (1999) Outpatient minimally invasive parathyroidectomy: a combination of sestamibi-SPECT localization, cervical block anesthesia, and intraoperative parathyroid hormone assay. Surgery 126(6):1016–1021; discussion 1021–1012
5. Inabnet WB, Fulla Y, Richard B, Bonnichon P, Icard P, Chapuis Y (1999) Unilateral neck exploration under local anesthesia: the approach of choice for asymptomatic primary hyperparathyroidism. Surgery 126(6):1004–1009; discussion 1009–1010
6. Lo Gerfo P (1998) Local/regional anesthesia for thyroidectomy: evaluation as an outpatient procedure. Surgery 124(6):975–978; discussion 978–979
7. Inabnet WB, Shifrin A, Ahmed L, Sinha P (2008) Safety of same day discharge in patients undergoing sutureless thyroidectomy: a comparison of local and general anesthesia. Thyroid 18(1):57–61. doi:10.1089/thy.2007.0148
8. Williams M, Lo Gerfo P (2002) Thyroidectomy using local anesthesia in critically ill patients with amiodarone-induced thyrotoxicosis: a review and description of the technique. Thyroid 12(6):523–525. doi:10.1089/105072502760143926
9. Snyder SK, Roberson CR, Cummings CC, Rajab MH (2006) Local anesthesia with monitored anesthesia care vs general anesthesia in thyroidectomy: a randomized study. Arch Surg 141(2):167–173. doi:10.1001/archsurg.141.2.167
10. Shih ML, Duh QY, Hsieh CB, Liu YC, Lu CH, Wong CS, Yu JC, Yeh CC (2010) Bilateral superficial cervical plexus block combined with general anesthesia administered in thyroid operations. World J Surg 34(10):2338–2343. doi:10.1007/s00268-010-0698-7
11. Gozal Y, Shapira SC, Gozal D, Magora F (1994) Bupivacaine wound infiltration in thyroid surgery reduces postoperative pain and opioid demand. Acta Anaesthesiol Scand 38(8):813–815
12. Cai HD, Lin CZ, Yu CX, Lin XZ (2012) Bilateral superficial cervical plexus block reduces postoperative nausea and vomiting and early postoperative pain after thyroidectomy. J Int Med Res 40(4):1390–1398
13. Egan RJ, Hopkins JC, Beamish AJ, Shah R, Edwards AG, Morgan JD (2013) Randomized clinical trial of intraoperative superficial cervical plexus block versus incisional local anaesthesia in thyroid and parathyroid surgery. Br J Surg 100(13):1732–1738. doi:10.1002/bjs.9292
14. Steffen T, Warschkow R, Brandle M, Tarantino I, Clerici T (2010) Randomized controlled trial of bilateral superficial cervical plexus block versus placebo in thyroid surgery. Br J Surg 97(7):1000–1006. doi:10.1002/bjs.7077
15. Spanknebel K, Chabot JA, DiGiorgi M, Cheung K, Curty J, Allendorf J, LoGerfo P (2006) Thyroidectomy using monitored local or conventional general anesthesia: an analysis of outpatient surgery, outcome and cost in 1,194 consecutive cases. World J Surg 30(5):813–824. doi:10.1007/s00268-005-0384-3
16. Biertho L, Chu C, Inabnet WB (2003) Image-directed parathyroidectomy under local anaesthesia in the elderly. Br J Surg 90(6):738–742. doi:10.1002/bjs.4175
17. Joseph D, John DA (2011) Thyroid surgery performed under local anesthesia and same-day surgery. In: Thyroid cancer. CRC Press, West Palm Beach, pp 249–269. doi:10.1201/b10945-16
18. Pandit JJ, Satya-Krishna R, Gration P (2007) Superficial or deep cervical plexus block for carotid endarterectomy: a systematic review of complications. Br J Anaesth 99(2):159–169. doi:10.1093/bja/aem160

19. Hakl M, Michalek P, Sevcik P, Pavlikova J, Stern M (2007) Regional anaesthesia for carotid endarterectomy: an audit over 10 years. Br J Anaesth 99(3):415–420. doi:10.1093/bja/aem171
20. Rosenblatt MA, Abel M, Fischer GW, Itzkovich CJ, Eisenkraft JB (2006) Successful use of a 20% lipid emulsion to resuscitate a patient after a presumed bupivacaine-related cardiac arrest. Anesthesiology 105(1):217–218
21. Masters RD, Castresana EJ, Castresana MR (1995) Superficial and deep cervical plexus block: technical considerations. AANA J 63(3):235–243

# Robotic Thyroidectomy

# 12

William S. Duke and David J. Terris

## 12.1 Remote Access Robotic Thyroidectomy Techniques

Refinements in operative techniques and improvements in surgical instruments have revolutionized modern surgery, leading to minimally invasive procedures and a population of patients who expect safe, efficacious surgery with minimal cosmetic impact. This drive to improve cosmetic outcomes has become especially important in thyroid surgery, where the incision is traditionally prominently exposed on the anterior neck. While minimally invasive techniques have been described to reduce the visible neck scar, remote access thyroidectomy procedures completely remove the incision from the anterior neck and move it to a distant, concealed location.

Remote access thyroid surgery was initially described using endoscopic instrumentation. The surgical robotic platform was incorporated into remote access thyroid surgery in 2009 [1], creating the remote access robotic-assisted thyroidectomy and making the cosmetic benefits available to selected patients throughout the world. The two approaches most commonly performed are the robotic axillary thyroidectomy (RAT) and the robotic facelift thyroidectomy (RFT) (Fig. 12.1). While RAT is still utilized in certain Asian markets, it has been associated with a number of complications in Western patient populations [2–5], and has largely been abandoned in many of the centers in the United States where it was first introduced [6, 7]. The RFT approach, however, has enjoyed an improved safety profile and overcomes many of the limitations of RAT.

W.S. Duke, MD • D.J. Terris, MD, FACS (✉)
Department of Otolaryngology Head and Neck Surgery, Georgia Regents University, 1120 Fifteenth Street, BP-4109, Augusta, GA 30912-4060, USA
e-mail: wduke@gru.edu; dterris@gru.edu



C.P. Lombardi, R. Bellantone (eds.), *Minimally Invasive Therapies for Endocrine Neck Diseases*, DOI 10.1007/978-3-319-20065-1_12

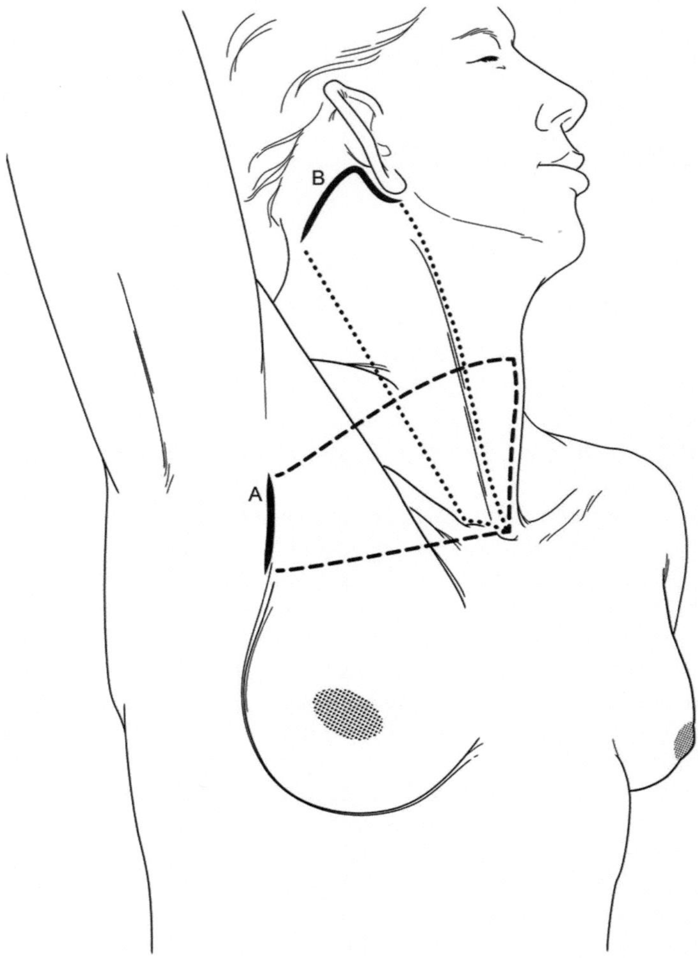


**Fig. 12.1** Comparison of the RAT and RFT approaches. *Dashed* and *dotted lines* show the extent of dissection for each procedure. *A* robotic axillary thyroidectomy (RAT), *B* robotic facelift thyroidectomy (RFT) (From Duke and Terris [22] © 2013 Georgia Regents University)

### 12.1.1 RAT Technique

The remote access robotic axillary thyroidectomy procedure has been extensively described [1, 2, 8, 9] and though it has undergone some modifications since its initial description, a generalized overview of the technique is presented here. The patient is placed supine on the operating table and the ipsilateral arm is extended at the shoulder and secured to an armrest. Flexing the elbow may minimize the risk of brachial plexus or ulnar nerve injury [2]. A 5–6 cm vertical incision is marked in the anterior axilla. A second 1 cm working port may be created on the patient's chest

2 cm above the nipple line and 2 cm off the midline, though many surgeons now omit this extra incision and introduce all the instruments through the axilla.

The axillary incision is continued down to the fascia overlying the pectoralis major muscle. Dissection proceeds across the pectoralis major to the midline and superiorly above the clavicle. The sternocleidomastoid muscle (SCM) is identified and the space between the sternal and clavicular heads of the SCM is developed. The sternal head is retracted ventrally to expose the strap muscles, avoiding injury to the internal jugular vein or its tributaries. The strap muscles are elevated off the thyroid gland from the sternal notch to the superior pole and across the midline, dividing the omohyoid muscle if necessary to improve access. The surgical field is maintained with a fixed retractor system.

The robot console is then introduced on the opposite side of the operating table. A 30° downward facing camera is inserted through the axillary incision. Harmonic shears (Ethicon Endosurgery Inc., Cincinnati, OH) are placed in the dominant arm, and ProGrasp forceps (Intuitive Surgical, Sunnyvale, CA) and a Maryland grasper are placed in the nondominant arms.

Using robotic assistance, the gland is retracted inferiorly, and the superior vascular pedicle is transected with the Harmonic device. Soft tissue attachments and vessels along the lateral and inferior aspect of the gland are divided and the gland is rotated medially. The recurrent laryngeal nerve (RLN) and parathyroid glands are identified and preserved. The isthmus and ligament of Berry are divided and the lobe is removed. Removal of the contralateral lobe through the same incision may be accomplished in select cases by performing a subcapsular dissection between the thyroid and the trachea to identify the contralateral RLN and remove the gland. A surgical drain is placed prior to wound closure, and patients are generally admitted for inpatient observation.

### 12.1.2 RFT Technique

The remote access robotic facelift thyroidectomy procedure has also been described in detail [10, 11]. A transverse anterior cervical incision is marked in a natural neck crease while the patient is sitting in an upright neutral position in the preoperative holding area in the unlikely event that conversion to an open procedure is necessary. The patient is positioned just off-center of the operating table toward the side to be operated on, with the top of the patient's head level with the top of the operating table.

A propofol infusion is used to maintain general anesthesia, allowing rapid titration of the anesthetic depth. A short-acting muscle relaxant may be used to facilitate intubation, but no paralytics should be used during the dissection. The patient is intubated with an EMG endotracheal tube (ETT) to permit intraoperative laryngeal nerve monitoring. GlideScope (Verathon Inc, Bothell, WA) visualization is useful during intubation so that proper positioning of the EMG electrodes can be confirmed by the surgeon. A straight extension attached to the anesthesia circuit limits tension on the tubing, and a 3-way stop-cock valve connected to the $CO_2$ return tubing

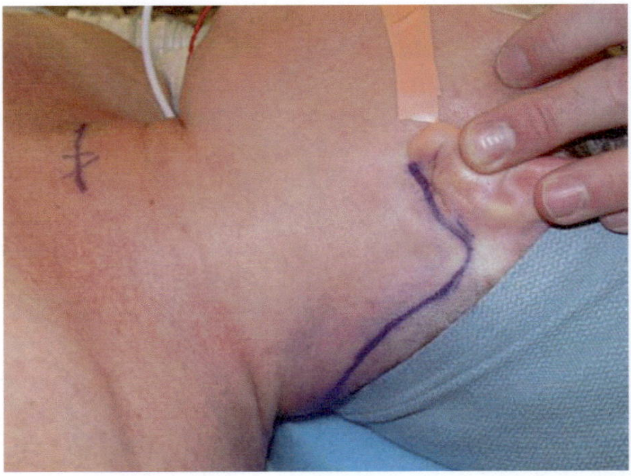

**Fig. 12.2** The robotic facelift thyroidectomy incision (From Terris et al. [11])

prevents kinking of this tube. The patient's arms are tucked at their sides and secured with wide silk tape. No safety straps are attached to the table above the patient's waist because they interfere with placement of the retractors. The bed is rotated 180° and patient's head is turned 20–30° towards the contralateral side, with the face supported by soft towels. Taping the anesthesia circuit to the operating table prevents any excessive tension which might cause the endotracheal tube to twist or migrate.

The occipital hairline is shaved back 1 cm and the facelift incision is marked. The incision begins in the postauricular crease near the inferior extent of the earlobe. It continues superiorly and then posteriorly into the shaved region of the occipital hairline in a gentle curve behind the auricle (Fig. 12.2). This placement ensures the incision will be completely concealed once the hair grows back. The incision is continued as far posteriorly and inferiorly as necessary to ensure adequate exposure.

A subplatysmal flap is developed and continued until the SCM is identified. A series of landmarks are then encountered as dissection continues anteriorly and inferiorly along the SCM. The great auricular nerve (GAN) is identified first, followed by the external jugular vein and the anterior border of the SCM. The external jugular vein is generally preserved, though it may be divided if necessary to improve exposure. Dissection continues along the anteromedial border of the SCM to the clavicle. Visualization during the deeper portions of the dissection is facilitated by placing the operating table in reverse Trendelenburg and rotating it away from the surgeon.

The omohyoid is identified, and a muscular triangle bounded by the anterior border of the SCM, the superior border of the omohyoid and the posterior border of the sternohyoid is defined. The strap muscles are retracted ventrally to expose the superior pole of the thyroid gland and the superior vascular pedicle is isolated. To limit the amount of robotic manipulation required, the lobe is mobilized as much as possible at this time. A modified Chung retractor (Marina Medical, Sunrise, FL) is fixed to the contralateral side of the table to retract the strap muscles ventrally.

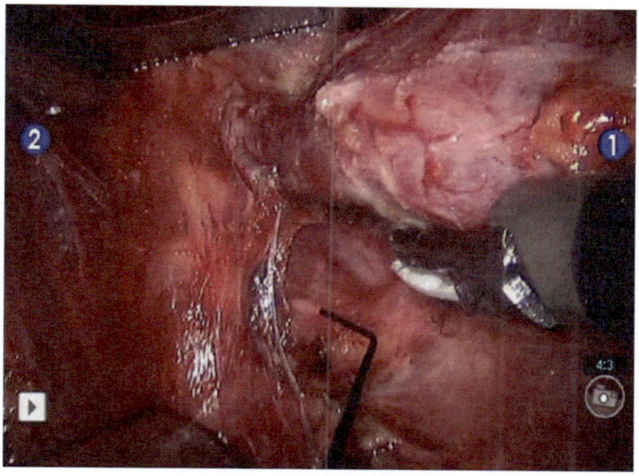


**Fig. 12.3** The recurrent laryngeal nerve is identified and electrically stimulated during the robotic facelift thyroidectomy (From Terris et al. [10])

A Singer hook (Medtronic, Jacksonville FL) attached to a Greenberg retractor (Codman & Shurtleff, Inc., Raynham, MA) is secured to the ipsilateral side of the table and used to retract the SCM.

The robotic console is then positioned near the opposite side of the operating table, with the pedestal angled 30° away from the table. Fine positioning adjustments are more easily accomplished by moving the table rather than by moving the robot console. The camera arm with a 30° down facing endoscope is positioned along the long axis of the modified Chung retractor. The camera arm is nearly fully extended so the hinges of the camera arm will not collide with the other arms. A Harmonic device is placed in the dominant arm and a Maryland grasper is used in the nondominant arm.

The robotic portion of the procedure begins by dividing the superior vascular pedicle with the Harmonic device. The superior thyroid pole is retracted inferiorly and ventrally, exposing the inferior constrictor muscle and preserving the superior laryngeal nerve. The superior parathyroid gland is identified on the posterior aspect of the thyroid and preserved. The RLN is then identified laterally as it courses under the inferior constrictor (Fig. 12.3). Tracing the nerve inferiorly exposes the ligament of Berry. The middle thyroid vein is divided. With the nerve under direct visualization, the ligament is transected with the Harmonic device and the thyroid isthmus is divided. The inferior parathyroid gland is preserved, and the inferior vessels are transected with the Harmonic device. Any remaining soft tissue attachments to the thyroid are divided and the specimen is removed.

The robotic cart is removed. The surgical field is irrigated and Surgicel (Ethicon, Inc., Somerville, NJ) is placed into the thyroid bed. The incision is approximated using buried interrupted deep dermal 4-0 Vicryl sutures (Ethicon, Inc., Somerville, NJ). The skin edges are sealed with tissue adhesive and ¼ inch Steri-Strips (3M Corporation, St. Paul, MN) placed horizontally along the incision. No drains are utilized. Deep extubation is recommended to minimize coughing or straining on emergence from anesthesia.

## 12.2 Indications for Remote Access Robotic Thyroid Surgery

Patients interested in remote access robotic assisted thyroid surgery place a high premium on cosmetic outcomes. Either for personal or professional reasons, they are highly motivated to avoid a visible neck scar, and they must be willing to accept the potential disadvantages of these procedures, such as a longer operative time, a prolonged recovery course, and procedure-specific risks not generally associated with other types of thyroid surgery. Candidates should be counseled that these procedures are not minimally invasive and are not "scarless." The scars associated with these procedures are usually longer than those of anterior cervical approaches; they are just concealed in remote locations. Finally, patients must be willing to accept the unlikely but possible chance that conversion to an anterior approach may be required.

### 12.2.1 RAT Patient Selection

There is no uniform set of selection criteria for the RAT [2, 5]. The procedure was initially described in patients with benign nodules ≤5 cm and malignant lesions ≤2 cm [1, 8]. Early exclusion criteria included prior neck surgery, "severe" Graves' disease, extrathyroidal extension of malignant disease, multiple lateral neck nodal metastases, nodal extracapsular spread or lesions in the dorsal aspect of the thyroid [8]. Patients with substernal or retropharyngeal extension have also been excluded [4].

While RAT is primarily performed for unilateral disease, total thyroidectomy [1, 2, 8, 12] as well as central and lateral neck dissections has been reported with this approach [1, 8, 13]. Potential candidates for lateral neck dissection have metastatic disease limited to 1 or 2 nodes in a single nodal basin and no evidence of extracapsular spread [13].

### 12.2.2 RFT Patient Selection

Unlike RAT, RFT selection criteria have been formalized to maximize the likelihood of operative success and minimize the risk of complications [11]. Patients should be generally healthy and able to tolerate general anesthesia for several hours. Patients should not be morbidly obese, although a slightly thicker layer of subcutaneous tissue does help protect the integrity of the soft tissue flap. There should be no prior history of neck surgery or radiation.

The disease being assessed should also meet specific criteria to be considered appropriate for RFT [11]. The thyroid lesion should be appropriate for unilateral surgery, such as an enlarging or symptomatic benign nodule or a follicular lesion of undetermined significance. The largest nodule should not exceed 4 cm in its greatest dimension, and there should be no thyroiditis or prior history of thyroid compartment surgery. Finally, there should be no substernal component, and no evidence of a high-grade malignancy such as extrathyroidal extension of the lesion or concerning lymphadenopathy.

## 12.3 Experience and Complications

### 12.3.1 RAT Outcomes

RAT outcomes have been reported for thousands of patients, mostly in Asia. The mean operative times reported for RAT range from 115 to 168 min [1, 8, 14, 15]. While this operative time is longer than for conventional open surgery [16], the overall hospital length of stay is shorter with remote access robotic thyroidectomy than with conventional open surgery [16].

The completeness of surgical resection with RAT appears similar to that achieved with conventional open surgery. A recent systematic review comparing RAT to open thyroidectomy showed no difference in the postoperative thyroglobulin levels between these two groups [16], while another study reported no abnormal $^{131}$I uptake levels in patients undergoing total thyroidectomy by RAT followed by postoperative radioactive iodine therapy [17].

Like all remote access procedures, RAT subjects patients to surgical risks that are not commonly seen in anterior cervical approaches. Complications such as hemorrhage, brachial plexus neuropathy, chyle leak, Horner's syndrome, conversion to an open procedure and tracheoesophageal injury have been reported [2, 4, 8, 14]. Temporary RLN injury has been reported in 0.7–8 % of cases [14, 15], with a permanent RLN injury rate of 0.4 % [14]. Hematoma occurs in up to 2.6 % of cases [15]. Temporary hypocalcemia is seen in up to 41 % of cases [15, 16].

### 12.3.2 RFT Outcomes

A morphometric analysis in cadaver models revealed that the RFT approach required 38 % less dissection than RAT [18]. Another study comparing the early RFT and RAT experiences found that the mean operative time for the first 10 RFT procedures was 156.9 min compared to 196 min for RAT [19]. While the differences in this small series did not reach statistical significance, the operative time in the RFT group compared favorably with early reports of the robotic axillary approach [8, 20] and steadily shortened throughout the study period, while the robotic axillary times remained stable. All patients treated with the axillary approach experienced chest wall numbness, while hypesthesia of the great auricular nerve distribution was ubiquitous in the RFT population.

Though results have been published for 22 RFT procedures in 18 patients [10, 11, 21], more than 60 procedures have been successfully completed at our institution. In all but the first patient, RFT was completed on an outpatient basis without a drain, and both concurrent bilateral and staged completion procedures have been performed [11]. There were two cases of small seromas and one incidence of transient vocal fold weakness, all of which resolved without intervention. No patients have experienced hypocalcemia and there have been no conversions to an anterior approach. No major or permanent complications have been reported with RFT. This experience has been repeated in at least 4 centers, with more than 100 procedures accomplished to date.

## 12.4 Management of Complications

All the potential complications inherent in conventional thyroid surgery exist in the robotic thyroidectomy approaches. Recurrent laryngeal nerve injury, hypocalcemia, hemorrhage, and injury to visceral structures such as the trachea and esophagus can occur regardless of the approach, and while the management of these conditions in robotic thyroid surgery is generally the same as in the anterior approaches, several potential complications deserve specific discussion.

Inadvertent tissue injury may occur due to several factors. Despite its many advantages, robotic thyroid surgery removes the haptic feedback from the tissue and instruments that the surgeon would receive in conventional surgery. Along with this decreased tactile feedback, much of the dissection is performed with an advanced energy device, which may stay hot for some time after each use. Aggressive dissection with these devices, especially right after they have been used to divide tissue, may injure delicate structures such as the recurrent laryngeal nerve. While it does not substitute for anatomic awareness and meticulous technique, intraoperative nerve monitoring may be useful for these cases.

Upper extremity injuries to the shoulder and brachial plexus have been reported with RAT [2–4]. These injuries most likely occurred as a result of excessive shoulder rotation or nerve compression. The risk of injury may be reduced by obtaining a history of any prior shoulder limitations or surgery, flexing the elbow rather than extending the arm straight above the head, and making sure the arm is appropriately padded. These injuries are generally treated conservatively or with physical therapy. Transient hypesthesia in the great auricular nerve distribution is ubiquitous in RFT patients, and occurs regardless of whether the nerve is preserved or divided. Patients should be informed about this side effect, and reassured that sensation returns with time [10].

Though significant bleeding during thyroid surgery is rare, the source is generally easily accessible in anterior approaches. However, due to the remote access nature of these procedures, bleeding during robotic thyroidectomy can be especially problematic, and great care should be taken to minimize this risk. Should bleeding occur, it can often be controlled with surgical clips or advanced energy devices, though conversion to an anterior approach may be necessary [4].

Finally, as with any equipment, the surgical robot is subject to malfunction or system failure. Though this rarely occurs, the operative team should have a thorough understanding of the proper setup, use, and troubleshooting algorithm of the system. Proper system function should be confirmed before the procedure begins, and patients should be counseled of the risk of conversion to an open procedure.

## References

1. Kang SW, Jeong JJ, Yun JS et al (2009) Robot-assisted endoscopic surgery for thyroid cancer: experience with the first 100 patients. Surg Endosc 23:2399–2406
2. Kuppersmith RB, Holsinger FC (2011) Robotic thyroid surgery: an initial experience with North American patients. Laryngoscope 121:521–526
3. Landry CS, Grubbs EG, Morris GS et al (2011) Robot assisted transaxillary surgery (RATS) for the removal of thyroid and parathyroid glands. Surgery 149:549–555

4. Kandil EH, Noureldine SI, Yao L, Slakey DP (2012) Robotic transaxillary thyroidectomy: an examination of the first one hundred cases. J Am Coll Surg 214:558–566
5. Lin HS, Folbe AJ, Carron MA et al (2012) Single-incision transaxillary robotic thyroidectomy: challenges and limitations in a North American Population. Otolaryngol Head Neck Surg 147(6):1041–1046
6. Perrier N (2012) Why I, have abandoned robot-assisted transaxillary thyroid surgery. Surgery 152:1025–1026
7. Inabnet WB (2012) Robotic thyroidectomy: must we drive a luxury sedan to arrive at our destination safely? Thyroid 22:988–990
8. Kang SW, Lee SC, Lee SH et al (2009) Robotic thyroid surgery using a gasless, transaxillary approach and the da Vinci S system: the operative outcomes of 338 consecutive patients. Surgery 146:1048–1055
9. Seybt M, Kuppersmith RB, Holsinger FC, Terris DJ (2010) Robotic axillary thyroidectomy: multi-institutional clinical experience with the daVinci. Laryngoscope 120(Suppl 4):S182
10. Terris DJ, Singer MC, Seybt MW (2011) Robot facelift thyroidectomy: II. Clinical feasibility and safety. Laryngoscope 121:1636–1641
11. Terris DJ, Singer MC, Seybt MW (2011) Robotic facelift thyroidectomy: patient selection and technical considerations. Surg Laparosc Endosc Percutan Tech 21(4):237–242
12. Berber E, Siperstein A (2011) Robotic transaxillary total thyroidectomy using a unilateral approach. Surg Laparosc Endosc Percutan Tech 21:207–210
13. Kang SW, Lee SH, Ryu HR et al (2010) Initial experience with robot-assisted modified radical neck dissection for the management of thyroid carcinoma with lateral neck node metastasis. Surgery 148:1214–1221
14. Ryu HR, Kang SW, Lee SH et al (2010) Feasibility and safety of a new robotic thyroidectomy through a gasless, transaxillary single-incision approach. J Am Coll Surg 211(3):e13–e19
15. Tae K, Ji YB, Cho SH et al (2012) Early surgical outcomes of robotic thyroidectomy by a gasless unilateral axillo-breast or axillary approach for papillary thyroid carcinoma: 2 years' experience. Head Neck 34:617–625
16. Jackson NR, Yao L, Tufano RP, Kandil EH (2014) Safety of robotic thyroidectomy approaches: meta-analysis and systematic review. Head Neck 36(1):137–143
17. Kang SW, Park JH, Jeong JS et al (2011) Prospects of robotic thyroidectomy using a gasless transaxillary approach for the management of thyroid carcinoma. Surg Laparosc Endosc Percutan Tech 21:223–229
18. Singer MC, Seybt MW, Terris DJ (2011) Robot facelift thyroidectomy: I. Preclinical simulation and morphometric assessment. Laryngoscope 121:1631–1635
19. Terris DJ, Singer MC (2012) Qualitative and quantitative differences between 2 robotic thyroidectomy techniques. Otolaryngol Head Neck Surg 147(1):20–25
20. Stevenson CE, Gardner DF, Grover AC (2012) Patient factors affecting operative times for single-incision trans-axillary robotic-assisted (STAR) thyroid lobectomy: does size matter? Ann Surg Oncol 19:1460–1465
21. Terris DJ, Singer MC (2012) Robotic facelift thyroidectomy: facilitating remote access surgery. Head Neck 34:746–747
22. Duke WS, Terris DJ (2014) Alternative approaches to the thyroid gland. Endocrinol Metab Clin N Am 43:459–474

# Minimally Invasive Video-Assisted Parathyroidectomy (MIVAP) 13

Carmela De Crea, Gerardo D'Amato, Emanuela Traini, Marco Raffaelli, and Celestino Pio Lombardi

## 13.1 Introduction

Bilateral neck exploration (BNE) with identification of four parathyroid glands and removal of all hyperfunctioning tissue has been considered the "gold standard" for the treatment of primary hyperparathyroidism (pHPT), achieving a cure in more than 95 % of cases with a complications rate generally less than 3 % [1].

During the last three decades, the improved preoperative localization studies [2] and the introduction in the clinical practice of intra-operative PTH (IO-PTH) assay [3] led to the development of the targeted approaches to parathyroidectomy [4].

The application of the endoscopic techniques to neck surgery during the late 1990s further contributed to the development of minimally invasive parathyroidectomy [5]. From a theoretical point of view, beyond the obvious better cosmetic outcome deriving from shortening the skin incision, other potential advantages of minimally invasive parathyroidectomy include decreased postoperative pain and complications rate, because of less extensive dissection. Indeed, several reports have demonstrated that the focused techniques are safe and effective as standard BNE, with potential advantages of less postoperative hypocalcemia, shorter operative time, earlier discharge, better cosmetic result, and reduced postoperative pain [6–9]. On the basis of these results, minimally invasive parathyroidectomy is nowadays considered a safe and cost-effective procedure to treat selected patients with sporadic pHPT, especially in patients with positive preoperative localization studies [10].

Minimally invasive (or focused or targeted or selective) parathyroidectomy encompasses several techniques, including open approaches (open minimally

C. De Crea (✉) • G. D'Amato • E. Traini • M. Raffaelli • C.P. Lombardi
Unità Operativa di Chirurgia Endocrina e Metabolica,
Università Cattolica Del Sacro Cuore, Roma, Largo Agostino Gemelli, 8,
Rome, RM 00168, Italy
e-mail: carmela.decrea@rm.unicatt.it; dinodamato@gmail.com;
emanuela.traini@rm.unicatt.it; marcoraffaelli@rm.unicatt.it; cp.lombardi@rm.unicatt.it



C.P. Lombardi, R. Bellantone (eds.), *Minimally Invasive Therapies for Endocrine Neck Diseases*, DOI 10.1007/978-3-319-20065-1_13

invasive parathyroidectomy; OMIP) [11], minimally invasive radio-guided parathyroidectomy (MIRP) [12], approaches that use the endoscope, such as video-assisted parathyroidectomy (VAP) [13–15] and purely endoscopic parathyroidectomy (EP) [5, 16–20].

The endoscopic and video-assisted procedures have the advantages not only of the targeted approach but also of endoscopic magnification, with the theoretical lowered risk of complications because of better view of the neck structures (recurrent laryngeal nerve and parathyroid glands).

Minimally invasive video-assisted parathyroidectomy (MIVAP) first described by Miccoli et al. [13] was introduced in our Department since 1998 [15]. Early after its description MIVAP gained a large worldwide acceptance in different surgical settings, due to its reproducibility and its similarity with the conventional technique for the parathyroidectomy [21–24].

In this chapter we describe the surgical technique, the indications, the results, and the advantages and disadvantages of MIVAP.

## 13.2 Surgical Technique

The operative technique has been previously described in detail [25]. The patient, under general or loco-regional anesthesia with cervical block [15, 25], is positioned in a supine position with the neck in slight extension.

A small (1.5 cm) skin incision is made between the cricoid cartilage and the sternal notch, in the midline. The skin incision is usually higher than in conventional surgery and can also be modulated in the neck on the basis of the preoperative ultrasound findings regarding the localization of the pathologic gland. The cervical *linea alba* is opened as far as possible. The thyroid lobe is separated from the strap muscles by small conventional retractors (Farabeuf retractors), which are also used to maintain the operative space. The thyroid lobe is medially retracted while the strap muscles are laterally retracted. The endoscope (5 mm – 30°) and the dedicated small surgical instruments (2 mm in diameter) are introduced through the single skin incision without using any trocar. The absence of any anchoring trocar allows the endoscope to move more freely depending on the site of dissection. The tip of the endoscope is usually oriented towards the head of the patient, but it can be re-oriented to expose and explore the upper mediastinum to look for mediastinal gland.

The first step of the procedure is to completely free the thyroid gland from the strap muscles to expose the parathyroid glands. After identifying the inferior (recurrent) laryngeal nerve in the involved side, usually where it crosses the inferior thyroid artery, a targeted exploration is performed to identify the abnormal gland preoperatively localized. The magnification (2–3 folds) of the endoscope allows easy identification of the nerve and of the parathyroid glands, if the principles of blunt and bloodless dissection are respected (Fig. 13.1).

Thanks to the central access, MIVAP allows contralateral parathyroid glands exploration through the same skin incision when necessary (suspicious of

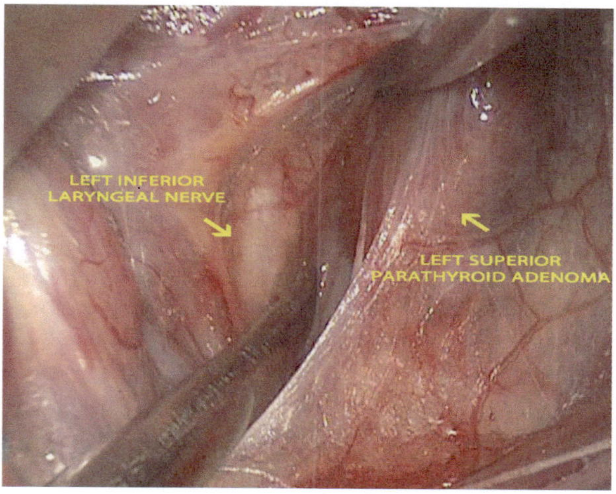


**Fig. 13.1** MIVAP: Left inferior laryngeal nerve and left superior parathyroid adenoma

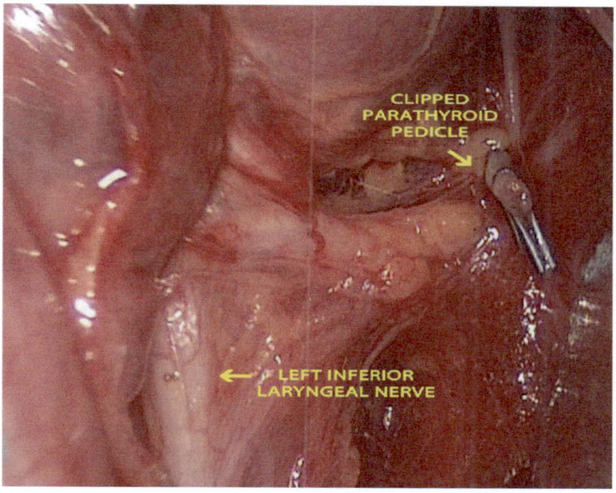


**Fig. 13.2** Operative field after left superior video-assisted parathyroidectomy

multiglandular disease because of inadequate IO-PTH decrease, two enlarged glands found at unilateral exploration, inadequate preoperative localization studies, etc.). Once identified, the parathyroid adenoma is bluntly dissected under endoscopic view using spatulas and a spatula shaped aspirator (Karl STORZ, Tuttlingen, Germany). The pedicle of the adenoma is usually clipped with titanium clips or tied with conventional ligature. After cutting the pedicle, the adenoma is extracted through the skin incision (Fig. 13.2). IO-PTH assay is used to confirm the removal of all pathologic parathyroid tissue. After checking for hemostasis the strap muscles and the platysma are closed. The skin is closed by a nonresorbable subcuticular running suture or by skin sealant. No drain is used.

## 13.3 Indications

Patients with sporadic pHPT in whom a single adenoma is suspected based on preoperative imaging studies (MIBI-scan and ultrasonography) are ideal candidates for MIVAP. Parathyroid adenoma larger than 3 cm is usually excluded because of the theoretical risk of capsular rupture and consequent parathyromatosis due to difficult dissection and extraction [26, 27].

At the beginning of the experience exclusion criteria included previous neck surgery, persistent or recurrent hyperparathyroidism, mediastinal adenomas, and concomitant large goiter. With the increasing experience, selection criteria for MIVAP have been widened. Patients with concomitant nodular goiter can undergo MIVAP if the usual inclusion criteria for the video-assisted thyroidectomy are met [28]. Moreover, in selected cases, patients with previous neck surgery or intrathymic/retrosternal adenomas can be selected for MIVAP. Because bilateral neck exploration is possible through the same access, MIVAP can be performed both in patients with suspected multiglandular disease and in patients with uncertain preoperative localization [27].

The rate of patients with sporadic pHPT who are candidates for MIVAP varies (37–71 %) [15, 26] due to different incidence of coexisting thyroid diseases that may require a conventional approach [15].

MIVAP has been proposed also for patients with four glands hyperplasia (i.e., familial pHPT and secondary and tertiary hyperparathyroidism) [21–30]. However, these indications, in our opinion, still need to be confirmed and validated by larger series and comparative studies.

## 13.4 Experience and Complications

Conversion rate is highly variable ranging from 0.9 % [15] to 25 % [31]. The more frequent indications to conversion are bleeding, inadequate IO-PTH decrease, false preoperative localization, difficult to localize/dissect the parathyroid adenoma(s), suspicious of malignancy, and ectopic localization of the pathologic gland. Proper patient selection and surgical team experience are able to lower the conversion rate even in regions with reported endemic goiters [15, 28].

Also the operative time strongly depend on surgical team skill and experience. Indeed, it has been demonstrated that the operative time decreases significantly with increasing experience and it is comparable or even shorter than that of conventional operation [15, 26, 32].

Several large retrospective series have reported on the short- and medium-term outcome of MIVAP. In 350 cases of MIVAP in 6 years, Miccoli et al. [26] reported a cure rate of 98.3 %. At a medium follow-up of 35.1 months, 4 patients had persistent disease due to false-positive IO-PTH. Complications occurred in 14 patients: 2.7 % transient hypocalcemia, 0.8 % permanent nerve palsy, and 0.3 % postoperative bleeding [26]. Others have reported similar results in smaller series [21, 23]. In our previous published series of 107 cases of MIVAP we reported a success rate of

98.1 % with persistent disease in 2 patients (1.9 %) [15]. We reported a 11.1 % rate of temporary hypocalcemia with no permanent hypoparathyroidism, and no other complications [15].

## 13.5 Advantages and Disadvantages

MIVAP presents some technical advantages compared with other endoscopic or video-assisted techniques [27]. First of all, this technique combines the advantages related to the endoscopic magnification with those due to its similarity with the conventional surgery. Indeed, the operative procedure reproduces all the steps of the open procedure. The excellent visualization of the neck structures due to the 2–3 fold endoscopic magnification permits easy identification of the laryngeal nerve and parathyroid glands. In a recently published prospective randomized trial, the mean time for adenoma localization was significant shorter for the group of patients who underwent MIVAP compared with patients operated on with an open minimally invasive technique [7].

Another merit of the technique is the possibility to perform a bilateral neck exploration when necessary through the same central access. This characteristic in part explains the very low conversion rate reported in different series [15, 26]. The possibility to perform a bilateral neck exploration produces two main effects on the restrictive inclusion criteria. Indeed, MIVAP can also be performed in case of unavailability of intra-operative PTH monitoring or in case of inadequate preoperative localization studies, because of the possibility to explore all the parathyroid sites [15, 33]. Another advantage of the central access is the possibility of associate thyroid resection, even bilateral, when necessary. Because of the high prevalence of multinodular goiter in some countries, this technical characteristic allowed experienced surgeons to increase the rate of patients eligible for a video-assisted procedure in selected patients. In our experience, with the high prevalence of goiter in Italian population, this allowed us to treat both thyroid and parathyroid diseases simultaneously in more than 30 % of the patients [28].

Moreover, the video-assisted access could imply a better cosmetic result and a less postoperative pain. Indeed, several comparative studies have demonstrated the advantages of MIVAP to reduce the postoperative pain, improve the cosmetic result and the patient satisfaction over both conventional and open non-endoscopic minimally invasive parathyroidectomy [7, 8].

Some criticisms about technical aspects for MIVAP still exist and are mainly related to the operative time. However, it has been demonstrated in large retrospective series [15, 26] and also in small comparative, randomized trials [7] that the operative time does not represent a limit.

Another technical problem is the number of members of the surgical team. The fact that two assistants are necessary to accomplish the MIVAP can represent an important concern for the application and diffusion of the procedure, at least in some surgical setting.

On the other hand, the main technical limitation of MIVAP is still represented by the volume of parathyroid adenoma and of the eventually associated goiter.

Dissection and extraction of large adenomas through a small incision can result in capsule rupture with the theoretical risk of parathyromatosis [15]. In contrast, previous neck surgery and the absence of a clear preoperative localization are not contraindications for MIVAP.

## 13.6 Avoiding Complications

In spite several reports have demonstrated that thyroid and parathyroid procedure are safely performed by residents operating under supervision and newly established surgical consultant, there is a significant inverse relationship between the number of procedures performed and the complication rate [34]. In other words patient volumes and surgical skill play an important role in reducing complications rate, as in other fields of surgery.

Obviously, lower complications rate are obtained in third care referral centers, where dedicated surgical teams and well-trained endocrine surgeons are provided and hospital facilities allow adopting all the measures and tools known by the medical community as the gold standard for patients treatment.

When the procedure is performed under optimal conditions combined with meticulous operative skill by surgeons who have been adequately trained, the incidence of complication should be at a minimum [34]. Nonetheless, complication may occur, not only because of surgical errors, but also for factor related to the patients or the disease itself.

### 13.6.1 Postoperative Hematoma

Data from the literature concur to demonstrate that the rate of postoperative major bleeding requiring surgical revision after video-assisted parathyroidectomy approaches the 0 % and only a few cases have been reported [15, 26, 34]. Even in absence of any significant difference in terms of postoperative complications in the published comparative studies [27], it could be inferred that the limited dissection, which characterizes these techniques, has the potential benefit to reduce the risk of this complication. These results could be biased by strict selection criteria for these procedures and the possible reduction of the postoperative bleeding could be related to the absence of other possible risk factors. Postoperative bleeding could be prevented by eliminating the cause in the majority of the patients. A meticulous surgical technique and hemostasis are mandatory to avoid or reduce the risk of this complication.

### 13.6.2 Recurrent Laryngeal Nerve Injury

A review of endocrine malpractice litigation, found that about 54 % of the adverse involved thyroid and parathyroid surgery and that about 79 % of these claimed surgical complications involved recurrent laryngeal nerve injury [34]. The risk of lesion of recurrent laryngeal nerve exists in all neck dissection. Individual mechanism of injury include stretch of traction, compression, or crush (i.e., ligature entrapment, hematoma formation), and thermal, electrical, and severing injuries (complete or partial transaction) [34]. Moreover, some conditions expose at a higher risk of nerve injury (i.e., lack of identification of recurrent laryngeal nerve during surgery, bilateral surgery, surgery for malignant diseases, previous neck surgery, longer operative times or greater blood loss, reoperation for bleeding). The knowledge of mechanism of injury and risk factors of recurrent laryngeal nerve palsy should thus help in its prevention. Because of the broad spectrum of anatomical variations, the identification of the recurrent laryngeal nerve can be difficult in some cases. The most important rule to follow during thyroid and parathyroid surgeries is that no structure should be cut until the recurrent laryngeal nerve is identified. Following this rule, recurrent laryngeal nerve injury, and in particular transection injury will be rare.

### 13.6.3 Hypocalcemia and Hypoparathyroidism

Postoperative hypocalcemia is one of the most common, complications of parathyroid surgery. Moreover, after RLN palsy permanent hypoparathyroidism accounts for the largest category of thyroidectomy related claims [34]. Temporary hypocalcemia has been reported to occur in 0–35 % of patients after parathyroidectomy, with permanent hypoparathyroidism resulting in 0–2.2 % of patients after successful parathyroidectomy [34].

Temporary symptomatic hypocalcemia is common after successful parathyroidectomy, despite minimally invasive and focused approaches have reduced its incidence when compared with bilateral neck exploration. Indeed, the targeted approaches to parathyroidectomy have the important advantage to avoid manipulation of normal glands and so to ensure normal parathyroid function postoperatively. In this setting, postoperative hypocalcemia is usually self-limiting and related to normal glands inhibition by the hyperfunctioning one and to the existence of a hungry bone syndrome. However, symptoms of hypocalcemia are frequently observed, even in absence of biochemical hypocalcemia. These symptoms are usually self limiting and moderate and resolve spontaneously within weeks. Some authors propose prophylactic of oral calcium administration to all patients who undergo parathyroidectomy, in order to avoid their manifestation and consequent anxiety and to adopt a short-stay procedure (ambulatory or same day discharge) [34]. On the contrary, definitive hypoparathyroidism is virtually impossible in the case of focused parathyroidectomy. On the other hand, bilateral neck exploration brings the possibility to injure also normal parathyroid glands, especially if biopsy is obtained to confirm the parathyroid origin of the identified structures. In such condition, patients are at risk of clinically relevant hypocalcemia and should not be selected for outpatient surgery. Permanent hypoparathyroidism after initial exploration occurs in only 0–0.5 % of patients after initial exploration for sporadic primary hyperparathyroidism [34], but is far more frequent in the case of operation for parathyroid hyperplasia, especially in patients undergoing total parathyroidectomy plus autotransplantation.

## References


1. Duh QY (1997) Surgical approach to primary hyperparathyroidism (bilateral approach). In: Clark OH, Duh QY (eds) Textbook of endocrine surgery. WB Saunders, Philadelphia
2. Mazzeo S, Caramella D, Lencioni R et al (1996) Comparison among sonography, double-tracer subtraction scintigraphy, and double phase scintigraphy in the detection of parathyroid lesions. AJR Am J Roentgenol 166:1465–1470
3. Irvin GL, Carneiro DM (1999) Rapid parathyroid hormone assay guided exploration. Oper Tech Gen Surg 1:18–27
4. Palazzo FF, Delbridge LW (2004) Minimal-access/minimally invasive parathyroidectomy for primary hyperparathyroidism. Surg Clin North Am 84:717–734
5. Gagner M (1996) Endoscopic subtotal parathyroidectomy in patients with primary hyperparathyroidism. Br J Surg 83:875
6. Bergenfelz A, Lindblom P, Tibblin S et al (2002) Unilateral versus bilateral neck exploration for primary hyperparathyroidism: a prospective randomized trial. Ann Surg 236:543–551
7. Barczyński M, Cichoń S, Konturek A et al (2006) Minimally invasive video-assisted parathyroidectomy versus open minimally invasive parathyroidectomy for a solitary parathyroid adenoma: a prospective, randomized, blinded trial. World J Surg 30:721–731
8. Miccoli P, Bendinelli C, Berti P et al (1999) Video-assisted versus conventional parathyroidectomy in primary hyperparathyroidism: a prospective randomized study. Surgery 126:1117–1122
9. Westerdahl J, Bergenfelz A (2007) Unilateral versus bilateral neck exploration for primary hyperparathyroidism: 5-year follow up of a randomized controlled trial. Ann Surg 249:976–980
10. Bergenfelz AOJ, Hellman P, Harrison B et al (2009) Positional statement of the European Society of Endocrine Surgeons (ESES) on modern techniques in pHPT surgery. Langenbecks Arch Surg 394:761–764
11. Udelsman R, Donovan PI, Sokoll LJ (2000) One hundred consecutive minimally invasive parathyroid explorations. Ann Surg 232:331–339
12. Norman J, Chheda H (1997) Minimally invasive parathyroidectomy facilitated by intraoperative nuclear mapping. Surgery 122:998–1003
13. Miccoli P, Pinchera A, Cecchini G et al (1997) Minimally invasive, video-assisted parathyroid surgery for primary hyperparathyroidism. J Endocrinol Invest 20:429–430
14. Henry JF, Defechereux T, Gramatica L et al (1999) Minimally invasive videoscopic parathyroidectomy by lateral approach. Langenbecks Arch Surg 384:298–301
15. Lombardi CP, Raffaelli M, Traini E et al (2008) Advantages of a video-assisted approach to parathyroidectomy. ORL J Otorhinolaryngol Relat Spec 70:313–318
16. Yeung GH, Ng JW (1998) The technique of endoscopic exploration for parathyroid adenoma of the neck. Aust N Z J Surg 68:147–150
17. Cougard P, Goudet P, Bilosi M et al (2001) Videoendoscopic approach for parathyroid adenomas: results of a prospective study of 100 patients. Ann Chir 126:314–319
18. Ikeda Y, Takami H, Niimi M et al (2002) Endoscopic total parathyroidectomy by the anterior chest approach for renal hyperparathyroidism. Surg Endosc 16:320–322
19. Ikeda Y, Takami H, Sasaki Y et al (2000) Endoscopic neck surgery by the axillary approach. J Am Coll Surg 191:336–340
20. Ohshima A, Simizu S, Okido M et al (2002) Endoscopic neck surgery: current status for thyroid and parathyroid diseases. Biomed Pharmacother 56:48s–52s
21. Mourad M, Ngongang C, Saab N et al (2001) Video-assisted neck exploration for primary and secondary hyperparathyroidism. Surg Endosc 15:1112–1115

22. Hallfeldt KK, Trupka A, Gallwas J et al (2001) Minimally invasive video-assisted parathyroidectomy. Surg Endosc 15:409–412
23. Lorenz K, Miccoli P, Monchik JM et al (2001) Minimally invasive video-assisted parathyroidectomy: multiinstitutional study. World J Surg 25:704–707
24. Suzuki S, Fukushima T, Ami H et al (2002) Video-assisted parathyroidectomy. Biomed Pharmacother 56(Suppl 1):18s–21s
25. Bellantone R, Lombardi CP, Raffaelli M (2005) Encyclopédie Médico-Chirurgicale, Tecniche Chirurgiche – Chirurgia Generale. Paratiroidectomia mini-invasiva video-assistita. 46–465-A. Elsevier SAS, Paris, pp 1–18
26. Miccoli P, Berti P, Materazzi G et al (2004) Results of video-assisted parathyroidectomy: single institution's six-year experience. World J Surg 28:1216–1218
27. Lombardi CP, Raffaelli M, Traini E et al (2009) Video-assisted minimally invasive parathyroidectomy: benefits and long-term results. World J Surg 33:2266–2281
28. De Crea C, Raffaelli M, Traini E, Giustozzi E, Oragano L, Bellantone R, Lombardi CP (2013) Is there a role for video-assisted parathyroidectomy in regions with high prevalence of goitre? Acta Otorhinolaryngol Ital 33(6):388–392
29. Miccoli P, Minuto M, Cetani F et al (2005) Familial parathyroid hyperplasia: is there a place for minimally invasive surgery? Description of the first treated case. J Endocrinol Invest 28:942–943
30. Alesina PF, Hinrichs J, Kribben A et al (2010) Minimally invasive video-assisted parathyroidectomy (MIVAP) for secondary hyperparathyroidism: report of initial experience. Am J Surg 199:851–855
31. Hessman O, Westerdahl J, Al-Suliman N et al (2010) Randomized clinical trial comparing open with video-assisted minimally invasive parathyroid surgery for primary hyperparathyroidism. Br J Surg 97:177–184
32. Berti P, Raffaelli M, Materazzi G et al (2001) Parathyroïdectomie vidéo-assistée : corbe d'apprentissage. Ann Chir 126:772–776
33. Miccoli P, Berti P, Materazzi G et al (2008) Endoscopic bilateral neck exploration versus quick intraoperative parathormone assay (qPTHa) during endoscopic parathyroidectomy: a prospective randomized trial. Surg Endosc 22:398–400
34. Raffaelli M, Lombardi CP, Bellantone R, De Crea C, Lesnik D, Potenza A, Randolph G (2012) Avoiding complications in thyroid and parathyroid surgery. In: (a cura di): Watkinson JC, Gilbert RW (eds) Stell and Maran's textbook of head and neck surgery and oncology. Hodder Arnold, Londra, pp 474–493. ISBN 978-0-340-92916-2

# Endoscopic Parathyroidectomy

# 14

Nunzia Cinzia Paladino, Carole Guérin, Eveline Slotema, Ilaria Fabiola Franco, Jean François Henry, and Frédéric Sebag

## 14.1 Techniques

Primary hyperparathyroidism (PHPT) is the third most common endocrine disorder with highest incidence in women, in postmenopausal period. The treatment is essentially surgical with removal of a parathyroid adenoma or hyperplasic glands. Medical treatment could be indicated in specific conditions as : malignant hypercalcemia (transitory), persistent hypercalcemia as a result of surgical failure and/or for patients in whom surgery is not an option (comorbidities, advanced age). Experienced surgeons are estimated to identify an affected gland in more than 95 % of cases.

Since the first parathyroidectomy, performed by Mandl in 1925, bilateral cervical neck exploration with identification of all glands is the standard approach, recognizing that 15–25 % can have multiple abnormal glands [1–4]. This technique has been for many years the surgical treatment of choice of PHPT with excellent published results and cure rates of 95–99 % [5].

However, over the last 20 years, the treatment of PHPT has undergone a radical change through the development of new imaging techniques, which allow identifying preoperatively abnormal glands and intraoperative PTH assay to confirm complete resection of pathological parathyroid tissue [6, 7].

N.C. Paladino • F. Sebag (✉) • C. Guérin • E. Slotema • I.F. Franco • J.F. Henry
General, Endocrine and Metabolic Surgery, Hopital La Conception, Aix-Marseille University, 147 Boulevard Baille, 13385 Marseille, France
e-mail: nunzia.paladino@ap-hm.fr; n.paladino@tiscali.it; frederic.sebag@ap-hm.fr; carole.guerin@ap-hm.fr; eveline.slotema@ap-hm.fr; ilaria-franco@ap-hm.fr; jeanfrancois.henry@ap-hm.fr



C.P. Lombardi, R. Bellantone (eds.), *Minimally Invasive Therapies for Endocrine Neck Diseases*, DOI 10.1007/978-3-319-20065-1_14

Challenging the traditional exploration, limited parathyroid surgery has progressively emerged. This new approach is based on the fact that about 85 % of patients with sporadic PHPT have a single parathyroid adenoma and therefore systematic exploration of all four glands is not mandatory in all cases. In this context, it seems legitimate to reduce surgical stress and morbidity [5, 8, 9]. Excision of mediastinal adenomas by thoracoscopy was the first demonstration of the application of minimally invasive techniques in parathyroid surgery [10]. In 1982, the first alternative procedure was proposed by Tibblin; a unilateral exploration was performed with identification of an enlarged abnormal gland and an ipsilateral normal gland. The surgery consisted in the pathological gland removal and in the biopsy of normal gland. According to the authors the removal of one whole gland facilitated the evaluation of hyperplasia for the pathologist; the bilateral neck exploration was performed in case of multiglandular disease revealed at the histopathologic examination of the glands from the first explored side. Following introduction of intraoperative PTH quick-assay (IOPTH), the identification of the ispilateral gland was not performed systematically [5, 6]. The concept of unilateral exploration was reinforced with the development of improved localization studies [8, 11, 12]. In this context, Chapuis proposed focused unilateral approach performed under local anesthesia [13]. In 2002, a survey by International Association of Endocrine Surgeons (IAES) showed that 59 % of surgeons performed currently minimally invasive parathyroidectomy (MIP) [14, 15]. A recent survey of parathyroid surgeons shows that limited approach, at present is performed by 68 % of survey respondent, compared with only 11 % in the previous decade. Bilateral exploration is performed by 10 % of respondents, compared with 74 % only 10 years previously [8, 16]. Recently consensus statement of European Society of Endocrine Surgeons (ESES) emphasizes that minimally invasive approach is a safe and cost-effective procedure to treat selected patients with sporadic PHPT [15].

In recent years, many new techniques have been described:

- Minimally invasive radioguided parathyroidectomy (MIRP) [17, 18]
- Open minimally invasive parathyroidectomy (OMIP) (central or lateral mini-incision under local or general anesthesia) [14, 19–22]
- Minimally invasive video-assisted parathyroidectomy (MIVAP) [23, 24]
- Full endoscopic parathyroidectomy with gas insufflations (EP) [9, 14, 25–28]

There is no uniform agreement on the definition of a "minimally invasive approach" but in general it is related to surgical procedures that use access of 2.5–3 cm or less with minimal dissection and minimal surgical trauma [5]. This concept cannot be limited to the length of the skin incision but it must be extended to anatomical structures dissected during surgical procedure [9, 29].

Generally, minimally invasive parathyroidectomy (MIP) may be divided into two groups: mini-open approaches (OMIP) performed by direct vision through a small cervical incision, and techniques using the endoscope.

Either technique has two common threads:

- Limited incision compared to conventional open transverse cervical incision.
- Surgery is targeted to one specific parathyroid gland and in most cases the exploration of other glands is not performed or limited [30]. MIP has advantage of the target approach and endoscopic magnification that allows performing the same intervention through very minimal access.

Under the nomenclature "*endoscopic parathyroidectomy*" or video-assisted technique, we find appropriate to group all interventions for PHPT in which the surgeon uses an endoscope, either during the full intervention or a part of it. As already said, the first use of the endoscope in parathyroid surgery has been described for video-assisted thoracoscopy for excision of mediastinal parathyroid adenomas [10]. In these rare cases of major ectopia, the advantages to the patient were irrefutable. However, it is difficult to demonstrate the same advantages for all cervical approaches. Two studies comparing conventional parathyroid surgery to endoscopic techniques have clearly shown a diminution of postoperative pain and better cosmetic results with endoscopic techniques [23, 31]. The endoscope has the advantage to provide light and magnification resulting in an excellent view for the surgeons. By direct vision, through mini-incision, it is more difficult to obtain an adequate view [9]. Recent study presented at the European Association of Endocrine Surgeons (ESES) shows that more than half patients with PHPT can undergo totally lateral endoscopic parathyroidectomy with a 98 % cure rate. The complication rate is similar to conventional techniques [29]. Following, we describe the endoscopic techniques making a brief mention of minimally invasive techniques that have induced their development.

### 14.1.1 Minimally Invasive Radioguided Approach (MIRP)

The MIRP, with a nuclear probe similar to that used for sentinel node biopsy, is able to localize an adenoma and has the ability to ensure complete removal by comparing the count in the adenoma with the background radioactivity [14, 15].

Surgery can be performed within 3–4 h after injection of 99mTc-sestamibi and incision is realized near the site of localization adenoma by sestamibi scintigraphy and measurement of gamma emission on the skin. It is not necessary to use IOPTH. Intervention is completed when the activity of excised adenoma is 20 % more than the background activity. Results obtained with this technique are encouraging. It is evident that this technique requires a multidisciplinary collaboration and coordination work [17].

### 14.1.2 Open Minimally Invasive Parathyroidectomy (OMIP)

It can be performed under local and cervical block anesthesia or hypnosedation with advantage of prevent postoperative nausea, vomiting and risk of vocal cord injury caused by intubation.

This technique is carried out through a 2–4 cm incision and can involve use of radioguidance [9]. This category includes central and lateral mini-open approaches. The lateral mini-open approach is used for removing inferior parathyroid adenomas because of the anterior position of PIII. This technique consists in a 15 mm transverse incision on the anterior side of sternocleidomastoid muscle. After platysma muscle has been sectioned, a bayonet access is made between sternohyoid and sternocleidomastoid muscles, 2 cm below the cricoids cartilage. Inferior thyroid pole and thyrothymic ligament are mobilized to the skin. In our experience, mini-open parathyroidectomy is fast (it can be realized in less than 15 min without identification of recurrent laryngeal nerve) and it is the procedure of choice for inferior and superficial adenomas [9].

*The central approach* is now reserved for adenomas localized much inferiorly near the thymus, from a 15 mm transverse incision in the supra sternal notch. Through this incision, conventional instruments like retractors and dissectors are used to isolate the inferior parathyroid glands under the strap muscles, with video-assisted images of an endoscope (5 mm, 0 or 30°). All maneuvers are therefore performed without the use of the endoscope or need of gas insufflation. This dissection is anterior to the trachea mostly in the thymus and thyrothymic ligament, and does not necessitate identification of the recurrent laryngeal nerve which is posterior [9].

### 14.1.3 Minimally Invasive Video-Assisted Parathyroidectomy (MIVAP)

*Minimally invasive video-assisted parathyroidectomy* (*MIVAP*) is a gasless procedure carried out through a 15–20 mm transversal skin incision performed 2 cm above sternal notch. The working space is maintained with small conventional retractors. The strap muscles on the side of adenoma are retraced with a small conventional retractor; the other retractor is placed on the thyroid lobe which is retracted medially and lifted up. Dissection lobe is performed under direct vision and the procedure is performed partially with the 30° endoscope, 5 mm in diameter. The endoscopic magnification allows an easy identification of recurrent laryngeal nerve and other anatomical structures. Any drain is placed [32].

### 14.1.4 Endoscopic Minimally Invasive Parathyroidectomy (EMIP)

Pure endoscopic techniques are performed totally with the help of the endoscope, using a midline access between the strap muscles [25, 29, 33, 34] or a lateral access, on the anterior border of the sternocleidomastoid muscle (SCM), using the "back route" between the carotid sheaths laterally and the strap muscles medially [26]. Pure endoscopic techniques include a gas insufflation and three or four trocars [33].

Other endoscopic techniques employ an extracervical approach: axillary approach [20] and anterior chest approach [35]. These operations, less commonly used in Europe, have the advantage of leaving no scar in the neck area. Nevertheless they cannot reasonably be described as minimally invasive as they require more dissection than conventional open surgery.

The diffusion of EMIP is hindered by the need to familiarize with the use of an endoscope in the neck. The learning curve can be long and monitoring by experienced surgeon in these techniques is recommended. This explains that for many parathyroid surgeons the use of endoscope during MIP remains debatable.

Surgeons who use the endoscope in the surgical neck consider that EMIP have the main advantage of offering a view and a light that permit a safe dissection. In their opinion, the use of the endoscope should be particularly recommended when the recurrent laryngeal nerve is at risk during MIP. Thus, the use of an endoscope during MIP may be determined by location of parathyroid adenoma. When the gland is posteriorly located and therefore in close proximity to the recurrent laryngeal nerve the use of the endoscope may be recommended.

In this context, the role of preoperative imaging studies is essential. Every patient with sporadic PHPT is a potential candidate for minimally invasive parathyroidectomy. The choice of the approach (lateral or central) could rely on the preoperative imaging studies [33]. Totally endoscopic lateral parathyroidectomy was described by Jean François Henry et al. in 1999 and we describe as follows this surgical technique.

### 14.1.5 Lateral Endoscopic Parathyroidectomy

The patient is in supine position without hyperextension of the head to avoid tension in anterior cervical muscles. The relapse of these muscles is essential to obtain a good dissection space with low flow insufflations of carbon dioxide. A 12–15 mm transversal incision is performed on the anterior border of the SCM below the omohyoid muscle at the same level of thyroid isthmus; dissection is continued through this mini-incision towards prevertebral fascia. The omohyoid muscle is the higher landmark. The fascia connecting lateral portion of the strap muscles and the thyroid lobe with the carotid sheath was gently divided far enough to visualize the prevertebral fascia. Access to posterior surface of thyroid lobe is quick and easy. In order to enlarge the working space one or two small humid swabs are introduced, upward and downward, deeply into the initially created space. This surprisingly quick, efficient, and bloodless maneuver allows excellent exposure operative field. Once enough space has been created, three trocars are introduced respectively, a 10–12 mm trocar through the incision, and two 2.5 mm trocars above and below the first trocar on the line of the anterior border of the SCM; these two trocars are introduced by 2 mm guide stick and are placed at 4 cm above and below the main trocar (Fig. 14.1). A purse string suture is placed around the 12–15 mm transverse skin incision to prevent both gas leakage and the 10 mm trocar from slipping out of the wound. The purse-string suture is tightened around the trocar in which is inserted a 10 mm 0° endoscopic camera. Instruments consist of grasper, scissors, and cautery hook; their length is 25 cm (Fig. 14.2). After verification of the proper positioning of the instruments, carbon dioxide is insufflated to 8 mm Hg pressure, which allows to maintain

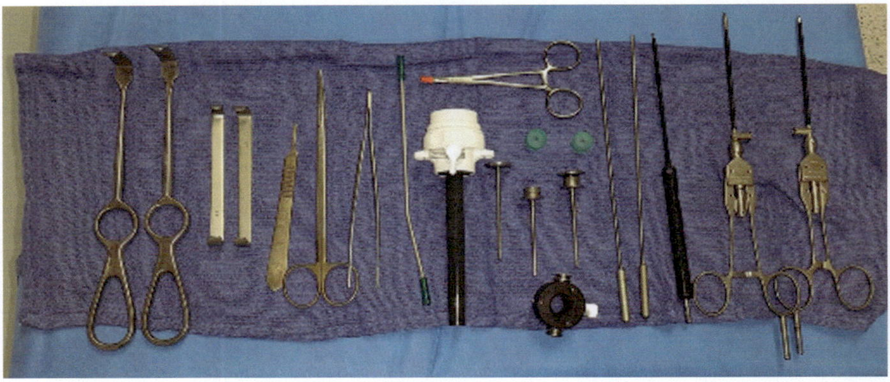

**Fig. 14.1** Instruments

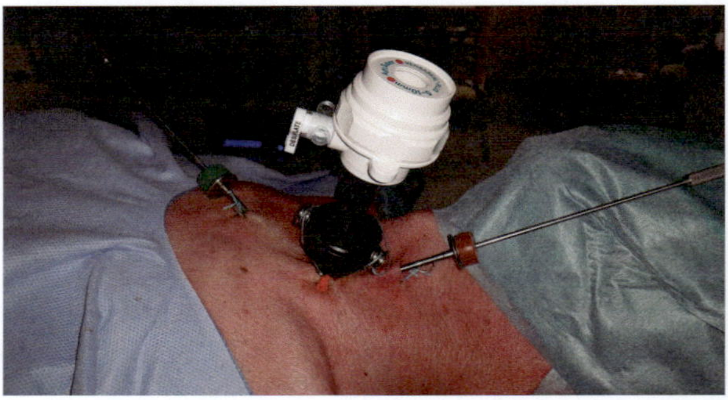

**Fig. 14.2** Trocars sites: three trocars are positioned on the line of anterior border of the SCM. Central trocar receive the 10-mm 0° endoscope and the other trocars are used for the 2-mm instruments

dissection space and to limit small bleeding. At this low pressure, there is no risk of subcutaneous emphysema or pneumomediastinum. The second step of surgical procedure is the endoscopic exploration. The assistant is devoted to endoscopic camera and surgeon begins the dissection after introducing instruments through two 2.5 mm trocars. The surgeon and assistant remain on the same side of adenoma. A monitor is placed in front of them. Immediately after introduction of the endoscope, with a minimal dissection all the anatomical structures can be easily identified. Esophagus, the inferior thyroid artery and recurrent laryngeal nerve are the landmarks. During this endoscopic dissection, ligatures or clip applications are not possible. The adenoma is progressively gently dissected from adjacent structures and more particularly from the recurrent laryngeal nerve. When its vascular pedicle is well isolated it is possible to coagulate and dissect endoscopically.

The third step of the procedure is performed once again without using the endoscope. After removing the three trocars the thyroid lobe is retracted medially and anteriorly and adenoma is visualized; it is extracted through the largest trocar site. If the vascular pedicle is not divided endoscopically, it can be well visualized and dissected after application of a clip without any difficulty. The adenoma is extracted from the neck directly through the incision. Drain is not necessary. Intraoperative nerve monitoring can be applied in this technique according to standard procedure (stimulation of vagus nerve and recurrent laryngeal nerve before, during, and after removal of adenoma). This approach is used principally for adenomas located behind the thyroid lobe. Skin is closed only with glue. Rapid IOPTH is used during surgery to confirm the success of procedure in all patients respectively at intubation time, incision, removal of adenoma, and 5, 15, and 30 min after adenoma excision. The reduction of more than 50 % of IOPTH is considered significant. All patients underwent pre and postoperative investigations of vocal cord movements. Serum calcium and phosphorus level and PTH are systematically evaluated on day 1 and day 8 and after 1 and 6 months after surgery. In our experience, the lateral approach is safe and effective. It is reserved for patients with sporadic PHPT, with a single adenoma well localized preoperatively and posteriorly located in the vicinity of inferior laryngeal nerve [26, 33, 34, 36, 37].

### 14.1.6 Robotic Transaxillary Parathyroidectomy

There is a little in literature regarding robotic parathyroidectomy however it is described as technically feasible in selected patients. Presence of a scar in the neck area remains an aesthetics concern for some patients, the majority of whom women, that has induced development of robotic transaxillary parathyroidectomy, especially in Asia. This technique, developed in South Korea for thyroid surgery in the late 2000 and by Ikeda [20] needs a learning curve and a team of endocrine surgeons proficient in use of the Robotic Da Vinci surgical system. The patient is supine with a gently extended neck and the ipsilateral arm extended at the shoulder and flexed at the elbow. Incision is made along the lateral border of the pectoralis major muscle. The subcutaneous flap is then dissected anteriorly to pectoralis fascia until the head of SCM. The sternal head and strap muscles are retracted anteriorly revealing a working space superficial to the thyroid. Instruments are introduced via the axillary incision. This technique poorly used in Europe and US, has received acclaim in Korea due to the higher rates of hypertrophic scarring and social stigma of cervical scar. A technical issue reported with robotic approach is related to the dissection of the subcutaneous flap that can be challenging in taller patients in whom the distance from the axilla to the sternal notch exceeds the limit of instruments. The risks of this technique are the following of which the last 3 are due to cervical hyperextension: vascular injury, tracheal perforation, transient ulnar nerve palsy, transient ipsilateral arm paralysis, and Horner's syndrome. Rate of transient inferior laryngeal nerve palsy remains debatable. According to authors the learning curve is steep [38, 39]. There remain issues regarding applicability of this approach to the general population in US while in Korea it has been successful. It is a very expensive technique: robotic system, regular maintenance fees, disposable equipment, costs associated to long anesthesia and operating times, and training surgeons. One potential drawback is multiglandular disease because whereas total thyroidectomy can be performed through a single axilla, bilateral parathyroid exploration required a bilateral axillary approach. The main advantage remains in the cosmetic outcome [39].

## 14.2 Indications

The key to successful MIP is careful patient selection and confident preoperative localization techniques [14]. Their development has been facilitated by improvement preoperative localization imaging such as 99mTc-sestamibi scintigraphy with single-positron emission computed tomography (SPECT), ultrasonography and intraoperative parathyroid hormone assays (IOPTH) [40, 41].

Particularly the three following conditions are more than wishful for minimally approach and especially for EMIP:

- Concordance between morphological and functional imaging studies able to identify pathological parathyroid.
- IOPTH able to confirm success of surgery with substantial fall in the PTH levels after adenoma excision. This is a highly accurate technique with a success rate of 95–98 %. Falling of more 50 % of maximum preexcision PTH level is considered significant but persistence more than 50 % after adenoma excision predicts the existence of secreting abnormal parathyroid tissue. In this case, it is necessary to continue surgical exploration. In our experience, it is determined at intubation, incision, removal of parathyroid adenoma, and 5, 15, and 30 min after excision [14, 42, 43].
- Specific surgical instruments.

Concordant positive imaging is necessary prelude for focused parathyroidectomy to confirm a solitary lesion [44]. For patients with suspicion of multiglandular parathyroid disease, a negative preoperative imaging, with concomitant goiter necessitating surgical treatment, previous neck surgery, familial hyperparathyroidism, lithium therapy, the bilateral neck exploration is the preferred surgical technique. The size of adenoma may be a limit but resection of large and slender adenomas more 3 cm is possible in particular when they develop in the posterosuperior mediastinum [34].

Also suspicion of parathyroid gland cancer is an absolute contraindication [30, 37]. There is a consensus that appropriate patient selection for single gland disease is the key of successful targeted parathyroidectomy. Generally these selected patients are 50–75 % of all patients with PHPT. According to our experience for totally endoscopic lateral approach this percentage is 56 % in a large series of 644 patients [29, 45].

Endoscopic parathyroidectomy has some advantages for several reasons:

- Extensive neck dissection is not required
- Most parathyroid lesions are small and benign
- Aesthetic result is satisfactory

The lateral endoscopic parathyroidectomy is the approach of choice for the posteriorly located parathyroid glands, especially for the superior parathyroid glands (P IV) when, as pathological, they tend to migrate posteriorly and to descend into the posterosuperior mediastinum. This approach seems also suitable for dissection of some inferior parathyroid glands (PIII) located at the posterior side of the inferior thyroid pole. In this situation, high volume adenomas tend to be in contact with the recurrent inferior laryngeal nerve. With this approach, it is easy to identify the recurrent laryngeal nerve and perform safe surgery [34].

## 14.3 Experience and Complications

According to our experience, endoscopic techniques have proved to be superior because they are able to show anatomical structures greater and better with optical magnification and light improvement than conventional open surgery. It is likely that with mini-incisions there is inadequate vision without endoscope and it is our belief that optimal conditions for exploration are not met, even if those surgeons use frontal lamps and surgical loops. At the beginning of our experience, we have listed permanent recurrent laryngeal nerve palsy for one patient; at that time, after endoscopic mobilizing and liberation of adenoma, the section of vascular pedicle was not totally endoscopic but with open approach; the thyroid lobe was retracted medially and anteriorly and vascular pedicle was sectioned openly after clipping. We believe that involved mechanism of injury was probably due to the damage occurred during extraction of parathyroid adenoma as vascular pedicle was dissected in the absence of endoscopic vision. Usually recurrent laryngeal nerve is properly identified during endoscopic surgical dissection. According to literature [46] that reports rates of nerve injury equal to 1–2 %, we have observed a reduction in recurrent nerve palsy when parathyroidectomy is fully endoscopic and especially after the use of intraoperative nerve monitoring (IONM). We believe that maneuvers of extraction can be dangerous as already described in the literature about minimally invasive thyroidectomy in which nerve recurrent palsy can occur during extraction of lobe from the mini-incision [47]. The monitoring of inferior laryngeal nerve has become a practice commonly used in thyroid surgery. There is no support to visualize nerve but allows to evaluate preoperative and per operative status and establish prognosis in case of occurrence of laryngeal nerve palsy (LNP). In the literature, it is reported a decrease of transient LNP with monitoring compared to only identification of nerve without use IONM [48–50]. The visualization of inferior laryngeal nerve remains the main factor preserving nerve function and decrease LNP [48]. In our experience, introduction of the use of IONM has facilitated the use of endoscopic lateral approach.

According to our experience, not all patients with PHPT are candidate for this surgical approach. The failures of this approach are observed in patients with multiglandular adenomas, supernumerary glands, major ectopia, previous thyroid/parathyroid surgery. Today the mortality of this surgery tends to zero. Morbidity is very low. Hospital stay rarely exceeds 48 h and scar results are excellent in most patients.

The demonstration of meaningful advantages for EMIP over OMIP is not easy. Despite the increasing interest in MIP over the last few years, there is no published prospective randomized series comparing the two techniques. It will be very difficult to challenge the results of both techniques as most advantages consist of subjective aspects, such as satisfaction of the scar and level of postoperative comfort. The potential advantage of EMIP is the greater and better surgical visualization provided with by the endoscope. Whether the endoscope is better than a pair of 2.5× or 3.5× magnifying loops to identify anatomical structures is difficult to prove. But EMIP offers not only a magnified view of anatomical details but it offers also a perfect lighting of the area of dissection. The quality of the light provided by the endoscope is undoubtedly superior to the one obtained with frontal lamps. In OMIP, surgical exploration is limited and hindered by the length of the skin incision: the shorter the skin incision, the more difficult the OMIP. This is particularly true for deep-located parathyroid adenomas in patients with large and short necks. This explains in general skin incisions of OMIP are longer than skin incisions of EMIP. OMIP requires an incision of at least 2.5–3 cm long. In EMIP, the length of the incision is determined by the size of the trocars only, that is 12–15 mm maximum for a 10 mm trocar or less than 10 mm for a 5 mm trocar. One can argue that pure EMIP, performed with gas insufflation, requires additional trocars but these trocars are 2.5 mm in section and do not leave any significant scar in the neck [33]. In our opinion, the main interest of using an endoscope is not that one can perform a parathyroidectomy through a small incision, but that one can perform a safe parathyroidectomy through a small incision [7].

Superior parathyroid glands are grouped at the posterior aspect of the thyroid lobe and when they are enlarged they always tend to migrate posteriorly and in a downward direction. Consequently, the superior parathyroid adenomas themselves or their pedicles are always in close proximity to the nerve.

The territory of inferior parathyroid glands is much more extensive. In 61 % of cases, they are situated at the level of the inferior pole of the thyroid lobes, on the posterior, lateral or anterior aspects. In 26 % of cases, they are situated in the thyrothymic ligament or in the upper, cervical portion of the thymus [33, 51]. Adenomas located at the posterolateral part of the inferior pole of the thyroid lobe tend to descend posteriorly and in a downward direction to acquire a paratracheal or a paraesophageal position. It is in these cases that they become intimate with the recurrent laryngeal nerve. Other inferior parathyroid adenomas remain located superficially in the neck or in the superior mediastinum. During their dissection, the nerve is not at risk as it runs more posteriorly. We need to know preoperatively when the nerve is at risk, that reinforces the role of imaging studies to localize deep-seated adenomas. Therefore both ultrasonography and sestamibi scan are very helpful. These two localization studies are complementary, particularly when adenomas are located at the level of the inferior thyroid pole. At this level, it is very important to differentiate deeply located adenoma from superficially located adenomas.

The lateral approach is the procedure of choice in most cases because it allows access to the posterior surface of ipsilateral thyroid lobe. The working space is easily created with minimal dissection and maintained with low pressure of CO2 at 8 mmHg. We have not observed subcutaneous emphysema or pneumomediastinum. The lateral approach also permits a complete exploration of all anatomical structures in retro-thyroidal area from the superior vascular pedicle to the posterosuperior mediastinum. It is therefore indicated in all cases where the parathyroid adenoma is located posteriorly, as glands slide along the prevertebral plane next to the lateral esophageal border, usually for heavy superior parathyroid glands. The lateral approach is also indicated for inferior parathyroid glands located posterior to the inferior thyroid poles. This approach permits an easy and excellent identification of the laryngeal inferior nerve in contact with the adenoma and therefore allows a safe dissection. Surgeons with limited experience or in case of large adenomas (>3 cm) can encounter major difficulties that may lead to capsular rupture and local seeding of parathyroid adenomatous cells. In this case, the conversion is recommended [52].

## 14.4 Management of Complications

In case of complications, endoscopic parathyroidectomy can be converted. Hessman et al. in his series of 68 patients undergone to EMIP reported a conversion rate of 25 %. The causes were bleeding, difficulties in adenoma localization, and difficult dissection [5]. In our experience, conversion rate is 13 % among 365 patients. The causes were adenoma not found even if preoperative localized, insufficient fall of IOPTH, sestamibi and ultrasonography false positive results, difficult dissection, and multiglandular disease [45].

### Conclusions

In the past two decades, the approach for parathyroidectomy has undergone a major shift from bilateral cervical exploration to a focused approach [8]. Several studies reported success and cure rates of focused approaches similar to that of bilateral cervical exploration [40]. However, minimally invasive and focused approaches are associated with significant reduction in complication rates, incision length, operative time, and length of hospital stay [40]. Once contraindications have been eliminated, all patients with sporadic primary HPT can be considered candidates for MIP. Contrary to open surgery in which the surgeon relying on himself can have a success rate of more of 95 %, video-assisted surgery depends on special surgical instruments, rapid PTH assay and preoperative imaging concordance. Among many minimally invasive techniques applied to parathyroidectomy, the video-assisted technique has the main advantage to offer magnification images able to permit a precise and careful dissection with minimal risks. The use of the endoscope could be recommended when the parathyroid adenoma becomes intimate with the recurrent laryngeal nerve, when the adenoma is located in the retro-thyroidal area. In our opinion, mini-open approaches using a skin incision of less than 2.5–3 cm should be used only when there is no need to identify the nerve during the dissection, when the adenoma is superficially located in the neck.

Minimally invasive surgery requires competent and experienced surgeon. We think that pure endoscopic techniques allow a wider exposure of cervical structures than video-assisted gasless techniques. In addition, insufflation with CO2 creates a working space in which anatomical structures can be identified without distortion caused by mechanic retraction. In our opinion, the endoscopic lateral approach [45] provides the best access to the posterior aspect of the thyroid lobe. It permits a complete exploration of all anatomical elements of the retro-thyroidal area from the superior pedicle to the posterosuperior mediastinum. It is therefore applicable in all cases where the parathyroid adenoma is located posteriorly. Today the parathyroid surgeon is dependent upon the quality and the adequate interpretation of preoperative imaging to make a judicious choice for different procedures of MIP. Once contraindications have been eliminated, all patients with sporadic primary HPT can be considered candidates for MIP. The endoscopic parathyroidectomy has excellent results regarding hospital stay, postoperative time, and cosmetic results. This approach should not be opposed to conventional parathyroidectomy and should be reserved for patients with sporadic PHPT, with a single adenoma clearly localizated preoperatively. It has the main advantage of magnified view that permits a precise and careful dissection with minimal risks and it is particularly suitable for adenomas located posteriorly in the neck [52].

## References

1. Mandl F (1926) Klinisches und Experimenteles zur Frage der lakalisierten und generalisiereten Osteitis Fibrosa. Arch Klin Chir 143:1
2. Delbridge LW, Palazzo FF (2007) First parathyroid surgeon: Sir John Bland-Sutton and the parathyroids. ANZ J Surg 77(12):1058–1061
3. Fraser WD (2009) Hyperparathyroidism. Lancet 374(9684):145–158
4. Inabnet WB et al (2002) Targeted parathyroidectomy in the era of intraoperative parathormone monitoring. World J Surg 26(8):921–925
5. Hessman O et al (2010) Randomized clinical trial comparing open with video-assisted minimally invasive parathyroid surgery for primary hyperparathyroidism. Br J Surg 97:177–184
6. Tibblin SA et al (1982) Unilateral parathyroidectomy in hyperparathyroidism due to single adenoma. Ann Surg 195(3):245–252
7. Van Heerden JA, Grant CS (1991) Surgical treatment of primary hyperparathyroidism: an institutional perspective. World J Surg 15(6):688, 692
8. Wang TS et al (2014) Techniques of parathyroid exploration at North American endocrine surgery fellowship programs: what the next generation is being taught. Am J Surg 207(4): 527–532
9. Henry JF, Thakur A (2010) Minimal access surgery – thyroid and parathyroid. Indian J Surg Oncol 1(2):200–206
10. Prinz RA et al (1994) Thoracoscopic excision of enlarged mediastinal parathyroid glands. Surgery 116:999–1004
11. Russel CF et al (1990) Scan-directed unilateral cervical exploration for parathyroid adenoma: a legitime approach? World J Surg 14:406–409
12. Seving AI et al (2010) Success of minimally invasive single-gland exploration using the quick intraoperative parathyroid assay. Acta Chir Belg 110(4):463–466
13. Chapuis Y et al (1993) Peroperative assay of parathyroid hormone 1–84. Is the unilateral approach under local anesthesia justified in surgery for primary hyperparathyroidism? Chirurgie 1993–1994 119(4):230–232
14. Sackett WR et al (2002) Worldwide trends in the surgical treatment of primary hyperparathyroidism in the era of minimally invasive parathyroidectomy. Arch Surg 137(9):1055–1059

15. Bellantone R et al (2011) Minimally-invasive parathyroid surgery. Acta Otorhinolaryngol Ital 31(4):207–215
16. Greene AB et al (2009) National trends in parathyroid surgery from 1998 to 2008: a decade of change. J Am Coll Surg 209(3):332–343
17. Norman J, Chheda H (1997) Minimally invasive parathyroidectomy facilitated by intraoperative nuclear mapping. Surgery 122:998–1004, 1007
18. Burkey SH et al (2002) Will directed parathyroidectomy utilizing the gamma probe or intraoperative parathyroid hormone assay replace bilateral cervical exploration as the preferred operation for primary hyperparathyroidism? World J Surg 26:914–920
19. Udelsman R et al (2000) One hundred consecutive minimally invasive parathyroid explorations. Ann Surg 232(3):331–339
20. Ikeda Y et al (2002) Direct mini-incision parathyroidectomy. Biomed Pharmacother 56(Suppl 1): 14s–17s
21. Agarwal G et al (2002) Minimally invasive parathyroidectomy using the 'focused' lateral approach. II. Surgical technique. ANZ J Surg 72(2):147–151
22. Stalberg P et al (2007) Minimally invasive parathyroidectomy and thyroidectomy–current concepts. Surgeon 5:301–308
23. Miccoli P et al (1999) Video-assisted versus conventional parathyroidectomy in primary hyperparathyroidism: a prospective randomized study. Surgery 126:1117–1122
24. Miccoli P et al (1997) Minimally invasive, video-assisted parathyroid surgery for primary hyperparathyroidism. J Endocrinol Invest 20(7):429–430
25. Gagner M, Rubino F (2004) Endoscopic parathyroidectomy. In: Schwartz AE, Pertsemlidis D, Gagner M (eds) Endocrine surgery. Marcel Dekker, New York, pp 289–296
26. Henry JF (1999) Endoscopic exploration. In: Van Heerden JA, Farley DR (eds) Operative technique in general surgery. Surgical exploration for hyperparathyroidism. WB Saunders, Philadelphia, pp 49–61
27. Gagner M (1996) Endoscopic parathyroidectomy. Br J Surg 83:87511–87521
28. Suzuki S et al (2002) Video-assisted parathyroidectomy. Biomed Pharmacother 56(suppl 1):18s–21s
29. Fouquet T et al (2010) Totally endoscopic lateral parathyroidectomy: prospective evaluation of 200 patients. ESES, Vienna presentation. Langenbecks Arch Surg 395(7):935–940
30. Papier A et al (2014) Bilateral neck exploration with intraoperative iPTH assay in patients not eligible for minimally invasive parathyroidectomy. Przegl Lek 71(2):66–71
31. Henry JF et al (2001) Video-assisted parathyroidectomy via lateral approach versus conventional surgery in the treatment of sporadic primary hyperparathyroidism. Results of a case–control study. Surg Endosc 15:1116–1119
32. Miccoli P et al (2003) Minimally invasive video assisted parathyroidectomy (MIVAP). EJSO 29:188–190
33. Henry JF et al (2008) Endoscopic parathyroidectomy: why and when? World J Surg 32(11):2509–2515
34. Henry JF, Sebag F (2006) Lateral endoscopic approach for thyroid and parathyroid surgery. Ann Chir 131(1):51–56
35. Okido M et al (2001) Video-assisted parathyroidectomy for primary hyperparathyroidism: an approach involving a skin-lifting method. Surg Endosc 15:1120–1123
36. Henry JF et al (2001) Indications and results of video-assisted parathyroidectomy by a lateral approach in patients with primary hyperparathyroidism. Surgery 130(6):999–1004
37. Henry JF et al (1999) Endoscopic parathyroidectomy via a lateral neck incision. Ann Chir 53(4):302–306
38. Lee J et al (2010) The learning curve for robotic thyroidectomy: a multicenter study. Ann Surg Oncol 18:226–232
39. Foley CS et al (2012) Robotic transaxillary endocrine surgery: a comparison with conventional open technique. Surg Endosc 26(8):2259–2266
40. Karakas E et al (2014) Initial surgery for benign primary hyperparathyroidism: an analysis of 1.300 patients in a teaching hospital. World J Surg 38(8):2011–2018

41. Padma KS et al (2013) Feasibility of rapid parathormone assay for enabling minimally invasive parathyroid excision. Indian J Surg 75(3):210–215
42. Irvin GL et al (1993) Clinical usefulness of an intraoperative "quick parathyroid hormone" assay. Surgery 114(6):1019–1022; discussion 1022–1023
43. Carneiro DM et al (2003) Comparison of intraoperative iPTH assay (QPTH) criteria in guiding parathyroidectomy: which criterion is the most accurate? Surgery 134(6):973–979; discussion 979–981
44. Philippon M et al (2014) Bilateral neck exploration in patients with primary hyperparathyroidism and discordant imaging results: a single-centre study. Eur J Endocrinol 170(5):719–725
45. Henry JF et al (2004) Endoscopic parathyroid surgery: results of 365 consecutive procedures. World J Surg 28:1219–1223
46. Kandil E et al (2009) Minimally invasive video-assisted thyroidectomy and parathyroidectomy with intraoperative recurrent laryngeal nerve monitoring. Int J Otolaryngol 2009:739798
47. Dionigi G et al (2012) Recurrent laryngeal nerve injury in video-assisted thyroidectomy: lessons learned from neuromonitoring. Surg Endosc 26(9):2601–2608
48. Périé S et al (2013) Value of recurrent laryngeal nerve monitoring in the operative strategy during total thyroidectomy and parathyroidectomy. Eur Ann Otorhinolaryngol Head Neck Dis 130(3):131–136
49. Barczy′nski M et al (2009) Randomized clinical trial of visualization versus neuromonitoring of recurrent laryngeal nerves during thyroidectomy. Br J Surg 96:240–246
50. Moroni E et al (2007) Intraoperative neuromonitoring of the recurrent laryngeal nerve. Experience of 1000 consecutive patients. G Chir 28:29–34
51. Akerstrom G et al (1984) Surgical anatomy of human parathyroid glands. Surgery 95:14–21
52. Henry JH, Sebag F (2011) Endoscopic parathyroidectomy. In: Clark OH, Duh QY, Kebebew E (eds) Textbook of endocrine surgery. Saunders, Philadelphia, pp 467–471, Chapter 51

# Minimally Invasive Video-Assisted Neck Dissection

# 15

Emanuela Traini, Luca Sessa, Carmela De Crea, Celestino Pio Lombardi, and Rocco Bellantone

## 15.1 Introduction

During the last decade minimally invasive video-assisted thyroidectomy (MIVAT) gained more and more consent among endocrine surgeons to treat selected patients with thyroid disorders requiring surgery.

The key of its success mainly lies in its close similarity to traditional surgery which has tempted also surgeons not used to laparoscopy.

The endoscope, indeed, represents only a tool that allows performing the traditional intervention through a very minimal skin incision [1–5] and guarantees, with its two- to threefold magnification, an excellent visualization of the delicate anatomical structures of the neck which must be preserved.

As described in detail in another chapter of this handbook, the indications for MIVAT changed in the course of time.

At the beginning of the experience, suspicious cytology and evidence of suspicious lymph node involvement represented a contraindication for a video-assisted approach.

Nonetheless, after an adequate period of development, validation and standardization of the technique we [6, 7], as well as other authors [8], have proposed MIVAT also for the treatment of patients with small "low-risk" papillary thyroid carcinoma (PTC) [9].

The excellent oncological results, in terms of adequacy of resection and safety, led some authors to progressively apply MIVAT also for the treatment of differentiated

E. Traini (✉) • L. Sessa • C. De Crea • C.P. Lombardi • R. Bellantone
Unità Operativa Di Chirurgia Endocrina E Metabolica,
Università Cattolica Del Sacro Cuore, Roma, Largo Agostino Gemelli, 8,
Rome, RM 00168, Italy
e-mail: emanuela.traini@rm.unicatt.it; lucasessa83@gmail.com;
carmela.decrea@rm.unicatt.it; cp.lombardi@rm.unicatt.it; rbellantone@rm.unicatt.it



C.P. Lombardi, R. Bellantone (eds.), *Minimally Invasive Therapies for Endocrine Neck Diseases*, DOI 10.1007/978-3-319-20065-1_15

thyroid carcinomas (DTCs), starting from the so-called "low-risk" tumours to the "intermediate-risk" ones, which now represent optimal targets for this approach [9].

The increasing experience in this field and the demonstration of the oncological completeness of the video-assisted approach in selected cases have convinced some authors to try a concomitant central compartment lymphadenectomy and to experimentally test a video-assisted approach for lateral compartment lymphadenectomy.

### 15.1.1 Video-Assisted Central Compartment Dissection (VA-CCD)

Central compartment lymph node metastases, often microscopic, are frequent in patients with PTC [6, 7, 9–12] and in RET gene mutation carriers [13]. Nonetheless, according to the current international guidelines prophylactic central compartment dissection in case of DTC is not mandatory and it should be performed only in case of suspicious lymph node involvement [11, 12].

A macroscopic preoperatively identified lymph node involvement in case of PTC has been always considered an absolute contraindication for a video-assisted approach.

However, it is difficult to assess, with accuracy, the status of central compartment in a preoperative setting and the unexpected intraoperative finding of VI level lymph node enlargement during thyroidectomy for cancer is rather frequent.

In these cases enlarged lymph nodes should be removed in order to clarify the node status and sometimes to obtain a node clearance.

Since the first application of MIVAT to treat DTCs with no preoperative evidence of lymph node involvement, several times we have faced enlarged lymph nodes which required to be removed.

After obtained a certain expertise with the technique and supported by the evidence of safety and completeness of oncological resection of the video-assisted approach [6, 7], we tried to carry out a VA-CCD in patients undergone MIVAT for PTC or suspicious thyroid nodules with unexpected intraoperative finding of lymph node enlargement.

In 2002, we reported the results of our preliminary experience [10] on 5 patients who underwent removal of enlarged central neck lymph nodes incidentally discovered during MIVAT for PTC. We decided to remove only enlarged lymph nodes for frozen section. The mean number of removed lymph nodes was $2.4 \pm 1.3$ (range 1–4). Frozen section examination showed inflammatory and reactive changes in all the examined nodes so we decided not to go on completing the central compartment lymphadenectomy. For what concerns operative time, lymph node dissection added about 15 min to the time required for thyroidectomy in all the cases. We registered two cases of transient postoperative hypocalcemia requiring calcium and vitamin D oral administration. No other complications occurred. Final histology confirmed the absence of metastases in the examined lymph nodes. Through this first experience VA-CCD demonstrated to be feasible and safe with no additional risks of complication and with additional advantages in terms of better cosmetic result and less postoperative discomfort.

When we judge the results of this preliminary experience, especially with respect to the operative time, the fact that it represented the first application of this approach to perform central node dissection should be taken into consideration. Indeed, a certain learning and training period to become confident with a new surgical technique is necessary. To date the time required to perform VA-CCD is nearly the same registered for open surgery.

After this preliminary report many other papers concerning the results of VA-CCD in case of patients with PTC [6, 7, 9, 14–17] and in RET gene mutation carriers [13] have been published. By the way, all of them represented the report of experiences of different centres on relatively small series of patients.

Despite these encouraging results, some experts remained hesitant in accepting MIVAT as valid option to treat thyroid cancer [18]. One of the criticisms raised against the video-assisted approach concerned just the possibility to guarantee a surgical completeness performing a systematic central compartment lymphadenectomy, when necessary [18].

The lacking, in literature, of comparative studies specifically addressing the oncological results of VA-CCD in comparison with the conventional procedure led us to compare two groups of patients with PTC and similar epidemiologic and pathologic features who underwent, respectively, video-assisted (52 cases) and conventional (52 cases) central neck node dissection [19].

The mean follow-up time was comparable. All the patients underwent the same postoperative management and therapeutic protocol as previously described in detail [7, 9, 10, 14].

In all the included cases the decision to perform the central neck node dissection relied on the surgeon's intraoperative assessment of the nodal status. Indeed all the patients were considered N0 (node-negative) according to the preoperative evaluation.

The incidence of node metastases was 50 % and 46 %, respectively, in video-assisted and conventional groups. No statistically significant differences were found between the two groups in terms of mean operative time, complication rate, lesion size and number of removed lymph nodes as well as in terms of number of the metastatic lymph nodes at histology. Also the comparative analysis of the follow-up data showed no significant differences between the two groups in terms of mean sTg levels off LT4 suppressive treatment and mean postoperative quantitative $^{131}$I neck uptake obtained prior to $^{131}$I ablation.

The results of this study confirmed previous knowledge about the safety of the video-assisted technique and clearly demonstrated that the completeness of surgical resection of the two groups was similar, regardless of the surgical approach.

The two techniques showed also the same results in terms of patient outcome at short-medium follow-up. Despite the results of this approach are encouraging, further controlled studies are necessary to evaluate the long-term results.

From a pure technical point of view it should be considered that the endoscope shows specific advantages. Indeed it allows meticulous exploration of the central compartment, and enables identification of even slightly enlarged lymph nodes that might be overlooked at open surgery. In other words the endoscope might make easier the identification of potentially metastatic lymph nodes during the video-assisted procedure.

This advantage might play a certain role if we think that, at the present moment, no imaging methods are available to preoperatively evaluate, with high accuracy, the central compartment lymph nodes involvement [20]. The most widespread imaging technique used to assess the node status in patients with PTC is ultrasonography, but it is operator-dependent and it can identify only a small portion of lymph nodes found at surgical exploration because of the small size of lymph nodes, the interference of the thyroid gland or for certain unfavourable anatomic situations (e.g. obese patients, short necks, etc.).

On the other hand the endoscope, with its optical magnification, guarantees a good exposure of the neck structures allowing for a careful dissection that is very important when dealing with structures at high risk of injury like inferior laryngeal nerves and parathyroid glands that are extensively exposed and dissected when the central neck lymphadenectomy is carried on.

The advantages that might be expected from VA-CCD are the same that have been already demonstrated for other video-assisted operations like MIVAT and minimally invasive video-assisted parathyroidectomy (MIVAP), described in other chapters of this book. These advantages are not only the cosmetic outcome but also the reduction of postoperative pain and analgesic requirements.

### 15.1.2 Video-Assisted Lateral Neck Dissection (VALNED)

Supported by the results of video-assisted approach for selected cases of DTC and encouraged by the results of VA-CCD we also evaluated the feasibility of a minimally invasive video-assisted approach to the functional lateral neck dissection (VALNED) in patients with PTC. We considered eligible two patients with low-risk PTC and lateral neck nodal metastases < 2 cm, without evidence of great vessels involvement. One patient underwent bilateral and one patient unilateral VALNED. The mean number of removed nodes was 25 per side. Both patients experienced transient hypocalcemia. No other complications were registered. No evidence of residual tissue or recurrent disease was found at follow-up [21]. These results are encouraging but it should be considered a preliminary experience that shows only the feasibility of the technique. For definitive conclusions, larger series and comparative studies are necessary.

## 15.2 Indications

An accurate patients' selection plays a relevant role to ensure the success of any video-assisted procedure, especially at the beginning of the experience.

At the present moment, ideal candidates for video-assisted approach are patients with small low-intermediate risk DTC and RET gene mutation carriers who have no preoperative evidence of lymph node metastases.

Among these, the results of the studies mentioned above demonstrated that VA-CCD can be carried out with equivalent outcomes of conventional operation if unexpected suspicious or simply enlarged lymph nodes are found out during MIVAT.

Since we are aware of the need to investigate patients' cohorts with longer follow-up to draw definitive conclusions about the capability of VA-CCD to guarantee an unequivocal node clearance, for the time being the overt lymph node involvement remains a contraindication for video-assisted procedure. Furthermore we consider mandatory the conversion in conventional approach when an accurate node clearance cannot be obtained.

Obviously to obtain the best results, with similar or even less complication rate than conventional intervention, a good patients selection is not sufficient. Surgeons, indeed, should be well trained in both endocrine and endoscopic surgery [22–24].

To date no indications may be expressed for VALNED that should be considered, for the time being, only an experience to test its feasibility.

## 15.3 Surgical Technique

VA-CCD represents the completion of MIVAT. Therefore the endoscopic instrumentation is the same. On this subject it should be stressed the crucial role of the camera and the importance of the availability of the Harmonic scalpel. The camera, in video-assisted techniques, is free from trocars fixing it in a stable position. As previously described for MIVAT and MIVAP, the camera is handled by an assistant who can change his position rotating the 30° degree camera in order to better expose all the sites the operator wants to explore, for example, the upper mediastinum, maintaining, at the same time, an optimal vision of laryngeal nerves and parathyroid glands during all the procedure (Fig. 15.1).

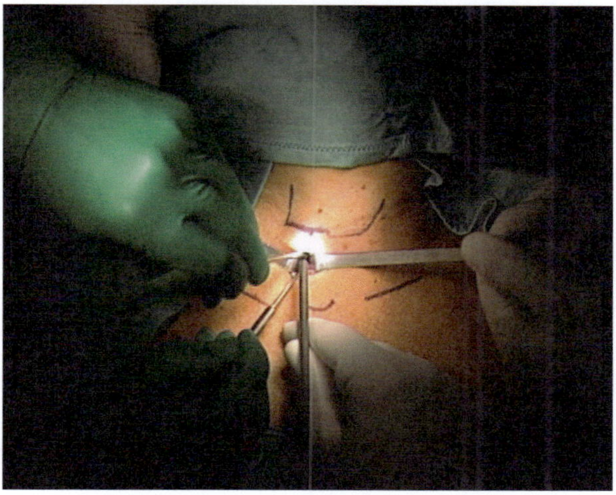

**Fig. 15.1** The camera is handled by an assistant who can rotate it in order to better expose the site of dissection

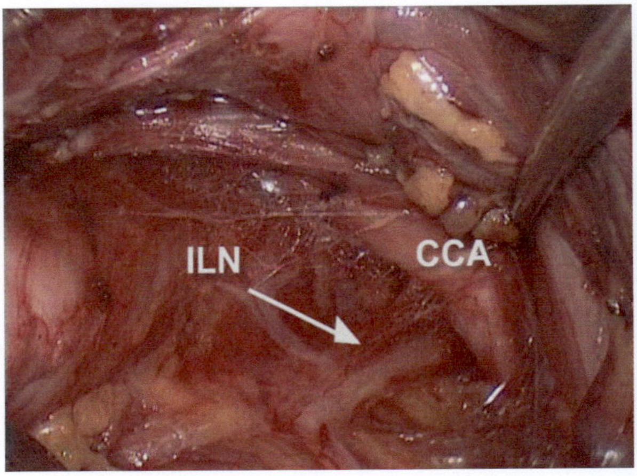


**Fig. 15.2** The magnification (two- to threefold) of the endoscope permits a quite easy identification of the nerves and parathyroid glands. *ILN* inferior laryngeal nerve; *CCA* common carotid artery

Harmonic scalpel is particularly useful when a VA-CCD is carried out because it can easily coagulate and cut all the lymphatic vessels, reducing the operating time and the risk of lymphatic leaks.

For what concerns the patient position and the composition of the surgical staff we refer to the chapter describing MIVAT.

For VA-CCD general anaesthesia with orotracheal intubation is required.

VA-CCD is accomplished, during MIVAT, through the same skin access, a small (1.5–2 cm) skin incision performed in the midline, usually just below (1 cm) the cricoid cartilage. Such a cranial position of the skin incision, that is of utmost importance to perform MIVAT because it permits a good exposure and a safe control of the superior vessels peduncle, does not represent an obstacle to approach the lymph nodes located in the upper mediastinum. In fact an optimal preparation of the upper and lower subcutaneous flaps, consents to open the cervical *linea alba* as far as possible and permits the small skin access to move on the deepest planes, under the skilled use of the retractors, letting the endoscopic instruments and the camera easily reach both the upper six level lymph nodes and the lower ones. In such a way it is possible to perform a complete VI level neck dissection removing all the lymph nodes and the fatty tissue from the bone hyoid superiorly, the innominate artery inferiorly, the pre-vertebral fascia dorsally, and between carotid arteries laterally [25].

The dissection is carried out by a blunt technique using the same two dedicated instruments called spatulas, previously mentioned for MIVAT. VA-CCD is carried out under endoscopic vision, selectively clipping and cutting, or directly cutting with an ultrasound knife system (Ultracision®), the lymphatic vessels. It is very important to accurately control the tip of the instrument to avoid any injury of the recurrent nerves and trachea. The magnification (two- to threefold) of the endoscope permits a quite easy identification of the nerves and parathyroid glands (Fig. 15.2).

Nonetheless, as highlighted above in our introduction, the endoscope enables the identification of enlarged lymph nodes and consequently not only influences the

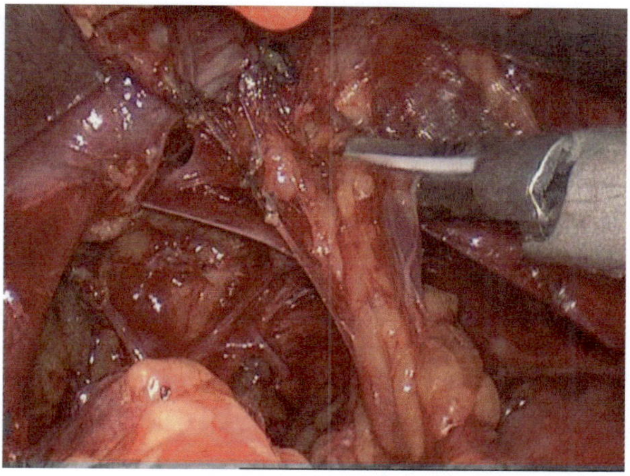

**Fig. 15.3** The endoscope enables the identification of enlarged lymph nodes allowing a more accurate dissection

surgeon's decision making but, during the procedure, allows a more accurate dissection (Fig. 15.3).

After checking the haemostasis the strap muscles are sutured along the midline as well as the platysma. The skin is closed by means of a not re-absorbable subcuticular running suture or by a skin sealant. Usually no drainage is left inside.

## 15.4 Personal Experience and Complications

A total of 161 VA-CCD were attempted between January 2000 and June 2014. No conversion to the conventional procedure was necessary.

Pathological studies showed DTC pT1 in 101 cases, pT2 in 6 cases and pT3 in 54 cases. Lymph node metastases were found in 79 patients (41 pT1, 2 pT2, 36 pT3).

Postoperative complications included 2 cases of transient (1.2 %) recurrent laryngeal nerve palsy, 63 cases of transient hypocalcemia (39.1 %) and 3 cases of definitive hypoparathyroidism (1.8 %). No definitive recurrent laryngeal nerve palsy, no postoperative hematoma and no wound infection occurred.

## References


1. Bellantone R, Lombardi CP, Raffaelli M et al (1999) Minimally invasive, totally gasless video-assisted thyroid lobectomy. Am J Surg 177:342–343
2. Miccoli P, Berti P, Bendinelli C et al (2000) Minimally invasive video-assisted surgery of the thyroid: a preliminary report. Langenbecks Arch Surg 385:261–264
3. Mourad M, Saab N, Malaise J et al (2001) Minimally invasive video-assisted approach for partial and total thyroidectomy: initial experience. Surg Endosc 15:1108–1111
4. Bellantone R, Lombardi CP, Raffaelli M et al (2002) Video-assisted thyroidectomy. J Am Coll Surg 194:610–614
5. Miccoli P, Berti P, Raffaelli M et al (2000) Minimally invasive video-assisted thyroidectomy. Am J Surg 181:567–570

6. Bellantone R, Lombardi CP, Raffaelli M et al (2003) Video-assisted thyroidectomy for papillary thyroid carcinoma. Surg Endosc 17:1604–1608
7. Lombardi CP, Raffaelli M, de Crea C et al (2007) Report on 8 years of experience with video-assisted thyroidectomy for papillary thyroid carcinoma. Surgery 142:944–951
8. Miccoli P, Elisei R, Materazzi G et al (2002) Minimally invasive video-assisted thyroidectomy for papillary carcinoma: a prospective study of its completeness. Surgery 132:1070–1074
9. Lombardi CP, Raffaelli M, De Crea C et al (2010) Video-assisted thyroidectomy for papillary thyroid carcinoma. J Oncol. doi:10.1155/2010/148542
10. Bellantone R, Lombardi CP, Raffaelli M et al (2002) Central neck lymph node removal during minimally invasive video-assisted thyroidectomy for thyroid carcinoma: a feasible and safe procedure. J Laparoendosc Adv Surg Tech A 12:181–185
11. Kebebew E, Clark OH (2000) Differentiated thyroid cancer: "complete" rational approach. World J Surg 24:942–951
12. Mirallié E, Visset J, Sagan C et al (1999) Localization of cervical node metastasis of papillary thyroid carcinoma. World J Surg 23:970–974
13. Miccoli P, Elisei R, Donatini G et al (2007) Video-assisted central compartment lymphadenectomy in a patient with a positive RET oncogene: initial experience. Surg Endosc 21:120–123
14. Miccoli P, Pinchera A, Materazzi G et al (2009) Surgical treatment of low- and intermediate-risk papillary thyroid cancer with minimally invasive video-assisted thyroidectomy. J Clin Endocrinol Metab 94:1618–1622
15. Wu CT, Yang LH, Kuo SJ (2010) Comparison of video-assisted thyroidectomy and traditional thyroidectomy for the treatment of papillary thyroid carcinoma. Surg Endosc 24:1658–1662
16. Seybt MW, Terris DJ (2010) Minimally invasive thyroid cancer surgery. Minerva Chir 65:36–43
17. Neidich MJ, Steward DL (2012) Safety and feasibility of elective minimally invasive video-assisted central neck dissection for thyroid carcinoma. Head Neck 34:354–358
18. Duh QY (2003) Presidential address: minimally invasive endocrine surgery – standard treatment of treatment or hype? Surgery 134:849–857
19. Lombardi CP, Raffaelli M, De Crea C et al (2012) Video-assisted versus conventional total thyroidectomy and central compartment neck dissection for papillary thyroid carcinoma. World J Surg 36:1225–1230
20. Mulla M, Schulte KM (2012) Central cervical lymph node metastases in papillary thyroid cancer: a systematic review of imaging-guided and prophylactic removal of the central compartment. Clin Endocrinol (Oxf) 76:131–136
21. Lombardi CP, Raffaelli M, Princi P et al (2007) Minimally invasive video-assisted functional lateral neck dissection for metastatic papillary thyroid carcinoma. Am J Surg 193:114–118
22. Miccoli P, Bellantone R, Mourad M et al (2002) Minimally invasive video-assisted thyroidectomy: multiinstitutional experience. World J Surg 26:972–975
23. Papavramidis TS, Michalopoulos N, Pliakos J et al (2010) Minimally invasive video-assisted total thyroidectomy: an easy to learn technique for skillful surgeons. Head Neck 32:1370–1376
24. Del Rio P, Sommaruga L, Cataldo S et al (2008) Minimally invasive video-assisted thyroidectomy: the learning curve. Eur Surg Res 41:33–36
25. Carty SE, Cooper DS, Doherty GM et al (2009) Consensus statement on the terminology and classification of central neck dissection for thyroid cancer. Thyroid 19:1153–1158

# Minimally Invasive Surgical Techniques: Critical Appraisal and Future Perspectives

16

Paolo Miccoli and Gabriele Materazzi

## 16.1 Parathyroidectomy

The possibility of very limited accesses to parathyroid adenomas on one side and the necessity of wide accesses in case of extensive explorations for hyperplasias, recurrent diseases, and carcinoma on the opposite side, has mostly limited the diffusion of endoscopic approaches to hyperparathyroidism (HPT), both primary and secondary. In fact, still the majority of surgeons do favor the so-called minimally invasive parathyroidectomy, which is characterized by an open targeted operation through a small incision [1]. In spite of this reluctance towards the use of endoscopy or other related techniques the minimally invasive parathyroidectomy (MIVAP) [2], which is probably the most widespread endoscopic technique [3], is used by several surgeons throughout the world [4]. Other endoscopic techniques lost most of their appeal either because they implied long insufflations of the neck [5] or because they only offered the chance of exploring one side of the neck due to their lateral access [6].

Moreover, other modalities of treatment have appeared recently such as high intensity focused ultrasound (HIFU) based on the capacity of an ultrasound beam to focus on a target and thus provoking a thermal necrosis of tissues. This technique has already been utilized for several pathologies such as prostate, uterus, pancreas, liver, etc. [7]. This same technique was also attempted in thyroid nodules [8], but the impossibility of having a histological information on these potentially malignant

P. Miccoli, MD (✉)
Department of Surgery, University of Pisa, Pisa, Italy
e-mail: paolo.miccoli@dc.unipi.it

G. Materazzi, MD
Department of Surgery, University of Pisa, Pisa, Italy

Dipartimento di Patologia Chirurgica, Medica, Molecolare e dell'Area Critica, Via Paradisa n 2, Pisa 56124, Italy
e-mail: gmaterazzi@yahoo.com



C.P. Lombardi, R. Bellantone (eds.), *Minimally Invasive Therapies for Endocrine Neck Diseases*, DOI 10.1007/978-3-319-20065-1_16

tumors limited very much its diffusion. In fact the parathyroid adenomas, having a very high probability of being benign (at least over 95 %), seemed very good candidates for this kind of nonsurgical treatment of primary HPT, where in most of the cases a single adenoma is involved in the disease [9]. Besides, the idea of treating both PHPT and secondary PHT with nonsurgical techniques had already been successfully established by some AA: the most popular being radiofrequency thermal ablation [10], ethanol injection [11], and ultrasound-guided laser thermal ablation [12]. All these technologies proved to be effective but they were used only sporadically in the treatment of HPT [9–12]. Alternatively, HIFU, which had proved to be so effective in treating some tumors of parenchymal organs, raised a great expectation in the field of parathyroid adenomas (PA), at least in their sporadic form [9].

In a pilot study set up by our Group [13] though, it was certainly possible to demonstrate the effectiveness of the procedure, but its safety was far from being ascertained: in fact, although the necrosis of the tissue was evident, and so was the stop of the hyper secretion of parathyroid hormone, also evidenced by both quick parathyroid hormone assay (qPTHa) and postoperative sestamibi scan in 3 out of 4 cases, a transient palsy of recurrent nerve was present. The latter lasted for few days, but it was considered as an intolerable complication rate and the study was interrupted. In spite of this disappointing result it cannot be excluded that with an appropriate refinement of this technique, when applied to PA, its side effects could be easily minimized. The problem of the relevant transmission of heat linked with any of the energy devices quoted above is consistent with the proximity of the recurrent nerve to PAs and cannot be by-passed, but some expedients could certainly improve the results in a significant way. A new assessment of the quantity of energy used on parathyroid tissue is necessary together with a better selection of patients: in order to reach this goal, it would be necessary to work out with more accuracy the presumed distance between adenoma and nerve, perhaps selecting only few inferior and anterior adenomas. Another issue to reduce the amount of energy could be to increase the number of sessions so as to use less energy during each application [13].

Once the criticism towards these minimally invasive techniques in parathyroid surgery has been expressed, the question to be addressed is: Can these approaches be considered still valid for the treatment of PHPT and which are their limitations? No doubt that all the nonsurgical approaches find a very limited application: probably they will remain an option only in cases where severe contraindications for surgery do exist; an example might be serious cardio vascular or respiratory diseases in elderly patients or advanced neoplastic patients who can sometimes present with a PHPT. Also serious renal insufficiency cases can occur with SHPT and even more with Tertiary HPT and these could be good candidates for such alternative techniques [10].

A further consideration though must be done for the general indications in PHPT surgery: most of the patients are now referred to the surgeon with a very clear indication and, above all, with a very accurate preoperative localization: which with a high degree of probability means the patient presents a sporadic adenoma [14] and no extensive exploration will be necessary. Then the effort to minimize the invasiveness of the surgery in all these cases, which besides represent the large majority of patients, has been widely justified, also making the standard open parathyroidectomy easily accessible for any surgeon: no doubt this operation can be performed through a small incision, using a lateral focused access, possibly facilitated by the use of qPTHa and this explains why it has been so successful [1, 2].

Considering this background, what might be the role today for MIVAP? In fact this is an operation which needs a learning curve [15] and a certain familiarity with the endoscopic procedures. According to the opinion of several AA [16–18] though, some important advantages are still evident in MIVAP. One of the most important to us is the possibility of exploring both sides [19] since this operation uses a central neck access; although this necessity quite rarely occurs, a bilateral exploration can prove to be of paramount importance in few selected cases. Also the possibility of performing the operation under local anesthesia makes MIVAP highly challenging when the surgeon has to choose a minimally invasive parathyroidectomy [20].

In conclusion, this operation which also has the great merit of having opened the way to all endoscopic surgery of the neck, after more than 20 years of life seems to be far from being abandoned, and, I would say, is here to stay.

## 16.2 Thyroidectomy

Traditional thyroidectomy is realized through a transverse cervical incision (Kocher's incision), and is associated with a very low morbidity and mortality rate. However, the scar remaining after the procedure, in such an exposed area as the neck, is disliked by many patients, also considering the main target of thyroid diseases: the female population. Therefore, in the early 1990s, after the introduction of laparoscopic/endoscopic surgery, which changed very quickly the attitude of many surgeons towards their operative behavior, countless new mini invasive techniques were soon proposed for almost any field of surgery and it was not difficult to imagine that endocrine surgery would not escape this fate.

The first report of an endoscopic parathyroidectomy was in 1996 by Gagner [5], even though a totally endoscopic approach soon appeared too technically demanding if compared to the simple standard parathyroidectomy. One year later, minimally invasive video-assisted parathyroidectomy [MIVAP], a gasless video-assisted technique firstly described in Italy [3], showed optimal results in a large series, concerning cosmetic and postoperative outcome. Following these encouraging results obtained by MIVAP, surgeons were pushed to try the same access and the same technique also for operations on thyroid [21] and first series of patients successfully undergone minimally invasive video-assisted thyroidectomy (MIVAT) were published [22]. In the mean time and for the following 10 years, several surgeons from different parts of the globe, aiming to give patients best cosmetic result a postoperative course, continued to devise and propose different endoscopic approaches for thyroid removal, describing remote accesses from axilla [23], breast [24], retroauricolar, or even mouth [25, 26].

In the last 5 years, also robotic thyroidectomy, both transaxillary and retroauricolar were described and they seemed to make improvements to the previous approaches by the endoscopic access, although with higher costs, longer operative time, and risk of new complications [27].

Attempting to classify all the approaches proposed for thyroidectomy in recent years, both minimally invasive and cosmetic, we could divide into two main classes: cervical and extracervical or "remote."

About cervical approach, the endoscopic approach proposed by Gagner and later by Henry has not been successful and were quickly abandoned. They were purely endoscopic, lateral approaches, based on Co2 insufflations. MIVAT instead, gasless technique, has been successful and spread among surgeons thanks to the low difficulty of execution, low cost and optimal cosmetic result combined with short and good postoperative course.

Briefly MIVAT can be described as follows: the patient is placed in a supine position without extension of the neck. A 1.5 cm incision is performed two fingers above the sternal notch. The midline is opened for 2–3 cm and strap muscles are dissected from the thyroid lobe and loaded by a small retractor. Once the thyroid lobe is completely freed from the strap muscles, larger retractors, "army-navy" type, are inserted in order to maintain the operative space during the entire procedure. At this point a 5 mm 30° endoscope is introduced together with other endoscopic instruments and the procedure becomes totally endoscopic. All vessels are sectioned by means of energy device (ultrasonic, radiofrequency) except vessels very close to the nerve when, in order to avoid thermal injuries, disposable titanium clips are preferred. Recurrent nerve and parathyroids can be easily identified and dissected thanks to the magnification of the endoscope.

Once the thyroid lobe is completely freed and all critical structures identified and preserved, it is delivered starting from its upper pole. Then, under direct vision, the Berry's ligament is sectioned and the lobe is completely freed and resected. Drainage is avoided. The midline is closed with a single stitch and skin glue is used for the wound.

MIVAT is indicated in patients with nodules less than 3 cm and thyroid volume less than 25 ml. This allows treating patients with small multinodular goiters, nodules microfollicolari, graves, toxic adenomas, and even low-risk papillary carcinomas. Numerous publications demonstrate that MIVAT is a safe technique, with excellent cosmetic results and excellent postoperative course. Moreover, MIVAT has proven effective in the treatment of papillary carcinoma, as demonstrated by comparative studies between traditional thyroidectomy and MIVAT. In these studies the clearance at thyroid bed level and outcome of patients undergoing these two different techniques were the same. Two main studies from Pisa clearly demonstrated the efficacy of MIVAT for papillary carcinoma. The first one is a prospective randomized study [28]: 35 patients with low-risk papillary carcinoma were allotted, 16 were operated on with MIVAT (group A), and 19 with conventional technique (group B). One month after surgery thyroglobulin (Tg) serum level was measured and a whole body scintigraphy (WBS) with $I^{131}$ was performed in all patients and no statistically significant difference in the results between the two groups was found.

The second prospective study [29] involved 221 patients with a papillary carcinoma smaller than 30 mm, treated by MIVAT or traditional thyroidectomy. After a mean follow-up of 5 years there were no statistically significant differences between the two groups in terms of age, sex, and mean follow-up. No differences in serum Tg and TSH levels and 131-I neck uptake were observed between the two groups of patients and no statistical difference was found between cured and not cured PTC patients at the end of follow-up. Same rates of hypoparathyroidism and/or recurrent laryngeal nerve palsy were recorded. These results after 5-year follow-up clearly suggest that MIVAT is a safe and effective technique in the treatment of low and intermediate risk papillary carcinomas.

The limits in the indications represented by thyroid volume and diameter of the nodules are probably the greatest limit of MIVAT, which in fact can only be performed in 15 % of patients with thyroid disease.

Despite this, MIVAT represents the most minimally invasive endoscopic technique performed in the western countries, as demonstrated by numerous publications that have appeared in the literature in recent years.

During the last 2 years more than 30 papers dealing with MIVAT appeared in the indexed literature, while 18 papers were published during 2008 and 11 during 2007. These data witness the great interest for video-assisted surgery of thyroid among the surgeons and how it became widespread, not only in Europe but also in the United States. According to Terris, "the technique most widely practiced in North America is ... MIVAT as originally described by Miccoli" [30]. When dealing with this operation several outcomes might be considered in order to critically appraise its results: Sgourakis et al. [31], for example, distinguished between primary and secondary outcomes: among the first ones they put adverse events and cosmesis, while among the second ones operative time, early and late postoperative time were considered. Others took also on account the hospital stay length. An attempt will be done in this chapter to examine the overall results as they emerge both from the most recent literature and from our personal experience.

To the best of our knowledge only two main reviews [31, 32] have been published aiming to give an evidence-based information on MIVAT: both of them are concordant on a statistical significance in favor of MIVAT versus traditional thyroidectomy when cosmesis and postoperative pain are examined. As far as adverse events are concerned it appears evident in these, as in almost all the papers dealing with MIVAT, that a statistical significance is impossible to reach due to the very low number of complications, in particular recurrent nerve palsies and hypoparathyroidism. In spite of the lack of a statistical significance though, all authors are concordant on the absolute safety of this procedure with respect to conventional surgery.

By then we can assume that the main advantages of this surgery are represented by a dramatic improvement of cosmetic outcome and a significant reduction of postoperative distress. The latter was recently demonstrated also via an evaluation of the increase of some biochemical mediators such as TGF-beta which correlate with post surgical pain [33], thus giving an objective demonstration of what had already been ascertained through the assessment of subjective pain scores (visual and numeric analogue scales) in several papers [31, 32, 34]. The first one is not just the result of minimizing the length of the incision; the possibility of avoiding the surgical drainage and the absence of skin sutures brilliantly substituted by cyanoacrylate glue, both concur to determine an excellent aesthetical sequel. As a further repercussion of the surgical trauma cutback, the diffusion of this and similar techniques contributed enormously to the ever increasing attitude to treat surgical thyroid diseases on an outpatient basis. Recently, in particular in the United States, most of the patients undergoing MIVAT are discharged on the same operative day: in some series up to more than 90 % of the cases [35, 36].

Among remote accesses, transaxillary is probably the most widely performed, especially in the eastern countries. Ikeda and Takami in 1999–2000 were the first to describe the feasibility of endoscopic thyroidectomy via an entirely camouflaged axillary incision [23]. They used a 3 cm skin incision in the medial folds of the axilla and a tunnel was made to expose the thyroid bed. Operation was performed by means of two trocars and a flexible endoscope. Carbon dioxide insufflation at 4 mmHg was used to maintain the working space.

Ishii described another extracervical approach which consisted in circum-mammary incisions and it was called "breast approach" (BA) [24]. Later on in 2002, Shimazu and colleagues modified the BA incorporating an axillary incision. This method was termed the "axillo-bilateral-breast approach" (ABBA) [37]. This technique eliminated the parasternal incision used in BA and the group reported a shorter operative time and better cosmetic result comparing with BA. Choe and colleagues found that total thyroidectomy via this approach with three ports was difficult. They presented the bilateral axillo-breast approach (BABA) [38] for improved visualization for total thyroidectomy by adding a contralateral axillary port.

Some studies comparing endoscopic techniques to conventional thyroidectomy demonstrated less postoperative pain, shorter hospital stays, and higher patient satisfaction with cosmesis, voice, swallowing, although outcomes such as surgical trauma, capsular disruption, and the introduction of new surgical complications have not been extensively studied [39–41].

Certainly, application of Robot to these techniques added further advantages and ameliorated all these approaches. Chung described in 2007 Transaxillary robotic thyroidectomy (RATT) [42] and now thousands of operations have been performed in Asia. Robotic thyroidectomy eliminates the necessity of gas insufflation and gets great advantage from 3D vision, use of fine and precise tools, ergonomy, and safety of ultrasonic dissector. In Europe RATT is performed in few centers. In Pisa we have operated 150 patients till now. Results are good, but costs and operative time are higher comparing both MIVAT and traditional thyroidectomy.

One of the problems that limited the diffusion of these thyroid procedures was initially represented by the exact definition of the two terms: "minimally invasive" and "endoscopic" Actually not all endoscopic thyroidectomies can be considered minimally invasive. Among the endoscopic accesses only those implying a direct cervical approach are minimally invasive; all those which are based on an extracervical access can certainly be considered as "cosmetic" or "scarless in the neck," but not minimally invasive. Moreover, axillary and breast accesses at their very onset could only be proposed for hemythyroidectomies, so limiting further the application of these techniques. Moreover, these techniques are even more time consuming reaching operative times which are as long as 160–280 min, according to the last reports in literature. Such operative times might hardly rival those of MIVAT or conventional thyroidectomy which, in expert hands, are more or less equivalent and are considered as the standard for this surgery in most of the Hospitals.

Although MIVAT is getting more and more widespread, it is important to keep on studying more advanced mini invasive surgical procedures on thyroid provided we are able to conjugate innovation with safety. Certainly robotic surgery constitutes a great opportunity for endoscopic surgery and it has gained a great favor in the recent years: in the field of thyroid surgery unfortunately the use of robot is only compatible with an extracervical access, which is far from being minimally invasive; the operation was initially performed through an axillary access and a further incision on the upper thorax area far enough from the cervical area to be not visible in a normally dressed woman. The operation was called cosmetic because in most of the eastern countries a scar in the neck is considered highly undesirable. More recently though the operation has been proposed through a unique axilla incision, thus reducing significantly postoperative pain: we perform ourselves this latter robotic procedure and can witness that the operation is very well tolerated and well accepted by patients who can be discharged two days after surgery. Besides the development of the so-called "single access" surgery, certainly will help technology to explore the possibility of using the robot also through single small incisions such as the one used by MIVAT and MIVAP, but also by other pediatric operations. Another future development of MIVAT might be a further extension of its indications, in particular the possibility of performing lateral lymphadenectomies through the same central incision: actually some preliminary results have already been published in literature [43] but the patients' recruitment is very difficult since the cases with small papillary carcinomas fulfilling the criteria to undergo MIVAT very rarely present with a lateral compartment lymph node involvement necessitating a lymphadenectomy.

Another interesting access proposed by German authors is the sublingual access, called "Trans Oral Video Assisted Thyroidectomy" (TOVAT) [44]. This procedure could be virtually defined as minimally invasive since the access is in the cervical area: it basically mimics the embryological pathway of the thyroid gland from its primitive site at the basis of the tongue to its final position in the neck. It might leave no scar in the cervical visible area and is a development of the so-called natural orifices trans endoscopic surgery( NOTES), but, in spite of this, its invasiveness is far from being reduced and several objections could be raised [45] against this access: through a 5 mm incision, as described by the authors, it would be very difficult to remove most of the thyroid lesions necessitating a surgical treatment, the haemostatic devices used in this operation hardly might guarantee a safe division of most of the upper pedicles of the thyroid glands and finally it is arguable that it is ethically correct to injure an intact mouth pavement to operate on a gland so easily accessible through the skin.

## References

1. Kunstmann JW, Udelsman R (2012) Superiority of minimally invasive parathyroidectomy. Adv Surg 46:171–189
2. Udelsman R, Akerström G, Biagini C, Duh QY, Miccoli P, Niederle B, Tonelli F (2014) The surgical management of asymptomatic primary hyperparathyroidism: proceedings of Fourth International Workshop. J Clin Endocrinol Metab 99:3595–3606

3. Miccoli P, Cecchini G, Conte M et al (1997) Minimally invasive video-assisted parathyroid surgery for primary hyperparathyroidism. J Endocrinol Invest 20:429–430
4. Lorenz K, Miccoli P, Monchick JM, Düren M, Dralle H (2001) Minimally invasive video-assisted parathyroidectomy: multiinstitutional study. World J Surg 25:704–707
5. Gagner M (1997) Endoscopic parathyroidectomy and thyroidectomy. Semin Laparosc Surg 4:235–240
6. Henry JF, Defechereux T, Gramatica L, de Boissezon C (1999) Minimally invasive videoscopic parathyroidectomy by lateral approach. Langenbecks Arch Surg 384:298–301
7. Sofuni A, Moriyasu F, Sano T, Yamada K, Itokawa F, Tsuchiya T, Tsuji S, Kurihara T, Ishii K, Itoi T (2011) The current potential of Hi intensity focused ultrasound for pancreatic carcinoma. J Hepatobiliary Pancreat Sci 18:295–303
8. Esnault O, Rouxel A, Le Nestour E, Gheron G, Leenhardt L (2010) Minimally invasive ablation of a toxic thyroid nodule by high-intensity focused ultrasound. AJNR Am J Neuroradiol 31:1967–1968
9. Kovatcheva RD, Vlahov JD, Shinkov AD et al (2010) High-intensity focused ultrasound to treat primary hyperparathyroidism: a feasibility study in four patients. AJR Am J Roentgenol 195:830–835
10. Carrafiello G, Laganà D, Mangini M et al (2006) Treatment of secondary hyperparathyroidism with ultrasonographically guided percutaneous radiofrequency thermoablation. Surg Laparosc Endosc Percutan Tech 16:112–116
11. Stratigis S, Stylianou K, Mamalaki E et al (2008) Percutaneous ethanol injection therapy: a surgery-sparing treatment for primary hyper- parathyroidism. Clin Endocrinol (Oxf) 69:542–548
12. Adda G, Scillitani A, Epaminonda P et al (2006) Ultrasound-guided laser thermal ablation for parathyroid adenomas: analysis of three cases with a three-year follow-up. Horm Res 65: 231–234
13. Ambrosini CE, Cianferotti L, Picone A, Torregrossa L, Segnini G, Frustaci G, Cetani F, Basolo F, Marcocci C, Miccoli P (2011) High-intensity focused ultrasound as an alternative to the surgical approach in primary hyperparathyroidism: a preliminary experience. J Endocrinol Invest 34:655–659
14. Mihai R, Barczynski M, Iacobone M, Sitges-Serra A (2009) Surgical strategy for sporadic primary hyperparathyroidism an evidence-based approach to surgical strategy, patient selection, surgical access, and reoperations. Langenbecks Arch Surg 394(5):785–798
15. Berti P, Materazzi G, Picone A, Miccoli P (2003) Limits and drawbacks of video-assisted parathyroidectomy. Br J Surg 90:743–747
16. Lombardi CP, Raffaelli M, Traini E, De Crea C, Corsello SM, Bellantone R (2009) Video-assisted minimally invasive parathyroidectomy: benefits and long-term results. World J Surg 33:2266–2281
17. Barczynski M, Cichon S, Konturek A, Cichon W (2006) Minimally invasive video-assisted parathyroidectomy versus open minimally invasive parathyroidectomy for a solitary parathyroid adenoma: a prospective, randomized, blinded trial. World J Surg 30:721–731
18. Miccoli P, Berti P, Materazzi G, Massi M, Picone A, Minuto MN (2004) Results of video assisted parathyroidectomy: single-institutions' six year experience. World J Surg 28:1216–1218
19. Miccoli P, Berti P, Materazzi G, Ambrosini CE, Fregoli L, Donatini G (2008) Endoscopic bilateral neck exploration versus quick intraoperative parathormone assay [qPTHa] during endoscopic parathyroidectomy: a prospective randomized trial. Surg Endosc 22:398–400
20. Miccoli P, Barellini L, Monchik JM, Rago R, Berti PF (2005) Randomized clinical trial comparing regional and general anaesthesia in minimally invasive video-assisted parathyroidectomy. Br J Surg 92(7):814–818
21. Huscher C, Chiodini S, Napolitano C, Recher A (1997) Endoscopic right thyroid lobectomy. Surg Endosc 11:877
22. Miccoli P, Berti P, Conte M, Bendinelli C, Marcocci C (1999) Minimally invasive surgery for thyroid small nodules: preliminary report. J Endocrinol Invest 22:849–851
23. Ikeda Y, Takami H, Niimi M, Kan S, Takayama J, Sasaki Y (2001) Endoscopic thyroidectomy by the axillary approach. Surg Endosc 15:362–364
24. Ohgami M, Ishii S, Arisawa Y et al (2000) Scarless endoscopic thyroidectomy: breast approach for better cosmesis. Surg Laparosc Endosc Percutan Tech 10:1–4

25. Terris DJ, Singer MC (2012) Robotic facelift thyroidectomy: facilitating remote access surgery. Head Neck 34(5):746–747
26. Nakajo A, Arima H, Hirata M, Mizoguchi T, Kijima Y, Mori S, Ishigami S, Ueno S, Yoshinaka H, Natsugoe S (2013) Trans-Oral Video-Assisted Neck Surgery (TOVANS). a new transoral technique of endoscopic thyroidectomy with gasless premandible approach. Surg Endosc 27(4):1105–1110
27. Lee J, Chung WY (2013) Robotic surgery for thyroid disease. Eur Thyroid J 2(2):93–101
28. Miccoli P, Elisei R, Materazzi G (2002) Minimally invasive video assisted thyroidectomy for papillary carcinoma: a prospective study of its completeness. Surgery 132:1070–1073
29. Miccoli P, Pinchera A, Materazzi G, Biagini A, Berti P, Faviana P, Molinaro E, Viola D, Elisei R (2009) Surgical treatment of low- and intermediate-risk papillary thyroid cancer with minimally invasive video assisted thyroidectomy. J Clin Endocrinol Metab 94:1618–1622
30. Terris D, Angelos P, Steward D, Simental A (2008) Minimally invasive video assisted thyroidectomy: a multi-institutional North American experience. Arch Otolaryngol Head Neck Surg 134:81–84
31. Sgourakis G, Sotiropoulos C, Neuhäuser M, Musholt J, Karaliotas C, Lang H (2008) Comparison between minimally invasive video-assisted thyroidectomy and conventional thyroidectomy: is there any evidence based information? Thyroid 18:721–727
32. Miccoli P, Minuto MN, Ugolini C, Pisano R, Fosso A, Berti P (2008) Minimally invasive video assisted thyroidectomy for benign thyroid diseases: an evidence-based review. World J Surg 32:1333–1340
33. Miccoli P, Rago R, Massi M, Panicucci E, Metelli MR, Berti P, Minuto MN (2010) Standard versus video-assisted thyroidectomy: objective postoperative pain evaluation. Surg Endosc 24(10):2415–2417
34. Alesina PF, Rolfs T, Ruhland K, Brunkhorst V, Groeben H, Walz MK (2010) Evaluation of postoperative pain after minimally invasive video assisted and conventional thyroidectomy: results of a prospective study. Langenbecks Arch Surg 395(7):845–849
35. Lai SY, Walvekar RR, Ferris RL (2008) Minimally invasive video assisted thyroidectomy: expanded indications and oncologic completeness. Head Neck 30:1403–1407
36. Terris DJ, Moister B, Seybt MW, Gourin CG, Chin E (2007) Outpatient thyroid surgery is safe and desirable. Otolaryngol Head Neck Surg 137:362
37. Bärlehner E, Benhidjeb T (2008) Cervical scarless endoscopic thyroidectomy: axillo-bilateral-breast approach (ABBA). Surg Endosc 22(1):154–157
38. Lee KE, Kim E, do Koo H, Choi JY, Kim KH, Youn YK (2013) Robotic thyroidectomy by bilateral axillo-breast approach: review of 1,026 cases and surgical completeness. Surg Endosc 27(8):2955–2962
39. Wang C, Feng Z, Li J, Yang W, Zhai H, Choi N, Yang J, Hu Y, Pan Y, Cao G (2015) Endoscopic thyroidectomy via areola approach: summary of 1,250 cases in a single institution. Surg Endosc 29(1):192–201
40. Hyun K, Byon W, Park HJ, Park Y, Park C, Yun JS (2014) Comparison of swallowing disorder following gasless transaxillary endoscopic thyroidectomy versus conventional open thyroidectomy. Surg Endosc 28(6):1914–1920
41. Lee H, Lee J, Sung KY (2012) Comparative study comparing endoscopic thyroidectomy using the axillary approach and open thyroidectomy for papillary thyroid microcarcinoma. World J Surg Oncol 10:269
42. Hakim Darail NA, Lee SH, Kang SW, Jeong JJ, Nam KH, Chung WY (2014) Gasless transaxillary endoscopic thyroidectomy: a decade on. Surg Laparosc Endosc Percutan Tech 24(6):211–215
43. Miccoli P, Materazzi G, Berti P (2008) Minimally invasive video-assisted lateral lymphadenectomy: a proposal. Surg Endosc 22(4):1131–1132
44. Benhidjeb T, Wilhelm T, Harlaar J, Kleinrensink GJ, Schneider TA, Stark M (2009) Natural orifice surgery on thyroid gland: totally transoral video-assisted thyroidectomy (TOVAT): report of first experimental results of a new surgical method. Surg Endosc 23(5):1119–1120
45. Miccoli P, Materazzi G, Berti P (2010) Natural orifice surgery on the thyroid gland using totally transoral video-assisted thyroidectomy: report of the first experimental results for a new surgical method: are we going in the right direction? Surg Endosc 24(4):957–958

# Part IV

# Intraoperative Adjuncts

# Superior Laryngeal Nerve Monitoring 17

Gianlorenzo Dionigi, Cesare Carlo Ferrari, Alberto Mangano, Matteo Lavazza, Andrea Ieotta, Stefano Rausei, and Luigi Boni

## 17.1 Introduction

Interest on the surgical anatomy, neurophysiology, and pathology of the external branch of the superior laryngeal nerve (EBSLN) increased in last two decades. In fact, there is an increasing attentiveness from both clinician and patient for the possible consequence of EBSLN injury in thyroid and parathyroid surgery, such as postoperative altered frequency of voice, modified timber, deterioration in performance (high-pitched sounds), reduced voice quality projection, and extra effort to speak, more noticeably in the voice of professionals and women (Fig. 17.1).

IONM is increasingly performed in endocrine surgery due to a significant improvement of the technical aspects, devices (Fig. 17.2), and evidences evolutions (Table 17.1). The recent international standards guideline statement on EBSLN monitoring highlighted in detail the advantages of intraoperative neuromonitoring (IONM) for accurate, early, and definitive identification and preservation of the EBSLN during thyroidectomy [5]. The International Neural Monitoring Study Group (INMSG) suggests EBSLN monitoring in thyroidectomy [5]. Recent studies enhanced the utility of IONM research for precise EBSLN neurophysiologic data [43].

G. Dionigi, MD, FACS (✉)
1st Division of General Surgery, Department of Surgical Sciences and Human Morphology, Research center for Endocrine Surgery, School of Medicine, University of Insubria (Varese-Como), Via Guicciardini, 9, Varese 21100, Italy
e-mail: gianlorenzo.dionigi@uninsubria.it

C.C. Ferrari • A. Mangano • M. Lavazza • A. Ieotta • S. Rausei • L. Boni
1st Division of Surgery, Department of Surgical Sciences, Research center for Endocrine Surgery, University of Insubria (Varese-Como), Via Guicciardini, 9, Varese 21100, Italy



C.P. Lombardi, R. Bellantone (eds.), *Minimally Invasive Therapies for Endocrine Neck Diseases*, DOI 10.1007/978-3-319-20065-1_17

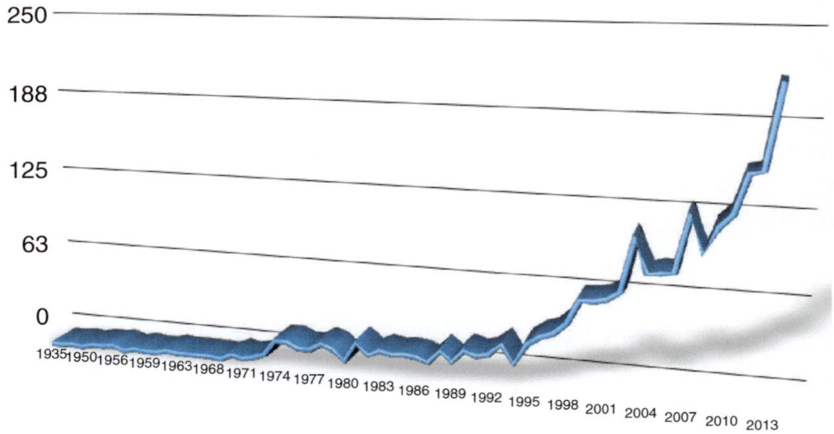


**Fig. 17.1** Total numbers of documents on EBSLN published by year (1935–2013)

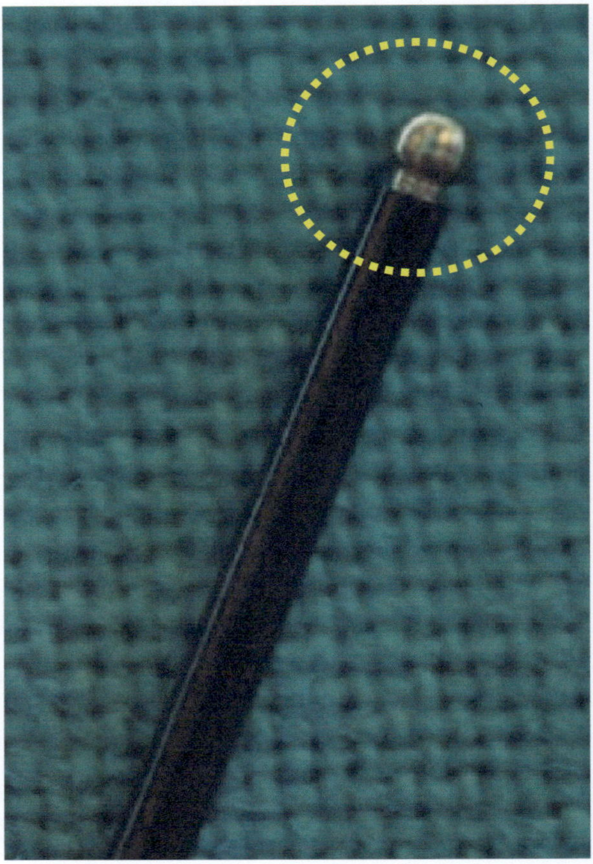

**Fig. 17.2** Atraumatic ball tip intraoperative nerve-monitoring probe stimulator for early EBSLN identification and confirmation

**Table 17.1** Reasons for increase usage of IONM

| |
|---|
| Noninvasive devices (endotracheal tube-based monitoring systems) |
| User-friendly systems |
| Randomized trials |
| Guidelines and standardization |
| Training courses |
| Medicolegal issues |
| Research |
| Societies recommendations |
| Commercial effort |

An unequivocal definition of EMG data from EBSLN monitoring is a prerequisite for correct definition of preserved nerve function, nerve stress and injury, recovery, and prognostication.

This chapter is a review of the evidence-based literature and the cumulative experience of the authors with EBSLN monitoring technique. EBSLN monitoring is our routine practice since 2007 [15] for both conventional and endoscopic procedures.

## 17.2 EBSLN Surgical Anatomy

EBSLN is one of the two main branches of the superior laryngeal nerve (SLN). It innervates the cricothyroid muscle (CTM) and the inferior pharyngeal constrictor muscle. Its anatomical position exposes it to damage risk during the dissection of the upper thyroid pole in the course of thyroidectomy procedures.

The SLN is the only nervous structure whose embryological development originates from the fourth pharyngeal arch. The thyroid, cricoid, arytenoid, corniculate, and cuneiform cartilages of the larynx are formed by the cartilaginous components of the fourth and sixth pharyngeal arches fused together. From the fourth arch develops also the cricothyroid muscle, the levator palatini muscle, and the constrictor of the pharynx, innervated by the different branches of the SLN [50].

The trunk of the SLN arises just caudal to the jugular foramen of the basicranium, branching from the vagus nerve or the nodose ganglion. It runs behind the carotid arteries descending in an anterior and medial direction toward the larynx [21, 22, 31]. The nerve splits into two branches nearly at the level of the superior cornus of the hyoid bone, averaging at 15 mm from its origin. The bifurcation often lies between the internal and the external carotid arteries. Both the branches exit from the carotid sheath about 20 mm below the bifurcation of the common carotid artery [25, 31, 40].

The internal branch of the superior laryngeal nerve (IBSLN) is always in a medial position relative to the lingual and facial arteries. It runs mainly parallel and medially to the superior laryngeal artery. It stays next to the pharyngeal wall, turns medially, caudal to the greater horn of the hyoid bone, passes behind the thyrohyoid muscle, and pierces the thyrohyoid membrane to get into the larynx [23].

EBSLN has many anatomical variants and knowing the variations in its course is fundamental for its identification during surgery. The diameter of the nerve is about 0.2 mm [31]. Its vascularization is supplied by the cricothyroid artery, branch of the superior thyroid artery (STA) [41]. After its branching, it crosses the medial border of the internal carotid artery (75 %) or runs posteriorly to the common carotid artery, lying medial to the cervical sympathetic ganglion [41].

Four different classifications for the position of the nerve have been proposed. Each of this classification uses different landmarks. Cernea classification [9] is the most commonly cited in the past and recent literature and it is simple and easy to be applied in the clinical practice.

### 17.2.1 Classifications

Cernea et al. [9] and Kierner et al. [33] describe the nerve path in relation to the STA, Friedman et al. [19] use as landmark the inferior constrictor muscle (ICM), and Selvan et al. [53] analyze the relationship between the entries of the nerve into the cricothyroid muscle, the superior thyroid vessels (STV), and the cricoid cartilage. Table 17.2 summarizes these classifications.

The Cernea et al.'s [9] classification divides EBSLN into type 1, that is, the nerve crosses the STA more than 1 cm above the margin of the superior thyroid pole (68 % in case of small goiter; 23 % in case of large goiter); type 2A, that is, the nerve crosses the STA <1 cm above the margin of the superior thyroid pole (18 % in case of small goiter; 15 % in case of large goiter); and type 2B, that is, when the nerve crosses the superior thyroid pedicle below the margin of the superior thyroid pole (14 % in case of small goiter; 54 % in case of large goiter).

Cernea 2A and 2B types are particularly frequent (15–55 %) and prone to be injured during the upper thyroid pedicle dissection and ligation.

Cernea classification is nowadays the most commonly used EBSLN surgical classification in the clinical practice and research, for its simplicity and ease of use.

### 17.2.2 The Sternothyroid–Laryngeal Triangle

Knowing this anatomical space, otherwise called Jolles space, is useful to find the EBSLN. The triangular region has the base at the bottom, represented by the upper edge of the superior thyroid pole; the medial margin is composed of the thyroid and cricoid cartilages, the pharyngeal constrictors and cricothyroid muscle, and the retracted sternothyroid muscle which normally lies above laterally. In the medial

**Table 17.2** EBSLN classifications

| Cernea et al. [9] |
|---|
| Type 1 → the nerve crosses the STA more than 1 cm above the margin of the superior thyroid pole (68 % in case of small goiter; 23 % in case of large goiter) |
| Type 2A → the nerve crosses the STA <1 cm above the margin of the superior thyroid pole (18 % in case of small goiter; 15 % in case of large goiter) |
| Type 2B → the nerve crosses the superior thyroid pedicle below the margin of the superior thyroid pole (14 % in case of small goiter; 54 % in case of large goiter) |
| Kierner et al. [33] |
| Type 1 → the nerve crosses the STA more than 1 cm above the margin of the superior thyroid pole |
| Type 2 → the nerve crosses the STA <1 cm above the margin of the superior thyroid pole |
| Type 3 → the nerve crosses the superior thyroid pedicle below the margin of the superior thyroid pole |
| Type 4 → the nerve crosses the STA immediately above the margin of the superior thyroid pole |
| Friedman et al. [19] |
| Type 1 → the nerve runs superficially or laterally to the inferior constrictor muscle for its whole course until it terminates in the cricothyroid muscle |
| Type 2 → the nerve penetrates the inferior constrictor muscle in its lower portion |
| Type 3 → the nerve goes under the superior fibers of the inferior constrictor muscle covered for the whole course |
| Selvan et al. [53] |
| Type 1a → the nerve lies 1 cm before the entry of the vessels into the gland or anterior/between the branches of the superior thyroid vessels and distant 3 cm from the cricoid cartilage (9 %) |
| Type 1b → the nerve lies 1 cm before the entry of the superior thyroid vessels into the gland but posterior to the vessels. The entry point is close to the anterior insertion of the cricothyroid muscle on the cricoid cartilage (3 %) |
| Type 2 → the nerve lies within 1–3 cm of the entry of the vessels into the gland or within 3–5 cm from the cricoid cartilage (68 %) |
| Type 3 → the nerve lies between 3 and 5 cm of the entry of the vessels into the gland or more than 5 cm from the cricoid cartilage (20 %) |

portion of the area, it is usually possible to find the EBSLN. The STV are located laterally and the STA between the vein and the nerve [42].

### 17.2.3 EBSLN Anastomoses

Another important aspect about the EBSLN is the presence of anastomoses between its trunk and the other nerves, particularly with the IBSLN and the recurrent laryngeal nerve (RLN). The connection between IBSLN and EBSLN runs through the thyroid foramen (an opening inside the thyroid cartilage) when present, often followed by the blood vessels [52]. The human communicating nerve (HCN) [61], also called pyriform nerve [51] or cricothyroid connection branch [38], is the anastomosis which connects the EBSLN to the RLN in one or both sides. Its position between these nerves suggests that it could be the nerve of the fifth branchial arch [51, 61]. It starts from the medial surface of the cricothyroid muscle and enters into the lateral surface of the thyroarytenoid (TA) muscle. Sometimes it is double branched, but more frequently it is a single trunk [38].

Depending on the position where the human communicating nerve joins the RLN, four variants of anastomoses have been described [38]:

- Type A → the HCN enters the RLN in correspondence to the inferior branch to the posterior cricoarytenoid muscle
- Type B → the HCN enters the RLN where the arytenoid branch originates
- Type C → the HCN enters the RLN where the lateral cricoarytenoid branch starts
- Type D → the HCN enters the last RLN into the branch to the thyroarytenoid (TA) muscle

This nerve is composed of sensory fibers, passing into the TA muscle to terminate near the cricoarytenoid joint in the subglottic mucosa, and motor fibers joining the RLN or entering the TA muscle directly [61].

## 17.3 Incidence of EBSLN Injury

The prevalence of EBSLN damage is hard to assess because, at this stage, there is too much intertrial methodological heterogeneity. Since vocal examination underestimates the incidence of neural damages and laryngeal postoperative exam can have inconsistent findings as well, CTM EMG is the only reliable way to diagnose EBSLN injury. Hence, the prevalence of such event ranges from 0 % to nearly 60 %. For all those reasons, EBSLN damage is considered the most commonly underestimated postoperative event [3, 5, 29, 32, 36, 46, 47]. However, higher intraoperative attention is given to the EBSLN (in particular during the dissection of the superior thyroid pole); the lower nerve damage rate is also reported. What is more, in recent years the increased use of IONM improved the neural detection rate and decreased the neural impairment rate [4, 5, 9, 18, 30].

Cernea et al., showed an incidence between 12 % and almost 30 % when the EBSLN was not identified during surgery [9, 10]. Jansson et al. reported a temporary EBSLN injury rate of almost 60 % and a permanent injury rate of almost 4 % when no EBSLN identification was achieved [29]. Additionally, a randomized trial showed that the distal ligation of the superior thyroid vascular branches without neural visual identification, if performed by experienced surgeons, seems to be a safe procedure, but there is a temporary EBSLN lesion prevalence superior to nerve identification technique (0.5 % vs. 0.8 %), and, of note, these authors did not report EMG definition of CTM function [6].

## 17.4 Diagnosis and Treatment of the EBSLN Injury

Clinical or endoscopic findings cannot accurately diagnose EBSLN dysfunctions, because they are often subclinical and widely variable (from loss of ability to produce high-pitched sounds to a deeper voice acquisition, from singing voice impairment to vocal tightness/weakness, or requiring extra effort in speaking) [5, 8, 48, 49, 55]. These symptoms may significantly affect the quality of life [12, 32]. Via the functional voice assessment, shortening of the maximum phonation time and lowering of the high tones and reduction of the vocal range can be detected. The effect of cricothyroid muscle dysfunction has controversial and variable effects at laryngoscopy exam [1, 5, 42, 56, 57, 60].

Since the clinical findings are often minimal and the laryngeal findings are heterogeneous, debatable, and not conclusive, EMG of the CTM (via percutaneous electrode placement into the muscle) is the most reliable way to detect EBSLN dysfunction (details of the technique are described in the guidelines) [5, 9, 59]. After temporary EBSLN damage (in case of paresis or unilateral paralysis), vocal quality improvement can follow; moreover residual muscular function can be implemented via vocal exercise. Notably, at this stage, when EBSLN damage is bilateral and complete, there is no effective way to restore dynamic pitch range [5]. Promising data were presented by El-Kashlan et al., who successfully performed selective cricothyroid muscle reinnervation (in a small sample with high vagal lesions). After reconstruction, all of these patients showed electromyographic and voice quality improvement [18].

IONM has been proposed for EBSLN test for postoperative prognostication. IONM is useful for intraoperative detection of nerve injury. Intraoperative electrical EBSLN testing at the end of the operation "*S2*" (Table 17.3) can serve for postoperative prognostication of the EBSLN function [5, 45]. At the end of the surgical operation, a positive cricothyroid twitch after stimulation of the EBSLN is a good evidence for functional EBSLN preservation, with a related low risk of intraoperative neural damage [5, 45]. It is mandatory to investigate the most cranial neural segment, above the region of the superior pole managed during surgery. Moreover, it is important to have accurate knowledge of the normal laryngeal and cricothyroid muscle anatomy to accurately assess the cricothyroid muscle twitch [5, 45].

**Table 17.3** Standardization of RLN and EBSLN monitoring

| |
|---|
| 1. L1 Preoperative laryngoscopy |
| 2. V1 Test vagus nerve before identification of RLN |
| 3. R1 Test RLN when it was identified at the tracheoesophageal groove |
| 4. S1 *EBSLN* stimulation at identification |
| 5. S2 *EBSLN* stimulation after STA ligation |
| 6. R2 Test RLN after it was completely dissected from Berry's ligament |
| 7. V2 Test vagus nerve after complete hemostasis |
| 8. L2 Postoperative laryngoscopy |

## 17.5 EBSLN Monitoring Technique

Standards for EBSLN management during thyroid surgery are detail knowledge of its anatomy, experience, training, visual identification, and exposure. EBSLN monitoring principles are similar to those of recurrent laryngeal nerve (RLN) monitoring, that is, IONM is an adjunct to meticulous technique and useful for EBSLN identification, confirmation, monitoring, functional verification, and exclusion of EBSLN proximity during dissection. Multiple surgical techniques have been reported to reduce the risk of injury to the EBSLN [5]: (1) ligation of the superior thyroid vascular branches under direct vision on the thyroid capsule without visual neural identification [6], (2) visual neural detection before superior thyroid pole vessel ligation [1], and (3) the use of either a nerve stimulator or intraoperative neuromonitoring for mapping and confirmation of the EBSLN identification [2, 4, 9, 10, 15, 20, 28, 30, 35].

### 17.5.1 Equipment and Setup

RLN and EBSLN share certain monitoring standards of equipment setup, endotracheal tube placement, anesthesia, and correct tube positioning verification tests [45]. Monitoring is set with event threshold of 100 mcV (150 mcV usually for RLN) and pulsatile stimulus duration of 100 mcs at 4 Hz [5]. We commonly use the intermitted IONM manual stimulator probe as dissecting instrument, disposable or reusable. We prefer the ball tip stimulator probe which is atraumatic during dissection (Fig. 17.2). On the other hand, stimulating electrodes may be monopolar or bipolar. Bipolar stimulator may be preferred to monopolar one for EBSLN monitoring due to its small nerve diameter, less stimulation artifacts, convergence, and precision of stimulation (Fig 17.3). Bipolar stimulator may provide the potential greater sensitivity [5]. If a bipolar device is used, the precise orientation of the anode and cathode stimulating electrodes placed on the nerve is of crucial importance. The bipolar probe may not be the best option for nerve mapping since the stimulation is more focal in comparison with the monopolar probe, which provides more diffuse current spread and may facilitate the mapping of a wider region [5]. The stimulator probe should be set at 1–2/3 mA. Stimulation is set with 2–3 mA for nerve identification, mapping, and dissection; with 1 mA for nerve confirmation, monitoring, *S1* and *S2* stimulation (Table 17.3). In particular, for confirmation of visually identified EBSLN, a 1 mA current should be preferred but higher values (up to 2 mA) should be used for EBSLN mapping. Multiple and heterogeneous different nerve-monitoring formats have been studied but for safety and simplicity reasons; endotracheal tube-based surface electrode systems are the most commonly used monitoring system [45]. De facto, endotracheal tube-based systems with a graphic monitor documentation are preferred for neural monitoring. New audio and graphic monitor IONM equipment must be preferred today to only audio monitors due to the possibility of print documentation, amplitude and latency quantification, storage/record, differentiation between signal and artifact, forensic issues, research, and justifications of surgical deliberations. In

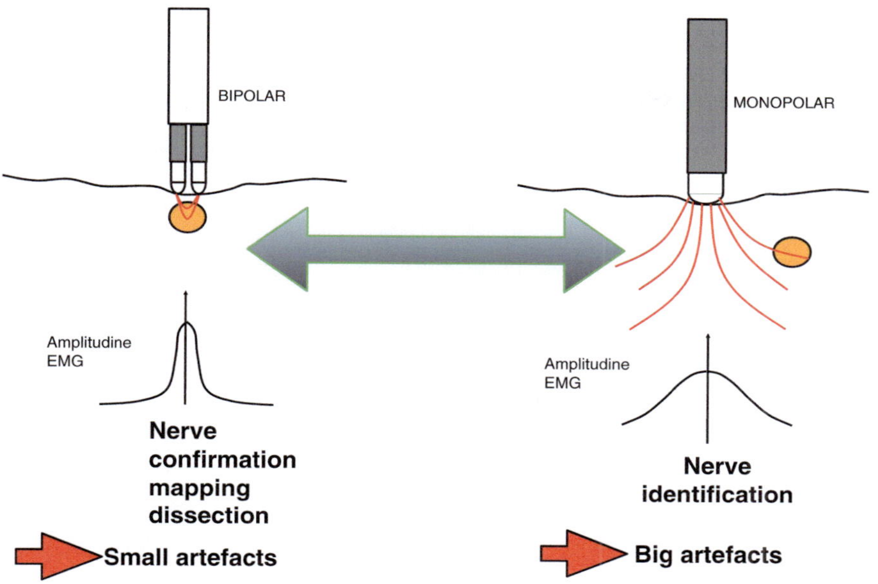


**Fig. 17.3** Intraoperative nerve-monitoring probes: bipolar vs. monopolar. Bipolar stimulator may be preferred to monopolar one for EBSLN monitoring due to its small nerve diameter, less stimulation artifacts, convergence, and precision of stimulation

fact, audio-only systems lack EMG response stimulation assessment (threshold, amplitude, latency, and waveform shape) [5, 45]. We routinely adopt EMG electrode surface endotracheal tube. Endotracheal EMG tube electrodes gain more popularity recently due to its availability, safety, noninvasive nature, ease of setup, ease of use, and the capacity to derive larger areas of evoked muscle potentials as for EBSLN monitoring. Finally, the SLN is the first branch of the vagal nerve after skull base exit; thus continuous monitoring (*C*-IONM) probe electrode cannot monitor EBSLN; however *C*-IONM may provide simultaneous and permanent monitoring of RLN during upper pole dissection.

An accurate surgical technique must be adopted to spare the cricothyroid muscle and the EBSLN. The EBSLN course must be visually identified and monitored in order to avoid neural damage when approaching the superior pole by identification of its course. For this reason, a perfect anatomical knowledge and the classification of the different EBSLN variations are mandatory [5]. In the avascular space between the superior pole and the cricothyroid muscle, a blunt dissection of the superior pole should be performed to obtain clear exposure of the sternothyroid–laryngeal triangle where the EBSLN is located (Fig. 17.4). In the vast majority of cases, there is no need for transverse division of the strap muscles if the thyroid has a normal size or it is only slightly enlarged. However, in cases of large masses or if a short neck is present, a partial division of the sternothyroid muscle may improve the surgical access. Moreover, a better exposure of the sternothyroid–laryngeal triangle can be achieved via gentle latero-caudal traction of the thyroid lobe [5]. The transverse

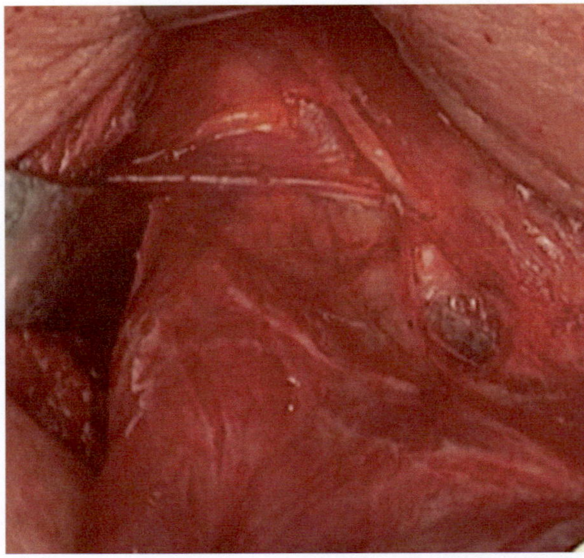

**Fig. 17.4** The sternothyroid–laryngeal triangle, otherwise called Jolles space, is useful to find the EBSLN. The triangular region has the base at the bottom, represented by the upper edge of the superior thyroid pole; the medial margin is composed of the thyroid and cricoid cartilages, the pharyngeal constrictors and cricothyroid muscle, and the retracted sternothyroid muscle which normally lies above laterally. In the medial portion of the area, it is usually possible to find the EBSLN

division of the cranial portion of the sternothyroid muscle should be performed with caution due to possible proximity of EBSLN. Previous stimulation/mapping is suggested to exclude *EBSLN* proximity with a stimulation set between 2 and 3 mA.

Via a blunt dissection, the superior thyroid vessels should be identified, and individual branches exposed [5]. Notably, transverse division of sternothyroid muscle (its superior edge) and a latero-caudal traction of the superior thyroid pole, followed by blunt dissection within the avascular plane of sternothyroid–laryngeal triangle, provide improved EBSLN exposure. The nerve is usually descending parallel to the superior thyroid artery and it is located on the inferior constrictor muscle before its termination within the cricothyroid muscle [5].

It is vital to visually search for the nerve, but of note, almost 20 % of EBSLNs cannot be visually identified because of their subfascial/intramuscular course [19, 34]. Selvan et al. have shown that in many cases, non-neural tissue can be misidentified for the EBSLN [53].

In modern monitored thyroidectomy, EBSLN visual identification and electrical IONM confirmation is defined as “S1” (Table 17.3). S1 is reference for EBSLN and STA dissection.

In all patients, the EBSLN should be visually identified and neural stimulation with the cricothyroid muscle (CTM) twitch assessment and glottis endotracheal EMG monitoring should be performed [5].

Non-neural fibers, vessels, and tendinous fibers can be mistaken for EBSLN. Visual EBSLN identification without IONM may be flawed. The IONM is useful in this stage for EBSLN confirmation: the absence of CTM twitch or EMG is the prerequisite.

In case of large goiters or in short necks, the superior thyroid pole dissection is more difficult and risky for the EBSLN because in such cases, the superior pole is more cranial and there is more adherence of the nerve to the thyroid [5]. Cernea et al. have documented that if the thyroid is >100 g, type 2B nerve incidence (which is more prone to damage) may rise to 54 % [9, 10]. Similarly, Furlan et al. found that a short neck and a large hemithyroid gland volume are risk factors for the EBSLN injury [24]. For those reasons, mass ligation technique should not be used, because it is unsafe for the EBSLN. Moreover, when energy-based device (EBD) is used, there is an additional risk of neural iatrogenic heat injury [14, 15]. In this way, IONM can be a valid adjunct to visualization [34]. Moreover, if a suture ligation or clip is applied near the EBSLN, and IONM suggests neural dysfunction, they must be removed, to avoid risk of permanent damage at this level.

The stimulator probe is useful for the management of the STA ligation. Mass ligation of the STA should be avoided. A 3 mm distance of safety is suggested to avoid collateral iatrogenic heat injury when using an energy-based device (EBD). Before STA ligature, stimulate at 2–3 mV the STA dorsally, medially, anteriorly, and laterally (i.e., 360°). In conventional IONM, there is a rule of the thumb that in case of cricothyroid twitch or signal at 2 mA stimulation, a nerve is to be proximal in about 2–3 mm. Cricothyroid twitch and EMG signal are reference for dissection and presence of the nerve in proximity. Thus, if stimulation of the STA that is to be divided is negative for EBSLN, this is true negative for absence of neural tissue in the pedicle. This maneuver excludes the EBSLN presence in the divided tissue by IONM. Again, this technique is useful as nearly 20 % of EBSLN cannot be visualized due to subfascial course or intraoperative bleeding. As a consequence, the STA is ligated. If EBD is used, we suggest protecting the cricothyroid muscle medially by sponge.

Again S2, the test of EBSLN at the end of operation, is assessed after complete STA ligation, thyroidectomy, and hemostasis. S2 must be ensured by the stimulation of the most cranial aspect of exposed EBSLN and it serves for postoperative prognostication. It is important in the operative notes to have a statement that mentions that the EBSLN was visualized and was intact (IONM) at the end of the procedure. We routinely insert S1 and S2 EMG data, together with L1, V1, R1, R2, V2, and L2 determinations. Finally, as a consequence of the variability of glottic EMG response (70–80 %), in 20–30 % of cases documentation, record, and storage of EBSLN EMG signal (S1 and S2) are not feasible.

### 17.5.2 Definitions of EBSLN Monitoring

- A *false-positive* stimulation (i.e., incorrect identification of the EBSLN) is a positive CTM twitch (with or without corresponding EMG response) in the case of non-neural shunt stimulation.
- This event is in some cases possible during neural mapping using a current of 2 mA: in order to assess the non-neural shunt stimulations, it is best to decrease

the current between 0.8 and 1 mA so that false-positive stimulation can be silenced [5].

- A *false-negative* stimulation (i.e., the EBSLN mistaken as non-neural tissue) occurs when there is no CTM twitch (and no relative EMG signal) after EBSLN stimulation. This event is most often related to a heterogeneous range of equipment malfunctioning due, for example, to neuromuscular blockage, low stimulating current, biologic liquids or tissue covering the stimulated nerve segment, or transient neuropraxia (e.g., due to stretch injury) [5].
- A *true negative* neuromonitoring result is when there is no CTM twitch after the stimulation of the non-EBSLN tissue [5].
- A *true positive* neuromonitoring result is when, after the stimulation of the ipsilateral nerve with 1 mA (in the presence or absence of the corresponding EMG response), correct identification of the EBSLN is confirmed via the CTM twitch [5].

## 17.6 Technique A

### 17.6.1 IONM of the EBSLN: Stimulation–CTM Twitch [5]

The principles highlighted in detail in the international standards guideline statement can be applied to the EBSLN stimulation and monitoring with few important differences [45]. The EBSLN should be visualized when possible and the surgical management of the superior pole should involve two neural monitoring steps [5]:

1. In order to get a true positive stimulation, the EBSLN must be stimulated as clearly present (through CTM visual twitch assessment or endotracheal glottic waveform if observable) cranially and medial to the superior pole pedicle [5]. Again, the first stimulation of the EBSLN is defined as S1 and is reference for the dissection (Fig. 17.5).

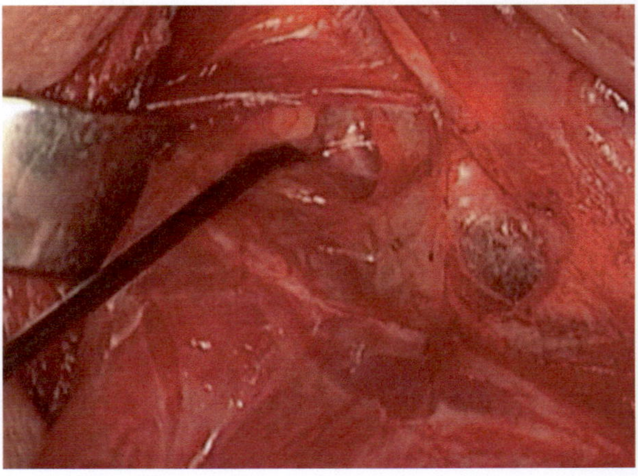

**Fig. 17.5** Identification by IONM of the EBSLN. In the avascular space between the superior pole and the cricothyroid muscle, a blunt dissection of the superior pole should be performed to obtain clear exposure of the sternothyroid–laryngeal triangle where the EBSLN is located

2. In order to get a true negative, it is important to check for the absence of neural tissue in the pedicle that is to be divided (i.e., no CTM visual twitch or endotracheal glottic waveform) [5]. Cricothyroid twitch and EMG signal are reference for dissection and presence of the nerve in proximity. Thus, if stimulation of the STA that is to be divided is negative for EBSLN, this is true negative for absence of neural tissue in the pedicle. This maneuver excludes the EBSLN presence in the divided tissue by IONM. Again, this technique is useful as nearly 20 % of EBSLN cannot be visualized due to subfascial course or intraoperative bleeding. As a consequence, the STA is ligated.

According to the International Neural Monitoring Study Group (INMSG), this sequence of neural monitoring data implements the preservation rate of the EBSLN. It has been shown that IONM can improve the identification rate of the EBSLN [2, 4, 10, 15, 20, 28, 30, 35]. Through those stimulation maneuvers, the EBSLN presence is effectively excluded and the surgical dissection is carried out more safely [5]. Notably, in a previous experience we showed in a randomized prospective study that the EBSLN identification rate in the IONM group was 84 % compared to 42 % in the non-IONM arm [15].

Lifante et al. also found, a greater rate of EBSLN detection during thyroidectomies under regional anesthesia, 65 % with neuromonitoring versus 33 % without [35].

Moreover, Barczynski et al., in a randomized controlled prospective trial of visualization versus neuromonitoring of the EBSLN, showed that the rate of EBSLN identification was improved via IONM (34 % without IONM versus 84 % with IONM). What is more, IONM reduced the prevalence of transient but not permanent EBSLN injury in a monitored versus non-monitored group [4].

Aina et al. used a nerve stimulator for identification of the EBSLN in more than 200 nerves at risk: the identification rate of the EBSLN was more than 95 % in primary thyroid surgery but in redo surgery was 65 % [2].

Selvan et al. showed a 100 % of EBSLN detection rate via nerve stimulation and EMG of the cricothyroid muscle, and, of note, many false positives were detected when visual identification alone was used prior to electrical stimulation [53].

Visual identification of the EBSLN without EMG confirmation may be misleading [5]. Nerve stimulation technique has the advantage of detecting all nerve types (including Cernea type 1 and types 2A and 2B which are most prone to surgical manipulation injury) [4].

INMSG recommend IONM use (with the stimulation current set at 1 mA) to assess EBSLN entrapment during each step of the superior pole dissection placing the stimulator probe between the tissue and the cricothyroid muscle. Visual neural identification can be confirmed via the application of probe directly on the nerve at the entry point into cricothyroid muscular fibers, i.e., *S1* [4].

To facilitate EBSLN detection, tissues should be stimulated parallel and underneath the laryngeal head of the sternothyroid muscle, which is a reliable landmark for EBSLN identification in its distal course before termination of the cricothyroid muscle [44].

**Table 17.4** Proposed algorithm for safe dissection of superior upper thyroid pole

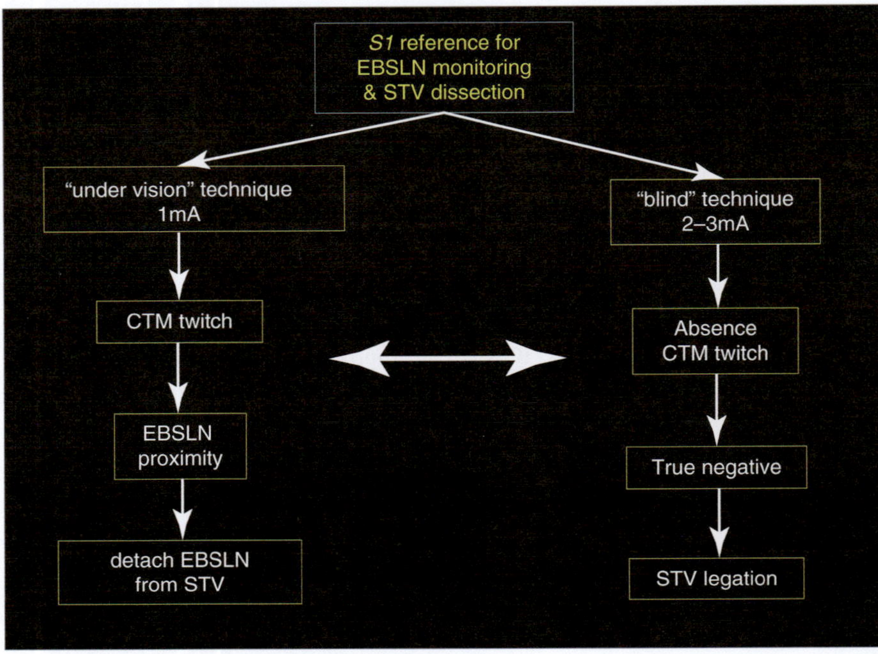


S1 is reference for EBSLN and STA dissection

Via neural monitoring for the EBSLN even when the EBSLN is not identified *de visu* (i.e., deep course into the inferior pharyngeal constrictor muscle fascia), if the nerve is mapped out (the current amplitude is increased from 1 to 2 mA), the EBSLN can be definitively identified [5, 45] (Table 17.4).

The laryngeal head of the sternothyroid muscle is an excellent landmark (the laryngeal head of the sternothyroid muscle, which inserts onto the thyroid cartilage lamina) for the EBSLN detection. A positive identification of the nerve should be confirmed by the CTM twitch (visualized as a triangular muscle profile on the anterolateral aspect of the cricoid cartilage), which in some cases can be also coupled with an auditory signal and an EMG response on the monitor. Moreover, after the superior thyroid pole dissection, the functional integrity of the nerve may be documented through electrical stimulation and a positive cricothyroid twitch response, i.e., *S2*. This technique is recommended for open thyroidectomy and also for MIVAT [5, 15]. Therefore, 100 % of EBSLNs can be identified using this technique (even those not *de visu* assessable). After the superior pole surgical approach, stimulation of the EBSLN superior and cranial to the region of superior pole vessel dissection can assess the ongoing EBSLN postoperative function [5].

## 17.7 Technique B

### 17.7.1 IONM of the EBSLN: Stimulation–Glottic EMG Signal [5]

In contrast to RLN, EBSLN monitoring is based on the assessment of cricothyroid twitch (present in all patients, 100 %) and electromyographic response which is present in 74–83 % of patients. The reason why EBSLN results in glottis identifiable waveform in only 80 % is unclear. The EMG response (74–83 %) variability may be due to several issues as (1) anatomy, i.e., the presence or absence of the human communicating nerve; (2) cooperation with anesthesiologist, i.e., correct EMG tube positioning; and (3) technology- and equipment-related limitations, i.e., the lack of capability nowadays to obtain larger areas of evoked muscle potentials (the need of newer electrode tube arrays). What is more, this EMG heterogeneity in EBSLN stimulation may also be linked to the fact that the EBSLN innervates primarily the anterior one-third of the cord, and its measurement may be very sensitive to endotracheal tube positioning. A lot of scientific and technological research is in progress to develop cutting-edge monitoring systems capable to record EMG in all cases during EBSLN EMG assessment [5]. Darr et al. [13] showed that IONM, with the use of the novel endotracheal tube (TriVantage EMG tube, Medtronic), can be safely used for EBSLN identification during thyroid surgery in 100 % of patients and the EBSLN EMG activity was assessed in 100 % of cases. Moreover, the standard monopolar stimulator and the novel bipolar stimulator probe produced comparable EMG data.

### 17.7.2 Normative Data of the EBSLN Monitoring

The generated waveform is of small amplitude and short latency and therefore may not be noted by monitoring software as a significant and recognizable event [5] (Fig. 17.6). Barczynski et al. recently showed, after a 1 mA stimulation of the EBSLN, that the mean amplitude of evoked potential detected by surface electromyography electrodes on the endotracheal tube was present in almost 75 % of the sample. Notably, the mean amplitude of evoked potential after RLN stimulation was superior to EBSLN stimulation [4]. Similar findings were recently showed by Randolph et al. in patient undergoing thyroid surgery. An EMG waveform following EBSLN stimulation was obtained in almost 80 % of the sample. The mean amplitude of the EBSLN amplitude was approximately one-third of the RLN, mean 250 mcV [43]. Since there is great heterogeneity in amplitude values (and influence of tube position on those values), it is crucial to determine what is the normal range of EBSLN monitoring [5]. Sritharan N. et al. recently published [54] an interesting paper with the aim to define the normative latency and amplitude of the RLN, vagus nerve, and EBSLN applying them to postsurgical neural function documentation. Those nerves showed individual different and unique electrophysiological characteristics that can be recorded as electrophysiological documentation of the existence of postresection neural function (Fig. 17.6).

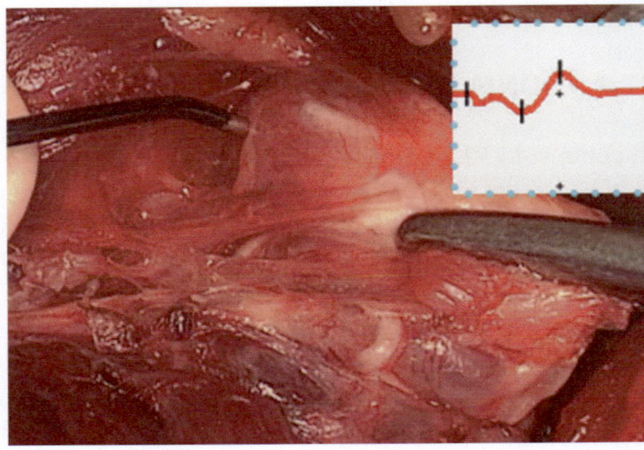

**Fig. 17.6** Positive identification of the EBSLN with cricothyroid muscle twitch and EMG signal. An EMG waveform following EBSLN stimulation is obtained in almost 80 % of cases. The mean amplitude of the EBSLN amplitude is approximately one-third of the RLN, mean 250 mcV

## Conclusion

A damage of the EBSLN is associated with cricothyroid muscle motility impairment, altering the high tone production ability, the voice, and frequency. This nerve is surgically relevant because of its proximity to the superior thyroid vessels [5, 37]. Notably, this nerve lies in close proximity to the superior pole vascular pedicle; for these reasons, these vessels must be carefully managed in order to avoid nerve injury [5, 37]. De facto, in just 15 % of the cases, the superior laryngeal nerve is located far from the superior pole vessels so that it is protected from surgical manipulation. EBSLN injuries can be avoided via a meticulous anatomic localization during the surgical dissection [10, 11, 58]. Actually, very often surgeons do not even attempt to identify this nerve before ligation of the upper pole vessels of the thyroid [37].

For the aforementioned reasons, there is an increasing trend to develop new technologies for EBSLN detection. Magnifying glasses are also available to identify and preserve the laryngeal nerves, hence keeping the morbidity at low levels [26]. Moreover, Berti et al. [7] reported a 65 % EBSLN detection rate in video-assisted thyroidectomy using an optical magnification visualization guidance via an endoscope. IONM has been proposed as an adjunct to the standard intraoperative *de visu* detection of the laryngeal nerves. IONM allows a reliable identification and neuromonitoring of the superior laryngeal nerves during neck surgery [15, 27, 28, 30, 53]. We showed that the EBSLN was more often detected in the IONM arm than in a control group without IONM (83.6 % vs. 42 %) [15].

There is currently the need for a standardized technique of EBSLN monitoring and anatomic detection. In particular, the standardization of IONM technique is relevant for many reasons: for technological safety, to obtain better surgical outcomes, to keep the obtained standards, for educational purposes, and for interoperability, repeatability, and ratification [16]. In order to monitor the EBSLN, the intact neural function of the entire EBSLN must be ensured via a stimulation of the most superior and caudal neural region exposed. On the contrary, indirect EBSLN stimulation via vagal nerve stimulation can be difficult to perform in routine surgical settings, since it requires more extensive surgical dissection; however it may be applicable when lateral compartment lymph node clearance is necessary [37]. The intact EBSLN function must be evaluated after thyroidectomy and hemostasis, i.e., *S2* stimulation. The SLN is the first branch of the vagal nerve after skull base exit; thus continuous monitoring (*C*-IONM) probe electrode cannot monitor EBSLN but *C*-IONM may provide simultaneous and permanent monitoring of RLN during upper pole dissection.

Recently Masuoka et al. [39] presented an interesting prospective randomized trial enrolling patient who underwent thyroid surgery for carcinoma. The visual and electro-stimulatory identification rate of the EBSLN was the primary end point. The changes in the postoperative voice performance were the secondary end point. In particular, 124 patients (203 nerves at risk) were enrolled in the IONM arm (even if the monitoring was not performed via an endotracheal tube with surface electrodes) and 128 patients (202 nerves at risk) in the conventional technique group using a simple nerve stimulator (Vari-Stim 3) to assess the CTM twitch. The authors concluded that IONM allowed an improved visualization rate (48.8 % vs. 17.8 %) and improved electro-stimulatory detection rate (5 times superior, i.e., 89.2 % vs. 17.8 %) in comparison with the conventional surgical technique. What is more, in the IONM arm, there was a reduction of patient complaining subjective voice impairment [39].

In conclusion, for all the aforementioned elements, IONM can provide multiple potential advantages in the EBSLN surgical management: clinically there is a better neural detection and monitoring, and it can provide additional advantages for legal, research, and educational aims [37].

Notably, stroboscopy is a mandatory step to evaluate if IONM reduces the EBSLN damage rate [15, 35, 53]. De facto, the neural functional impairment of the EBSLN during thyroidectomy is usually a rare event; for this reason, it is not easy to obtain an adequate statistical power. However, to perform well-powered studies is a mandatory step to get statistically supported data and to assess the role of new technologies/techniques in terms of detecting differences among the heterogeneous surgical approaches [17].

In order to better define and standardize the normative neural electrophysiological values of EBSLN, at this stage there is currently the urgent need for more in-depth studies investigating the electrophysiological and pathological aspects of the EBSLN. Once those aspects will be better clarified, a more standardized approach will be possible.

Hence, prospective randomized trials are needed for a better understanding of the role of IONM in the EBSLN surgery and for the standardization of the EBSLN IONM technique [17, 37].

## References


1. Adour KK, Schneider GD, Hilsinger RLJ (1980) Acute superior laryngeal nerve palsy: analysis of 78 cases. Otolaryngol Head Neck Surg 88:418–424
2. Aina EN, Hisham AN (2001) External laryngeal nerve in thyroid surgery: recognition and surgical implications. ANZ J Surg 71:212–214

3. Aluffi P et al (2001) Post-thyroidectomy superior laryngeal nerve injury. Eur Arch Otorhinolaryngol 258:451–454
4. Barczynski M et al (2012) Randomized controlled trial of visualization versus neuromonitoring of the external branch of the superior laryngeal nerve during thyroidectomy. World J Surg 36:1340–1347
5. Barczynski M et al (2013) External branch of the superior laryngeal nerve monitoring during thyroid and parathyroid surgery: International Neural Monitoring Study Group standards guideline statement. Laryngoscope 123(Suppl 4):S1–S14
6. Bellantone R et al (2001) Is the identification of the external branch of the superior laryngeal nerve mandatory in thyroid operation? Results of a prospective randomized study. Surgery 130:1055–1059
7. Berti P et al (2002) Visualization of the external branch of the superior laryngeal nerve during video-assisted thyroidectomy. J Am Coll Surg 195:573–574
8. Bevan K, Griffiths MV, Morgan MH (1989) Cricothyroid muscle paralysis: its recognition and diagnosis. J Laryngol Otol 103:191–195
9. Cernea CR et al (1992) Identification of the external branch of the superior laryngeal nerve during thyroidectomy. Am J Surg 164:634–639
10. Cernea CR et al (1992) Surgical anatomy of the external branch of the superior laryngeal nerve. Head Neck 14:380–383
11. Chuang FJ et al (2010) Surgical anatomy of the external branch of the superior laryngeal nerve in Chinese adults and its clinical applications. Head Neck 32:53–57
12. Crookes PF, Recabaren JA (2001) Injury to the superior laryngeal branch of the vagus during thyroidectomy: lesson or myth? Ann Surg 233:588–593
13. Darr EA et al (2014) Superior laryngeal nerve quantitative intraoperative monitoring is possible in all thyroid surgeries. Laryngoscope 124:1035–1041
14. Dionigi G et al (2012) The safety of energy-based devices in open thyroidectomy: a prospective, randomised study comparing the LigaSure (LF1212) and the Harmonic(R) FOCUS. Langenbecks Arch Surg 397:817–823
15. Dionigi G et al (2009) Neuromonitoring and video-assisted thyroidectomy: a prospective, randomized case-control evaluation. Surg Endosc 23:996–1003
16. Dionigi G, Dionigi R (2010) Standardization of intraoperative neuromonitoring of recurrent laryngeal nerve in thyroid operation: to the editor. World J Surg 34:2794–2795
17. Dionigi G et al (2013) Limits of neuromonitoring in thyroid surgery. Ann Surg 258:e1–e2
18. El-Kashlan HK et al (2001) Selective cricothyroid muscle reinnervation by muscle-nerve-muscle neurotization. Arch Otolaryngol Head Neck Surg 127:1211–1215
19. Friedman M, LoSavio P, Ibrahim H (2002) Superior laryngeal nerve identification and preservation in thyroidectomy. Arch Otolaryngol Head Neck Surg 128:296–303
20. Friedman M, Toriumi DM (1986) Functional identification of the external laryngeal nerve during thyroidectomy. Laryngoscope 96:1291–1292
21. Furlan JC (2002) Anatomical study applied to anesthetic block technique of the superior laryngeal nerve. Acta Anaesthesiol Scand 46:199–202
22. Furlan JC (2002) Sympathetic fiber origin of the superior laryngeal nerve and its branches: an anatomic study. Clin Anat 15:271–275
23. Furlan JC et al (2003) Surgical anatomy of the extralaryngeal aspect of the superior laryngeal nerve. Arch Otolaryngol Head Neck Surg 129:79–82
24. Furlan JC, Cordeiro AC, Brandao LG (2003) Study of some "intrinsic risk factors" that can enhance an iatrogenic injury of the external branch of the superior laryngeal nerve. Otolaryngol Head Neck Surg 128:396–400
25. Furlan JC et al (2002) Localization of the superior laryngeal nerve during carotid endarterectomy. Surg Radiol Anat 24:190–193
26. Gimm O et al (2002) An update on thyroid surgery. Eur J Nucl Med Mol Imaging 29(Suppl 2):S447–S452
27. Hurtado-Lopez LM et al (2005) Importance of the intraoperative identification of the external branch of the superior laryngeal nerve during thyroidectomy: electromyographic evaluation. Thyroid 15:449–454

28. Inabnet WB et al (2009) Neuromonitoring of the external branch of the superior laryngeal nerve during minimally invasive thyroid surgery under local anesthesia: a prospective study of 10 patients. Laryngoscope 119:597–601
29. Jansson S et al (1988) Partial superior laryngeal nerve (SLN) lesions before and after thyroid surgery. World J Surg 12:522–527
30. Jonas J, Bahr R (2000) Neuromonitoring of the external branch of the superior laryngeal nerve during thyroid surgery. Am J Surg 179:234–236
31. Kambic V, Zargi M, Radsel Z (1984) Topographic anatomy of the external branch of the superior laryngeal nerve. Its importance in head and neck surgery. J Laryngol Otol 98: 1121–1124
32. Kark AE et al (1984) Voice changes after thyroidectomy: role of the external laryngeal nerve. Br Med J (Clin Res Ed) 289:1412–1415
33. Kierner AC, Aigner M, Burian M (1998) The external branch of the superior laryngeal nerve: its topographical anatomy as related to surgery of the neck. Arch Otolaryngol Head Neck Surg 124:301–303
34. Lennquist S, Cahlin C, Smeds S (1987) The superior laryngeal nerve in thyroid surgery. Surgery 102:999–1008
35. Lifante JC et al (2009) A prospective, randomized trial of nerve monitoring of the external branch of the superior laryngeal nerve during thyroidectomy under local/regional anesthesia and IV sedation. Surgery 146:1167–1173
36. Lore JMJ et al (1998) Thirty-eight-year evaluation of a surgical technique to protect the external branch of the superior laryngeal nerve during thyroidectomy. Ann Otol Rhinol Laryngol 107:1015–1022
37. Mangano A, Dionigi G (2011) The need for standardized technique in intraoperative monitoring of the external branch of the superior laryngeal nerve during thyroidectomy. Surgery 149:854–855
38. Maranillo E et al (2003) Is the external laryngeal nerve an exclusively motor nerve? The cricothyroid connection branch. Laryngoscope 113:525–529
39. Masuoka H et al (2014) A prospective randomized study on injury of the external branch of the superior laryngeal nerve during thyroidectomy comparing intraoperative nerve monitoring and a conventional technique. Head Neck [Epub ahead of print]
40. Melamed H, Harris MB, Awasthi D (2002) Anatomic considerations of superior laryngeal nerve during anterior cervical spine procedures. Spine (Phila Pa 1976) 27:E83–E86
41. Monfared A, Gorti G, Kim D (2002) Microsurgical anatomy of the laryngeal nerves as related to thyroid surgery. Laryngoscope 112:386–392
42. Moosman DA, DeWeese MS (1968) The external laryngeal nerve as related to thyroidectomy. Surg Gynecol Obstet 127:1011–1016
43. Potenza AS et al (2013) Normative intra-operative electrophysiologic waveform analysis of superior laryngeal nerve external branch and recurrent laryngeal nerve in patients undergoing thyroid surgery. World J Surg 37:2336–2342
44. Randolph G (2013) SLN monitoring. Saunders/Elsevier, Philadelphia, pp 339–342
45. Randolph GW et al (2011) Electrophysiologic recurrent laryngeal nerve monitoring during thyroid and parathyroid surgery: international standards guideline statement. Laryngoscope 121(Suppl 1):S1–S16
46. Reeve TS et al (1969) The recurrent and external laryngeal nerves in thyroidectomy. Med J Aust 1:380–382
47. Rossi RL et al (1986) Current results of conservative surgery for differentiated thyroid carcinoma. World J Surg 10:612–622
48. Roy N et al (2009) An in vivo model of external superior laryngeal nerve paralysis: laryngoscopic findings. Laryngoscope 119:1017–1032
49. Roy N et al (2009) Exploring the phonatory effects of external superior laryngeal nerve paralysis: an in vivo model. Laryngoscope 119:816–826
50. Sadler TW (2012) Langman's medical embryology. Wolters Kluwer Health/Lippincott Williams & Wilkins, Philadelphia
51. Sanders I et al (1993) The innervation of the human larynx. Arch Otolaryngol Head Neck Surg 119:934–939

52. Sanudo JR et al (1999) An anatomical study of anastomoses between the laryngeal nerves. Laryngoscope 109:983–987
53. Selvan B et al (2009) Mapping the compound muscle action potentials of cricothyroid muscle using electromyography in thyroid operations: a novel method to clinically type the external branch of the superior laryngeal nerve. Ann Surg 250:293–300
54. Sritharan N et al (2015) The vagus nerve, recurrent laryngeal nerve, and external branch of the superior laryngeal nerve have unique latencies allowing for intraoperative documentation of intact neural function during thyroid surgery. Laryngoscope 125(2):E84–E89
55. Tanaka S, Hirano M, Umeno H (1994) Laryngeal behavior in unilateral superior laryngeal nerve paralysis. Ann Otol Rhinol Laryngol 103:93–97
56. Teitelbaum BJ, Wenig BL (1995) Superior laryngeal nerve injury from thyroid surgery. Head Neck 17:36–40
57. Tsai V et al (2007) Videostroboscopic findings in unilateral superior laryngeal nerve paralysis and paresis. Otolaryngol Head Neck Surg 136:660–662
58. Whitfield P, Morton RP, Al-Ali S (2010) Surgical anatomy of the external branch of the superior laryngeal nerve. ANZ J Surg 80:813–816
59. Woodson GE (1990) Respiratory activity of the cricothyroid muscle in conscious humans. Laryngoscope 100:49–53; discussion 53
60. Woodson GE et al (1998) Unilateral cricothyroid contraction and glottic configuration. J Voice 12:335–339
61. Wu BL et al (1994) The human communicating nerve. An extension of the external superior laryngeal nerve that innervates the vocal cord. Arch Otolaryngol Head Neck Surg 120: 1321–1328

# Recurrent Laryngeal Nerve Monitoring 18

Rahul R. Modi, Dipti Kamani, and Gregory W. Randolph

Thyroid surgery is unique in head and neck surgery in that both right and left cranial nerves are subject to risk in one surgical procedure. It is a well-known fact that unilateral vocal cord palsy can lead to voice changes sufficient enough to alter vocation especially in professional voice users, and may be accompanied by dysphagia and aspiration, whereas bilateral vocal cord paralysis may necessitate a tracheostomy [1]. Current reported rates for temporary vocal cord paralysis range anywhere between 1.4 and 38.4 % (average 9.8 %), whereas it ranges between 0 and 18.6 % (average 2.3 %) for permanent vocal cord paralysis [2]. Thus importance of ensuring functional integrity of the recurrent laryngeal nerve anatomy (RLN) during thyroid surgery cannot be overstated.

The current gold standard for prevention of injury to the RLN is visual identification of the nerve during surgery. Intraoperative nerve monitoring (IONM) is a useful supplement to this practice. The basic guiding principle of IONM is that a nerve that appears structurally intact and is surgically well preserved may not necessarily be functional. It may not be possible to visually identify thermal or stretch injuries to a nerve. This chapter reviews the principles, and application of monitoring techniques for RLN, utility of IONM as well as new advancements in the technique.

R.R. Modi
Division of Thyroid and Parathyroid Surgery, Department of Otolaryngology, Massachusetts Eye and Ear Infirmary, 243 Charles St, Boston, MA 02114, USA

Department of Otolaryngology – Head and Neck Surgery, Bharati Vidyapeeth Deemed University Medical College, Pune, Maharashtra, India
e-mail: Rahul_Modi@meei.harvard.edu

D. Kamani • G.W. Randolph (✉)
Division of Thyroid and Parathyroid Surgery, Department of Otolaryngology, Massachusetts Eye and Ear Infirmary, 243 Charles St, Boston, MA 02114, USA
e-mail: Dipti_kamani@meei.harvard.edu; Gregory_randolph@meei.harvard.edu



C.P. Lombardi, R. Bellantone (eds.), *Minimally Invasive Therapies for Endocrine Neck Diseases*, DOI 10.1007/978-3-319-20065-1_18

IONM has gained widespread acceptance as an essential adjunct to visual identification and is being used extensively. Interestingly, the use of IONM is more popular in centers enjoying a higher volume (>100 cases/year) of cases [3]. As experience with IONM is growing, its role in reducing vocal cord paralysis rates is slowly becoming apparent. Uniform use of standard techniques [4, 5] and protocols has led to a better understanding of the role of IONM during surgery. Organizations such as the American Academy of Otolaryngology and Head and Neck Surgery (AAOHNS), the American Thyroid Association (ATA), the American Association of Endocrine Surgery (AAES), the American Head and Neck Society (AHNS), the British Association of Endocrine and Thyroid surgeons, and the German Association of Endocrine Surgery have also endorsed the utility of IONM [6–10].

## 18.1 Applications of IONM

Although the utility of IONM in reducing incidence of vocal cord paralysis has been debated extensively in the literature, there is a definite trend towards reduction in the rate of vocal cord paralysis with use of IONM. The average rate of nerve paralysis with IONM was found to be 4.7 % and without the use of IONM was 5.7 % [3, 11–26]. Many individual studies have also established that IONM decreases temporary and permanent vocal cord paralysis rates in thyroid surgeries, especially in cases of retrosternal goiters, revision surgeries, and surgeries for thyroid cancer [27, 28]. Dralle et al. have showed that complications such as rate of vocal cord palsy are significantly less when IONM is used by low volume surgeons [3, 29]. Along with thyroid and parathyroid surgery, IONM is also useful for neck surgeries such as surgery for airway stenosis, carotid endarterectomy, anterior approaches to the cervical spine, and certain skull base procedures. Although the greatest advantage with nerve monitoring is in difficult thyroid operations, routine application has shown to steepen learning curves through greater experience in interpretation of the signal and troubleshooting system malfunction [4].

Routine use of IONM during surgery tends to benefit the surgeon in the following areas:

1. *Neural mapping*: Studies have reported nerve identification rates between 98 and 100 % with the use of IONM [4]. Linear stimulation along the paratracheal region can help map out the entire course of the nerve, this neural map can guide further dissection and visualization of the nerve. IONM is particularly useful during revision surgeries where it might be difficult to identify nerve in scar tissue and also in cases with distorted anatomy such as large goiters and invasive malignancies.
2. *Understanding pathologic states of RLN*: Electrophysiologic stimulation of a nerve invaded by malignancy may reveal significant residual electromyograhy (EMG) activity. This is possible even in the setting of a preoperative vocal cord paralysis. In a recently conducted study [30] by our unit, we found that out of the 12 patients with preoperative vocal cord paralysis due to invasive disease,

about a third still showed significant EMG activity. Resection of such a nerve during surgery may lead to additional dysphagia and aspiration. Surgical management of invaded nerve can be impacted by intraoperative EMG activity. Thus IONM can provide valuable insights in the functioning of invaded nerves which is otherwise not available with simple visual identification.

3. *Detection of intraoperative nerve injury and prognostication of nerve function:* Use of IONM during surgery allows the surgeon to predict the functional status of RLN with reasonable accuracy. This is the most important feature of IONM as it assists the surgeon in avoiding bilateral vocal cord paralysis in almost all the cases. There is evidence to suggest that visual identification alone is vastly insufficient to prognosticate postoperative RLN function. A study reviewing more than 3600 cases from the Scandinavian endocrine quality register reported that the surgeon was only able to predict injuries in 11.3 % of the nerves injured and that in fact only 16 % (1 out of 6) bilateral injuries were identified intraoperatively [31]. Similar results have been reported by Snyder et al. [15] Thus approximately 90 % of the injuries are not visually identifiable. In comparison, use of IONM is a highly precise neural function test and has negative predictive value of over 95 % [19, 20, 23, 33, 32]. Though the positive predictive value of IONM is lower and can be quite variable, this is related to how presumptive loss of signal is evaluated with respect to equipment troubleshooting. Universal and accurate definition of loss of signal and a better knowledge of normative neural monitoring parameters can greatly augment prognostic function of IONM [4, 34, 35]. The idea of postponing the surgery on opposite side in the setting of neural related loss of signal represents the greatest extension of neural prognostication ability of IONM. Evaluation after a loss of signal is further explored in the following section. Another reported indicator for nerve injury during IONM is frequent passive EMG activity. This might indicate a nerve under stress secondary to mechanical stretch or cautery injury and should prompt urgent evaluation of surgical maneuver [36–38]. However, in our experience this activity is a poor indicator of nerve injury and is also encountered when the patient is in a lighter plane of anesthesia.

## 18.2 Intraoperative Nerve Monitoring Standards

### 18.2.1 Introduction

Use of different electrodes, techniques, and output methods lead to incomparable results. Standardization of a technique ensures optimum utilization and comparable outcomes. The International Nerve Monitoring Study Group (INMSG) is a multidisciplinary international group of researchers with expertise in the field of neural monitoring as it pertains to thyroid and parathyroid surgery [4, 5]. These include surgeons, laryngologists, voice and laryngeal EMG specialists, and anesthesiologists. This group has suggested certain standards for IONM with a primary objective of improving quality of nerve monitoring and achieving comparable outcomes.

Technique of IONM, setup of the equipment, interpretation of loss of signal (LOS), and troubleshooting during IONM are the major areas addressed by these standards.

### 18.2.2 Technique: IONM

The INMSG recommends certain basic overarching elements, which form an integral part of any IONM technique. These elements are immensely helpful not only for verifying the functionality of the system and for neural mapping but also for providing accurate prognostic information for postoperative glottic function. These include the following:

1. Preoperative and postoperative laryngoscopy (L1 and L2)
2. Predissection and postdissection suprathreshold vagal stimulation (V1 and V2)
3. Predissection and postdissection suprathreshold RLN stimulation (R1 and R2)

Predissection suprathreshold vagal stimulation allows for verification of system functionality and improves upon the negative predictive value of IONM for RLN mapping, whereas postdissection suprathreshold vagal stimulation is the most accurate prognostic test available for postoperative glottic function and has been shown to have higher sensitivity, slightly higher specificity, higher positive predictive value, and slightly higher negative predictive value than for RLN stimulation in the prediction of vocal cord paralysis [4, 23]. This can be explained by the fact that stimulation distal to the site of injury on the RLN might demonstrate a false positive response while a postsurgical stimulation of the vagus nerve will alert the surgeon to the injury. The above mentioned elements can be noted in the form of L1, V1, R1 and R2, V2, L2.

### 18.2.3 The Equipment Setup

A basic setup of the neural monitoring equipment is shown in Fig. 18.1.

Various nerve monitoring formats are available for IONM. These include glottic observation [39–41], laryngeal palpation [21, 25, 42, 43], endotracheal tube–based surface electrodes [26, 44–50], postcricoid surface electrodes [51, 52], and many more. These can be audio only or ones that provide both audio and visual waveform information. The major drawback with audio only systems is that the information such as wave-form amplitude, latency, and morphology which may provide insights into the pathologic state of the nerve is unavailable. As our understanding of RLN electrophysiology improves this information may prove to be useful in surgical decision making. Also, at times, it might be difficult to differentiate between the signal and the artifact with audio-only systems. Currently, the most preferred neural monitoring equipment is an endotracheal tube–based system that includes a visual graphic documentation of the EMG waveform elicited from thyroarytenoid muscle

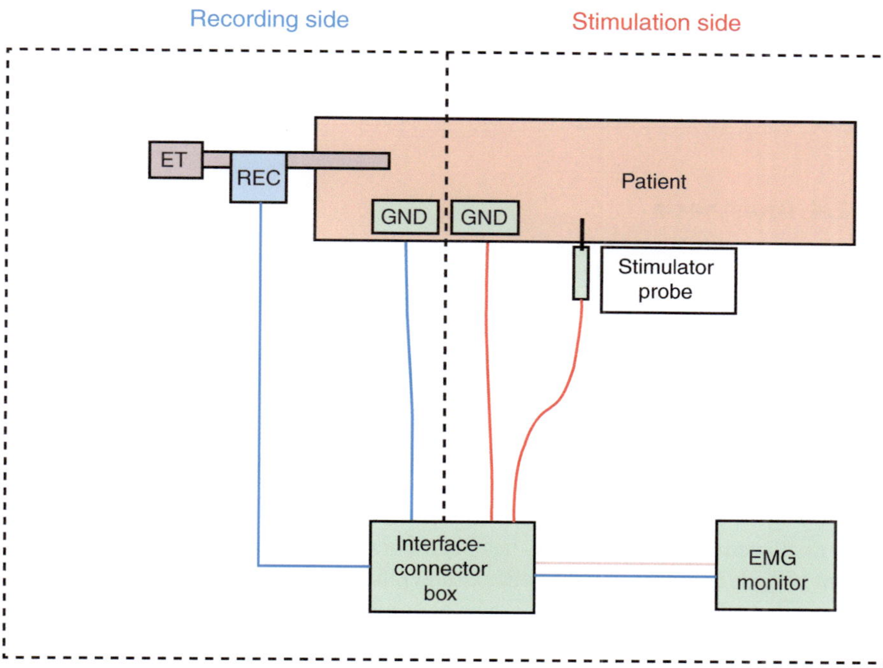


**Fig. 18.1** Basic IONM equipment setup *ET* endotracheal tube, *REC* recording electrodes, *GND* ground electrodes (Adapted from Randolph et al. [4] *permissions awaited*)

[53]. Prefabricated endotracheal tubes with paired stainless steel electrodes exposed at the level of the glottis or standard tubes with thin electrodes placed over the tube with adhesive pads can be used. Another option is to use needle electrodes instead of surface electrodes but these carry additional risk of injury to the cords, laceration or hematoma, and are less preferred.

Introduction of any technique comes with its own learning curve. Studies have suggested that optimum functioning of the IONM can be achieved after performance of 50–100 monitoring cases [4, 54]. Dionigi et al. [54] have reported that setup related problems can occur in up to 10 % of patients. The most common problem being that related to tube positioning and occurred in 53 % of the patients. Chiang et al. have shown that routine application of IONM can reduce setup related problems from 4.4 to 0 % [55]. Thus, adherence to a standard setup and tube placement algorithm reduces the occurrence of intraoperative problems. Ground electrodes are adhered to the shoulder or the sternum area. Poor grounding can cause a noisy baseline, making it difficult to interpret the EMG data. It is also important to keep the electrocautery unit more than 10 ft away from the neural monitoring unit to avoid electrical interference. Choice of the stimulating electrode depends upon its intended use. Monopolar electrodes are generally preferred for initial neural mapping, whereas bipolar electrodes may be more sensitive in stimulating a focal point on the nerve once it is identified. The major drawback with bipolar electrodes being that incorrect orientation of the anode (positive) and cathode (negative) relative to the nerve may give a false negative signal [56]. After the equipment is setup, care is taken to ensure that the recording side and the stimulation side circuitry is functional (Fig. 18.1).

### 18.2.4 Anesthesia

An important member of the team performing IONM is the anesthesiologist. A detailed discussion on special needs of anesthesia during nerve monitoring is imperative prior to surgery. It is important that long acting muscle relaxants are avoided during surgery to enhance the accuracy of the nerve monitoring system. Short acting muscle relaxants such as succinyl choline can be used for induction with the aim of recovering normal muscle twitch activity within minutes of intubation. A good way of ensuring optimum contact between the electrodes and the vocal cord is to select an endotracheal tube with the largest admissible size. Use of a drying agent and oral suctioning of any secretions are also helpful in this regard. Tube displacement of up to 6 cm has been documented during positioning of the patient [57]. It is thus prudent to check tube placement after final positioning. The gold standard for tube placement is visual confirmation [4]. Another reliable way of confirming tube positioning is identification of "respiratory variations." These are waveforms with amplitude between 30 and 70 μV which are observed in the small window of time when the effect of initial muscle relaxant wears off and the patient is in a lighter plane of anesthesia. They appear as coarsening of the baseline EMG activity and can be seen reliably in more than 90 % of the patients. In a recently concluded study, our unit found that presence of respiratory variations independently predicted a good evoked response intraoperatively and obviated the need of a repeat laryngoscopy in most patients [58]. Impedance checks for a higher overall impedance (more than 5 Ω) or an imbalance between the two sides (more than 1 Ω) is another good tactic for checking the robustness of the IONM circuitry. During the initial setup, the monitor is set at an event threshold of 100 μV and the stimulator probe at 2 mA for initial neural mapping. This can be reduced to 1 mA after the nerve is identified for a more focal stimulation and end of surgery prognostication. These levels have been reported to be extremely safe and no unfavorable effects have been reported [59]. In the surgical field, the stimulator probe is tested on the strap muscle first to look for a local muscle twitch and to confirm that the current is being reported back on the monitor. Prior to labeling any tissue as being truly negative (not the RLN), a predissection supra threshold vagal stimulation (V1) should be performed to obtain a true positive signal verifying the integrity of the IONM circuitry. The suprathreshold vagal stimulation utilizes 2 mA current and is usually performed effectively without direct vagal dissection by placing the stimulator probe between the jugular vein and carotid artery. The surgeon should also feel for a "laryngeal twitch" response from the laryngeal muscles by rolling the fingers on the side of the larynx. This response always accompanies a true positive signal.

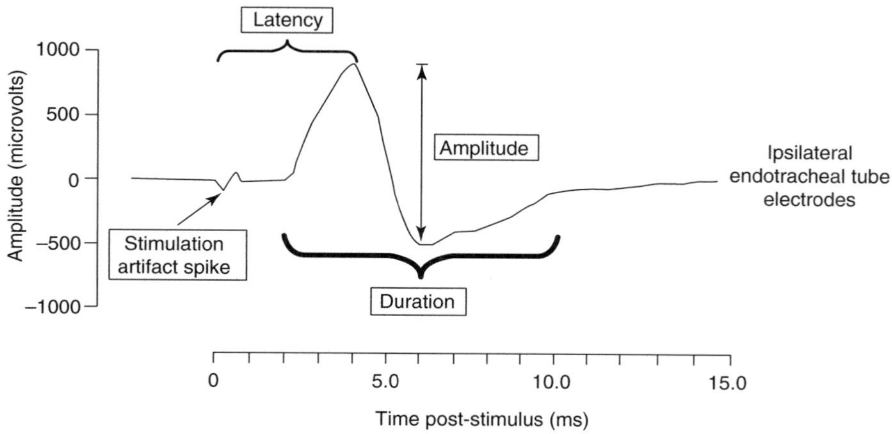


**Fig. 18.2** A typical triphasic evoked waveform captured during IONM with various parameters indicated (Adapted from Intraoperative monitoring: normative range associated with normal postoperative glottic function. Caragacianu et al. [59] permission awaited)

The human RLN and vagus nerve typically have biphasic or a triphasic waveform. Parameters such as amplitude and latency in the waveform can provide useful prognostic information regarding glottis function at the end of surgery. Amplitude is defined as the vertical height of the apex of the positive initial waveform deflection to the lowest point in the net subsequent opposite polarity phase of the waveform (Fig. 18.2). Interestingly, a study performed by Caragacianu et al. [59], reports that the strength of the stimulation current (1 mA vs. 2 mA) had no significant impact on the amplitude recorded. It also notes that a final amplitude of >250 μV recorded during postdissection vagal stimulation at 1 mA accurately predicts postoperative glottic function. However, currently there is a lack of consensus over the definition for latency. The INMSG defines latency as the time from the stimulation spike to the first evoked waveform peak [4]. Latencies recorded during intraoperative monitoring are distinctive and can differentiate artifacts from neural stimulated structures and also can be used to distinguish superior laryngeal nerve, vagus nerve, and RLN and also distinguish left from right vagus nerve easily.

## 18.2.5 Loss of Signal and Its Interpretation (Fig. 18.3)

Absence of EMG activity or loss of signal (LOS) during surgery should prompt a quick review of the IONM setup. The first response of the surgeon should be to feel for the laryngeal twitch response. If the response is present then the problem is likely to be on the recording side of the system while if the twitch response is absent then it is considered a stimulation side problem. Adherence to the accompanying algorithm (Fig. 18.3) can guide the surgeon to adopt a systematic approach towards

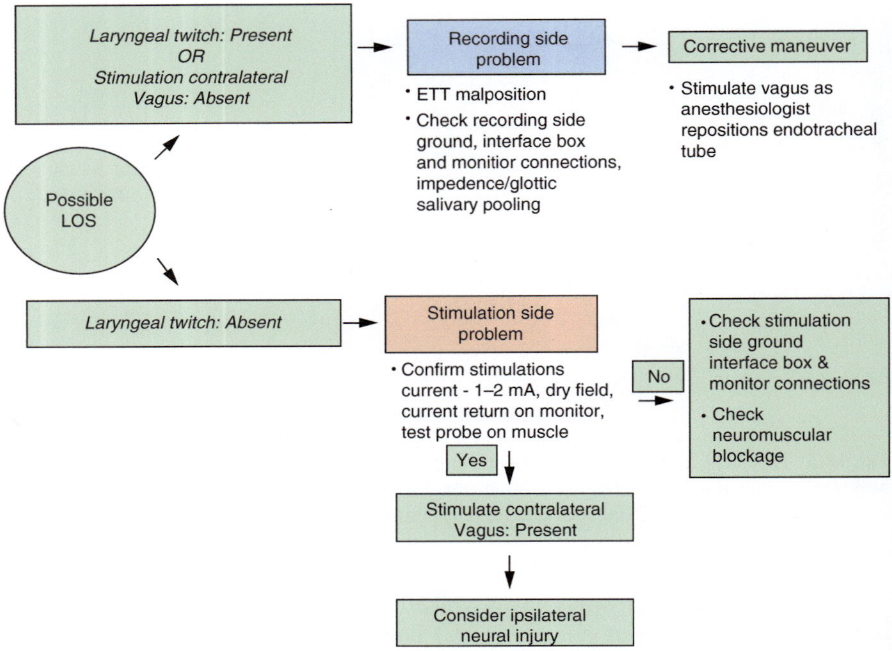


**Fig. 18.3** Intraoperative evaluation of loss of signal (*LOS*) standard (Adapted from Randolph et al. [4]. Permissions awaited)

managing such a scenario. A true loss of signal is currently defined only when the following conditions are met:

1. Presence of a satisfactory EMG (Amplitude >100 μV) prior to the event
2. No or low response (i.e., 100 μV or lower) with stimulation at 1–2 mA in a dry field
3. Absence of laryngeal twitch and/or glottis twitch on ipsilateral vagal stimulation

A true LOS strongly suggests a neural injury. Identification of the point of injury can allow the surgeon to guide further management of the injured nerve. Once the signal is lost, the surgeon can locate the point of injury by stimulating the RLN at the laryngeal entry point [60] and then proceeding proximally to identify the injured segment. If identified, segmental injuries are labeled as a Type 1 Injury. Sometimes, the whole course of the RLN and the vagus nerve is nonconductive, this is labeled as a global nerve injury and is defined as a Type II injury. Detection of LOS in a visually intact nerve is the most significant advantage of IONM, which can guide the surgeon in reconsidering surgery on the contralateral side and can prevent a potential bilateral cord paralysis [56].

### 18.2.6 Prognostic Testing Errors

Postdissection suprathreshold RLN and vagus stimulation is a reliable indicator of postoperative glottis function. As mentioned earlier, numerous studies have shown a high negative predictive value (>95 %) for the same. However, the following errors might occur while using IONM.

1. *False positive errors:* (Errors where there is an LOS intraoperatively but the nerve is functional postoperatively). These can occur in the following conditions
   (i) Stimulation of the nerve in a wet bloody field may yield a false positive LOS
   (ii) Equipment errors on the recording side (tube displacement, improper grounding of electrodes)
   (iii) Prolonged neuromuscular blockade
   (iv) Early neuronal recovery especially if the postoperative laryngoscopy is delayed by a few days
2. *False negative errors:* (Errors where there is a positive signal present at the end of the surgery stimulation of RLN but absence of nerve function postoperatively). Although uncommon, especially if IONM is performed in a systematic manner, these errors can occur due to:
   (i) Stimulation of the nerve distal to the site of injury. This error can be avoided by postdissection vagal stimulation.
   (ii) Endotracheal tube related injury such as laryngeal edema and dislocation of the arytenoid cartilage.
   (iii) Injury to the nerve after the final stimulation – during wound closure.
   (iv) In situations where there is an extralaryngeal branching of the RLN, a posterior branch injury may not be detected by IONM if postcricoid electrodes are not used. This may present as an abduction defect on laryngoscopy.

## 18.3 Promising Advances in IONM

### 18.3.1 Continuous Vagal Monitoring and Neural Injury Prevention

While IONM in its present format, is tremendously useful in assisting a surgeon, its greatest shortcoming is that it can only intermittently evaluate the functional integrity of the RLN, thus allowing the nerve to be at risk for injuries in-between stimulations [3, 31]. This could underlie the notion that, IONM, in its current format may have limited ability to prevent neural injury [31, 61, 62]. Continuous IONM (CIONM) with vagal nerve electrode provides a real-time EMG data by monitoring the entire vagus and RLN functional integrity uninterruptedly throughout the surgery. This real-time electrophysiological information from RLN obtained by

**Table 18.1** Mild and severe combined events

| | |
|---|---|
| Mild combined event (mCE): | Amplitude decrease of >50–70 % with a concordant latency increase of 5–10 % |
| Severe combined event (sCE): | Amplitude decrease of >70 % with a concordant latency increase of >10 % |

CIONM is extremely vital as it alerts the surgeon prior to the occurrence of irreversible neural damage and thereby evading a possible permanent injury to the RLN. CIONM is not associated with significant neural, cardiac, pulmonary, or gastrointestinal vagal side effects [63, 64].

CIONM, through adverse EMG changes, can alert a surgeon regarding an impending neural injury and allow the surgeons to prompt a corrective action to preserve nerve function by aborting maneuvers that lead to adverse EMG changes and thereby possibly preventing permanent vocal cord paralysis [65]. However, it is essential that, a surgeon is able to differentiate between true adverse events and artifacts as well as can isolate meaningful adverse events. Our group has identified mild (mCE) and severe combined events (sCE) by combining reduction in amplitude with increase in latency (Table 18.1). In our study, notably, mCE and isolated amplitude or latency changes were not associated with vocal cord paralysis, while a sCE denoted a typically reversible electrophysiologic event if the related surgical maneuver was aborted, otherwise sCE could lead to LOS (which typically is much less reversible) and to possible postoperative vocal cord paralysis. Thus, modification of surgical maneuver associated with sCE can prevent subsequent neural injury leading to postoperative vocal cord paralysis. However, surgeons should keep in mind that any IONM format is more useful for preventing impeding neural damage secondary to a stretch or compression injury than the neural damage due to an inadvertent neural transection injury [65].

### 18.3.2 Superior Laryngeal Nerve (SLN) Monitoring

RLN paralysis and hypoparathyroidism are the most common complications discussed when a thyroidectomy is planned but injury to external branch of SLN (EBSLN) can occur in up to 58 % of patients undergoing thyroid surgery [66]. EBSLN is at risk of injury during superior pole dissection and ligation of superior thyroid vessels. Injury to external branch of the SLN (EBSLN) results in cricothyroid muscle dysfunction and affects vocal projection and the ability to produce higher registers of the voice. While subtle, these voice changes can significantly impact professional voice users. The injury to EBSLN is difficult to identify intraoperatively as well as by postoperative laryngeal exam. Intraoperative visual identification of EBSLN is limited as 20 % of EBSLNs run a subfasical course [67]. IONM is now widely accepted as an adjunct to visual identification of the RLN, and can be similarly extended to EBSLN identification. Application of IONM should allow stimulation and identification of all EBSLNs including those visually unidentifiable subfascial EBSLNs mentioned earlier. Recently published guidelines on EBSLN monitoring emphasize that SLN monitoring is associated with higher rate of nerve identification as compared to visual identification alone [5]. The SLN monitoring utilizes the laryngeal head of the sternothyroid muscle as a useful landmark for identification of the EBSLN. The tissue parallel and underneath the laryngeal head of the sternothyroid muscle is stimulated to delineate distal course of EBSLN before it enters the cricothyroid muscle. A twitch in the cricothyroid muscle seen upon this stimulation is presently the most accurate way of EBSLN localization. For detailed review of technique and utility of EBSLN monitoring, the reader is requested to refer to the guidelines published by the INMSG [5]. It has been recently demonstrated that a specially designed electrode array incorporated on an endotracheal tube can facilitate quantifiable EMG response from the EBSLN in all patients [68].

### 18.3.3 Neural Monitoring and Staged Thyroidectomy in Thyroid Cancer Surgery: An Emerging Concept

The Concept of staging oncology surgeries has a longstanding history. Staged surgery was recommended by Dunhill, for severe toxic goiter in 1912 and by Lahey for severe hyperthyroidism in 1936 [69, 70]. Frazzell, in 1961, proposed a planned staging of surgeries where sacrifice of bilateral internal jugular veins was anticipated [71]. Extensive neck surgeries typically carry a higher risk of complications, and bilateral RLN paralysis being one of the most dreadful of all. Extensive neck surgeries are often necessary to address frequently encountered bilateral nodal metastases in thyroid cancers. By staging these surgeries, a surgeon may offset some of the associated complications, especially the temporary ones. RLN neuropraxia as well as parathyroid glands may recover functionally in the intervening period between the two stages of the surgeries.

While the aforementioned staged surgeries are typically planned preoperatively, often a surgeon intraoperatively faces a dilemma of proceeding to bilateral surgery or of staging the opposite side surgery. Usefulness of LOS as an intraoperative decision-making tool in such circumstances is slowly becoming evident. Dralle et al. found that 94 % of surgeons in Germany would stage a total thyroidectomy upon encountering a LOS during the surgery [72]. Goretski et al. have reported that when LOS was integrated in surgical decision making in bilateral surgeries, incidence of bilateral vocal cord paralysis reduced to zero from 17 % [73]. A surgeon should be aware that a detailed preoperative consent process is essential if staging of surgery is being envisioned as a possibility [74]. Our unit routinely performs staged surgery when patients present with extensive thyroid cancer with bilateral nodal disease. Our unpublished data from a series of patients undergoing planned staged surgery for advanced thyroid malignancy, reported zero percent permanent RLN paralysis and 3.3 % permanent hypoparathyroidism rate. Postoperatively thyroglobulin was undetectable in 90 % and averaged 0.8 ng/ml during a three-year follow-up.

### 18.3.4 Intraoperative Identification of Nonrecurrent Laryngeal Nerve

The nonrecurrent laryngeal nerve (NRLN) is an anatomical variant of RLN, presenting more commonly on the right side (0.5–1 % of all RLNs) than on the left side (0.04 %) [75, 76]. NRLN has no functional bearing, except that it makes the nerve more vulnerable to injury, especially when a surgeon is oblivious of its presence. Thus, knowledge of presence of NRLN prior to dissection in related cervical region is important in averting intraoperative injury to NRLN. An electrophysiologic algorithm of presence of positive EMG response to proximal stimulation of vagus at the superior border of thyroid cartilage and absence of EMG response to distal stimulation of vagus below the inferior border of 4th tracheal ring reliably identified all NRLNs in our series of NRLNs [30]. Brauckhoff et al. have also found similar utility of this vagal stimulation technique for NRLN identification [24]. The electrophysiological parameters like amplitude, latency, and threshold of right NRLN are similar to that of right RLN. Although, some research studies [77] suggest that a latency of less than 3.5 ms is a strong pointer of NRLN, further studies are merited before its acknowledgment as a conclusive indication of NRLN. Since no steadfast technique for preoperative acknowledgment or exclusion of NRLN exists, at the present time, aforementioned electrophysiologic algorithm represents a reliable tool to alert a surgeon regarding presence of NRLN prior to the dissection in the related cervical region.

## References


1. Munch S, deKryger L (2001) A piece of my mind. Moral wounds: complicated complications. JAMA 285(9):1131–1132
2. Jeannon JP, Orabi AA, Bruch GA, Abdalsalam HA, Simo R (2009) Diagnosis of recurrent laryngeal nerve palsy after thyroidectomy: a systematic review. Int J Clin Pract 63(4):624–629. doi:IJCP1875 [pii] 10.1111/j.1742-1241.2008.01875.x
3. Dralle H, Sekulla C, Haerting J, Timmermann W, Neumann HJ, Kruse E, Grond S, Muhlig HP, Richter C, Voss J, Thomusch O, Lippert H, Gastinger I, Brauckhoff M, Gimm O (2004) Risk factors of paralysis and functional outcome after recurrent laryngeal nerve monitoring in thyroid surgery. Surgery 136(6):1310–1322. doi:S0039606004005550 [pii] 10.1016/j.surg.2004.07.018 [doi]
4. Randolph GW, Dralle H, Abdullah H, Barczynski M, Bellantone R, Brauckhoff M, Carnaille B, Cherenko S, Chiang FY, Dionigi G, Finck C, Hartl D, Kamani D, Lorenz K, Miccolli P, Mihai R, Miyauchi A, Orloff L, Perrier N, Poveda MD, Romanchishen A, Serpell J, Sitges-Serra A, Sloan T, Van Slycke S, Snyder S, Takami H, Volpi E, Woodson G (2011) Electrophysiologic recurrent laryngeal nerve monitoring during thyroid and parathyroid surgery: international standards guideline statement. Laryngoscope 121(Suppl 1):S1–S16. doi:10.1002/lary.21119
5. Barczynski M, Randolph GW, Cernea CR, Dralle H, Dionigi G, Alesina PF, Mihai R, Finck C, Lombardi D, Hartl DM, Miyauchi A, Serpell J, Snyder S, Volpi E, Woodson G, Kraimps JL, Hisham AN, with the International Neural Monitoring Study G (2013) External branch of the superior laryngeal nerve monitoring during thyroid and parathyroid surgery: international neural monitoring study group standards guideline statement. Laryngoscope. doi:10.1002/lary.24301
6. Chandrasekhar SRG, Seidman MS, Rosenfeld R, Angelos P, Barkmeier-Kraemer J, Benninger MS, Blumin J, Dennis G, Hanks J, Haymart M, Kloos RT, Seals B, Schreibstein JM, Thomas

TM, Waddington C, Warren B, Robertson PJ (2013) American Academy of Otolaryngology Head and Neck Surgery clinical practice guidelines: improving voice outcomes after thyroid surgery. Otolaryngol Head Neck Surg 148(6 Suppl):S1–S37

7. Chen AY, Bernet VJ, Carty SE, Davies TF, Ganly I, Inabnet William B III, Shaha AR (2014) Thyroid 24(2):181–189. doi:10.1089/thy.2013.0291
8. Shindo ML, Caruana SM, Kandil E, McCaffrey JC, Orloff LA, Porterfield JR, Shaha A, Shin J, Terris D, Randolph G (2014) Management of invasive well-differentiated thyroid cancer: An American head and neck society consensus statement: AHNS consensus statement. Head Neck 36:1379–1390. doi: 10.1002/hed.23619
9. Scott-Coombes D, Kinsman R (2009) The British Association of Endocrine and Thyroid Surgeons (BAETS) Third National Audit Report. Oxfordshire: Dendrite Clinical Systems Ltd
10. Musholt TJ, Clerici T, Dralle H, Frilling A, Goretzki PE, Hermann MM, Kussmann J, Lorenz K, Nies C, Schabram J, Schabram P, Scheuba C, Simon D, Steinmuller T, Trupka AW, Wahl RA, Zielke A, Bockisch A, Karges W, Luster M, Schmid KW (2011) German Association of Endocrine Surgeons practice guidelines for the surgical treatment of benign thyroid disease. Langenbecks Arch Surg 396(5):639–649. doi:10.1007/s00423-011-0774-y
11. Cavicchi O, Caliceti U, Fernandez IJ, Ceroni AR, Marcantoni A, Sciascia S, Sottili S, Piccin O (2011) Laryngeal neuromonitoring and neurostimulation versus neurostimulation alone in thyroid surgery: a randomized clinical trial. Head Neck. doi:10.1002/hed.21681
12. Shindo M, Chheda NN (2007) Incidence of vocal cord paralysis with and without recurrent laryngeal nerve monitoring during thyroidectomy. Arch Otolaryngol Head Neck Surg 133(5):481–485
13. Robertson ML, Steward DL, Gluckman JL, Welge J (2004) Continuous laryngeal nerve integrity monitoring during thyroidectomy: does it reduce risk of injury? Otolaryngol Head Neck Surg 131(5):596–600. doi:S0194599804015724 [pii] 10.1016/j.otohns.2004.05.030 [doi]
14. Yarbrough DE, Thompson GB, Kasperbauer JL, Harper CM, Grant CS (2004) Intraoperative electromyographic monitoring of the recurrent laryngeal nerve in reoperative thyroid and parathyroid surgery. Surgery 136(6):1107–1115. doi:S0039606004005252 [pii] 10.1016/j.surg.2004.06.040 [doi]
15. Snyder SK, Hendricks JC (2005) Intraoperative neurophysiology testing of the recurrent laryngeal nerve: plaudits and pitfalls. Surgery 138(6):1183–1191; discussion 1191–1182. doi:S0039-6060(05)00553-2 [pii] 10.1016/j.surg.2005.08.027 [doi]
16. Hemmerling TM, Schmidt J, Bosert C, Jacobi KE, Klein P (2001) Intraoperative monitoring of the recurrent laryngeal nerve in 151 consecutive patients undergoing thyroid surgery. Anesth Analg 93(2):396–399, 393rd contents page
17. Jonas J, Bahr R (2006) Intraoperative neuromonitoring of the recurrent laryngeal nerve – results and learning curve. Zentralbl Chir 131(6):443–448. doi:10.1055/s-2006-955453
18. Kunath M, Marusch F, Horschig P, Gastinger I (2003) The value of intraoperative neuromonitoring in thyroid surgery–a prospective observational study with 926 patients. Zentralbl Chir 128(3):187–190. doi:10.1055/s-2003-38529
19. Hamelmann WH, Meyer T, Timm S, Timmermann W (2002) A critical estimation of intraoperative neuromonitoring (IONM) in thyroid surgery. Zentralbl Chir 127(5):409–413. doi:10.1055/s-2002-31982
20. Tomoda C, Hirokawa Y, Uruno T, Takamura Y, Ito Y, Miya A, Kobayashi K, Matsuzuka F, Kuma K, Miyauchi A (2006) Sensitivity and specificity of intraoperative recurrent laryngeal nerve stimulation test for predicting vocal cord palsy after thyroid surgery. World J Surg 30(7):1230–1233. doi:10.1007/s00268-005-0351-z
21. Echeverri A, Flexon PB (1998) Electrophysiologic nerve stimulation for identifying the recurrent laryngeal nerve in thyroid surgery: review of 70 consecutive thyroid surgeries. Am Surg 64(4):328–333
22. Eltzschig HK, Posner M, Moore FD Jr (2002) The use of readily available equipment in a simple method for intraoperative monitoring of recurrent laryngeal nerve function during thyroid surgery: initial experience with more than 300 cases. Arch Surg 137(4):452–456; discussion 456–457. doi:sne1016 [pii]

23. Dralle H, Sekulla C, Lorenz K, Brauckhoff M, Machens A (2008) Intraoperative monitoring of the recurrent laryngeal nerve in thyroid surgery. World J Surg 32(7):1358–1366. doi:10.1007/s00268-008-9483-2
24. Brauckhoff M, Walls G, Brauckhoff K, Thanh PN, Thomusch O, Dralle H (2002) Identification of the non-recurrent inferior laryngeal nerve using intraoperative neurostimulation. Langenbecks Arch Surg 386(7):482–487. doi:10.1007/s00423-001-0253-y
25. Gavilan J, Gavilan C (1986) Recurrent laryngeal nerve. Identification during thyroid and parathyroid surgery. Arch Otolaryngol Head Neck Surg 112(12):1286–1288
26. Dackiw AP, Rotstein LE, Clark OH (2002) Computer-assisted evoked electromyography with stimulating surgical instruments for recurrent/external laryngeal nerve identification and preservation in thyroid and parathyroid operation. Surgery 132(6):1100–1106; discussion 1107–1108. doi:10.1067/msy.2002.128483 [doi] S0039606002002593 [pii]
27. Chan WF, Lang BH, Lo CY (2006) The role of intraoperative neuromonitoring of recurrent laryngeal nerve during thyroidectomy: a comparative study on 1000 nerves at risk. Surgery 140(6):866–872; discussion 872–863. doi:S0039-6060(06)00478-8 [pii] 10.1016/j.surg.2006.07.017 [doi]
28. Barczynski M, Konturek A, Cichon S (2009) Randomized clinical trial of visualization versus neuromonitoring of recurrent laryngeal nerves during thyroidectomy. Br J Surg 96(3):240–246. doi:10.1002/bjs.6417
29. Dralle H et al (2004) What benefits does neural monitoring bring to thyroid surgery? Artz Krankenhaus 12:369–376
30. Kamani D, Randolph G, Potenza A, Cernea C (2013) Electrophysiologic monitoring characteristics of the recurrent laryngeal nerve preoperatively paralyzed or invaded with malignancy. Otolaryngol Head Neck Surg 149:682–688
31. Bergenfelz A, Jansson S, Mårtensson H, Reihnér E, Wallin G, Kristoffersson A, Lausen I (2007) Scandinavian quality register for thyroid and parathyroid surgery: audit of surgery for primary hyperparathyroidism. Langenbecks Arch Surg 392(4):445–451. doi:10.1007/s00423-006-0097-6
32. Chan WF, Lo CY (2006) Pitfalls of intraoperative neuromonitoring for predicting postoperative recurrent laryngeal nerve function during thyroidectomy. World J Surg 30(5):806–812. doi:10.1007/s00268-005-0355-8
33. Thomusch O, Sekulla C, Machens A, Neumann HJ, Timmermann W, Dralle H (2004) Validity of intra-operative neuromonitoring signals in thyroid surgery. Langenbecks Arch Surg 389(6):499–503. doi:10.1007/s00423-003-0444-9
34. Phelan E, Kamani D, Shin J, Randolph GW (2013) Neural monitored revision thyroid cancer surgery: surgical safety and thyroglobulin response. Otolaryngol Head Neck Surg 149(1):47–52. doi:10.1177/0194599813489662
35. Lorenz K, Sekulla C, Schelle J, Schmeiss B, Brauckhoff M, Dralle H (2010) What are normal quantitative parameters of intraoperative neuromonitoring (IONM) in thyroid surgery? Langenbecks Arch Surg 395(7):901–909. doi:10.1007/s00423-010-0691-5
36. Pearlman RC, Isley MR, Ruben GD, Sandler SC, Weisbaum B, Khan MA, Greene BS, Charles V, Shah A (2005) Intraoperative monitoring of the recurrent laryngeal nerve using acoustic, free-run, and evoked electromyography. J Clin Neurophysiol 22(2):148–152. doi:00004691-200504000-00009 [pii]
37. Prass RL, Luders H (1986) Acoustic (loudspeaker) facial electromyographic monitoring: Part 1. Evoked electromyographic activity during acoustic neuroma resection. Neurosurgery 19(3):392–400
38. Dong CC, Macdonald DB, Akagami R, Westerberg B, Alkhani A, Kanaan I, Hassounah M (2005) Intraoperative facial motor evoked potential monitoring with transcranial electrical stimulation during skull base surgery. Clin Neurophysiol 116(3):588–596. doi:10.1016/j.clinph.2004.09.013
39. Scheuller MC, Ellison D (2002) Laryngeal mask anesthesia with intraoperative laryngoscopy for identification of the recurrent laryngeal nerve during thyroidectomy. Laryngoscope 112(9):1594–1597. doi:10.1097/00005537-200209000-00011
40. Riddell V (1970) Thyroidectomy: prevention of bilateral recurrent nerve palsy. Results of identification of the nerve over 23 consecutive years (1946–69) with a description of an additional safety measure. Br J Surg 57(1):1–11

41. Premachandra DJ, Radcliffe GJ, Stearns MP (1990) Intraoperative identification of the recurrent laryngeal nerve and demonstration of its function. Laryngoscope 100(1):94–96. doi:10.1288/00005537-199001000-00019
42. James AG, Crocker S, Woltering E, Ferrara J, Farrar W (1985) A simple method for identifying and testing the recurrent laryngeal nerve. Surg Gynecol Obstet 161(2):185–186
43. Otto RA, Cochran CS (2002) Sensitivity and specificity of intraoperative recurrent laryngeal nerve stimulation in predicting postoperative nerve paralysis. Ann Otol Rhinol Laryngol 111(11):1005–1007
44. Brennan J, Moore EJ, Shuler KJ (2001) Prospective analysis of the efficacy of continuous intraoperative nerve monitoring during thyroidectomy, parathyroidectomy, and parotidectomy. Otolaryngol Head Neck Surg 124(5):537–543. doi:S0194-5998(01)37139-5 [pii] 10.1067/mhn.2001.115402 [doi]
45. Hemmerling TM, Schmidt J, Wolf T, Wolf SR, Jacobi KE (2000) Surface vs intramuscular laryngeal electromyography. Can J Anaesth 47(9):860–865
46. Lamade W, Meyding-Lamade U, Buchhold C, Brauer M, Brandner R, Uttenweiler V, Motsch J, Klar E, Herfarth C (2000) First continuous nerve monitoring in thyroid gland surgery. Chirurg 71(5):551–557
47. Timon CI, Rafferty M (1999) Nerve monitoring in thyroid surgery: is it worthwhile? Clin Otolaryngol Allied Sci 24(6):487–490. doi:coa292 [pii]
48. Horn D, Rotzscher VM (1999) Intraoperative electromyogram monitoring of the recurrent laryngeal nerve: experience with an intralaryngeal surface electrode. A method to reduce the risk of recurrent laryngeal nerve injury during thyroid surgery. Langenbecks Arch Surg 384(4):392–395. doi:93840392.423 [pii]
49. Barwell J, Lytle J, Page R, Wilkins D (1997) The NIM-2 nerve integrity monitor in thyroid and parathyroid surgery. Br J Surg 84(6):854
50. Eisele DW (1996) Intraoperative electrophysiologic monitoring of the recurrent laryngeal nerve. Laryngoscope 106(4):443–449
51. Marcus B, Edwards B, Yoo S, Byrne A, Gupta A, Kandrevas J, Bradford C, Chepeha DB, Teknos TN (2003) Recurrent laryngeal nerve monitoring in thyroid and parathyroid surgery: the University of Michigan experience. Laryngoscope 113(2):356–361. doi:10.1097/00005537-200302000-00028
52. Rea JL, Khan A (1998) Clinical evoked electromyography for recurrent laryngeal nerve preservation: use of an endotracheal tube electrode and a postcricoid surface electrode. Laryngoscope 108(9):1418–1420
53. Randolph GW, Shin JJ, Grillo HC, Mathisen D, Katlic MR, Kamani D, Zurakowski D (2011) The surgical management of goiter: part II. Surgical treatment and results. Laryngoscope 121(1):68–76. doi:10.1002/lary.21091
54. Dionigi G, Bacuzzi A, Boni L, Rovera F, Dionigi R (2008) What is the learning curve for intraoperative neuromonitoring in thyroid surgery? Int J Surg 6(Suppl 1):S7–S12. doi:S1743-9191(08)00188-X [pii] 10.1016/j.ijsu.2008.12.023 [doi]
55. Chiang FY, Lee KW, Chen HC, Chen HY, Lu IC, Kuo WR, Hsieh MC, Wu CW (2010) Standardization of intraoperative neuromonitoring of recurrent laryngeal nerve in thyroid operation. World J Surg 34(2):223–229. doi:10.1007/s00268-009-0316-8
56. Randolph G (2013) Surgical anatomy of recurrent laryngeal nerve. In: Randolph GW (ed) Surgery of the thyroid and parathyroid glands, 2nd edn. Saunders, Philadelphia
57. Yap SJ, Morris RW, Pybus DA (1994) Alterations in endotracheal tube position during general anaesthesia. Anaesth Intensive Care 22(5):586–588
58. Chambers KJ, Pearse A, Coveney J, Rogers S, Kamani D, Sritharan N, Randolph GW (2015) Respiratory variation predicts optimal endotracheal tube placement for intra-operative nerve monitoring in thyroid and parathyroid surgery. World J Surg 39(2):393–399. doi:10.1007/s00268-014-2820-8
59. Caragacianu D, Kamani D, Randolph GW (2013) Intraoperative monitoring: normative range associated with normal postoperative glottic function. Laryngoscope 123(12):3026–3031. doi:10.1002/lary.24195

60. Snyder SK, Lairmore TC, Hendricks JC, Roberts JW (2008) Elucidating mechanisms of recurrent laryngeal nerve injury during thyroidectomy and parathyroidectomy. J Am Coll Surg 206(1):123–130. doi:S1072-7515(07)01248-3 [pii] 10.1016/j.jamcollsurg.2007.07.017 [doi]
61. Beldi G, Kinsbergen T, Schlumpf R (2004) Evaluation of intraoperative recurrent nerve monitoring in thyroid surgery. World J Surg 28(6):589–591
62. Scott AR, Chong PS, Hartnick CJ, Randolph GW (2010) Spontaneous and evoked laryngeal electromyography of the thyroarytenoid muscles: a canine model for intraoperative recurrent laryngeal nerve monitoring. Ann Otol Rhinol Laryngol 119(1):54–63
63. Schneider R, Przybyl J, Pliquett U, Hermann M, Wehner M, Pietsch UC, Konig F, Hauss J, Jonas S, Leinung S (2010) A new vagal anchor electrode for real-time monitoring of the recurrent laryngeal nerve. Am J Surg 199(4):507–514. doi:10.1016/j.amjsurg.2009.04.036
64. Lamade W, Ulmer C, Seimer A, Molnar V, Meyding-Lamade U, Thon KP, Koch KP (2007) A new system for continuous recurrent laryngeal nerve monitoring. Minim Invasive Ther Allied Technol 16(3):149–154. doi:779591904 [pii] 10.1080/13645700701383241 [doi]
65. Phelan E, Schneider R, Lorenz K, Dralle H, Kamani D, Potenza A, Sritharan N, Shin J, Randolph WG (2014) Continuous vagal IONM prevents recurrent laryngeal nerve paralysis by revealing initial EMG changes of impending neuropraxic injury: A prospective, multicenter study. The Laryngoscope 124:1498–1505. doi:10.1002/lary.24550
66. Jansson S, Tisell LE, Hagne I, Sanner E, Stenborg R, Svensson P (1988) Partial superior laryngeal nerve (SLN) lesions before and after thyroid surgery. World J Surg 12(4):522–527
67. Lennquist S, Cahlin C, Smeds S (1987) The superior laryngeal nerve in thyroid surgery. Surgery 102(6):999–1008, doi:0039-6060(87)90328-X [pii]
68. Darr AE, Tufano R, Ozdemir S, Kamani D, Hurwitz S, Randolph GW (2014) Superior laryngeal nerve quantitative intraoperative monitoring is possible in all thyroid surgeries. Laryngoscope 124(4):1035–1041
69. Lahey FH (1946) Useful operative points in two patients with completely intrathoracic goiters. Lahey Clin Bull 5(2):34–40
70. Dunhill TP (1912) A discussion on partial thyroidectomy under local anaesthesia, with special reference to exophthalmic goitre: an address introductory to a discussion on the subject. Proc R Soc Med 5(Surg Sect):61–69
71. Frazell EL, Moore OS (1961) Bilateral radical neck dissection performed in stages. Experience with 467 patients. Am J Surg 102:809–814
72. Dralle H, Sekulla C, Lorenz K, Nguyen Thanh P, Schneider R, Machens A (2012) Loss of the nerve monitoring signal during bilateral thyroid surgery. Br J Surg 99(8):1089–1095. doi:10.1002/bjs.8831
73. Goretzki PE, Schwarz K, Brinkmann J, Wirowski D, Lammers BJ (2010) The impact of intraoperative neuromonitoring (IONM) on surgical strategy in bilateral thyroid diseases: is it worth the effort? World J Surg 34(6):1274–1284. doi:10.1007/s00268-009-0353-3
74. Dionigi G, Frattini F (2013) Staged thyroidectomy: time to consider intraoperative neuromonitoring as standard of care. Thyroid 23(7):906–908. doi:10.1089/thy.2013.0004
75. Fellmer PT, Bohner H, Wolf A, Roher HD, Goretzki PE (2008) A left nonrecurrent inferior laryngeal nerve in a patient with right-sided aorta, truncus arteriosus communis, and an aberrant left innominate artery. Thyroid 18(6):647–649. doi:10.1089/thy.2007.0284
76. Henry JF, Audiffret J, Denizot A, Plan M (1988) The nonrecurrent inferior laryngeal nerve: review of 33 cases, including two on the left side. Surgery 104(6):977–984, doi:0039-6060(88)90157-2 [pii]
77. Brauckhoff M, Machens A, Sekulla C, Lorenz K, Dralle H (2011) Latencies shorter than 3.5 ms after vagus nerve stimulation signify a nonrecurrent inferior laryngeal nerve before dissection. Ann Surg 253(6):1172–1177. doi:10.1097/SLA.0b013e3182128b9e

# Hemostatic Devices

# 19

Serafino Vanella, Anna Crocco, Emanuela Traini,
Celestino Pio Lombardi, and Marco Raffaelli

## 19.1 Introduction

Early surgical approaches for treatment of thyroid disorders were associated with high rates of mortality and morbidity due to hemorrhage, asphyxia, air embolism, and infection. It was not until the late 1800s after the advent of ether as anesthesia, antiseptic technique, and effective artery forceps allowed Theodor Kocher to perfect the technique for thyroidectomy. Kocher used the technique of precise ligation of the arterial blood supply to perform an unhurried, meticulous dissection of the thyroid gland, decreasing the morbidity and mortality associated with thyroid surgery to less than 1 % [1].

Hemostasis in surgery still represents a major challenge. Control of bleeding is particularly important for thyroid surgery, due to the narrow operating field, closeness of essential anatomic structures, and hypervascularization. In addition, intraoperative and postoperative bleeding, besides possible significant blood loss, are crucial factors determining the frequency of other surgical complications, as well as the prolongation of the length of surgery, thereby increasing the length of hospital stay and expenses. Various devices have been introduced in clinical practice to achieve a safe and faster hemostasis: electrosurgical devices use heat energy to denature proteins and the heating of the surgical field due to lateral dispersion may damage vital structures. In the recent years, research has been looking for new instruments with less thermal spread in the effort to reduce both operating time and complications. Many methods designed to maintain surgical hemostasis are presently used: ligation and suturing (threads, clips, staplers), coagulation

S. Vanella (✉) • A. Crocco • E. Traini • C.P. Lombardi • M. Raffaelli
Unità Operativa Di Chirurgia Endocrina E Metabolica, Università Cattolica Del Sacro Cuore, Roma, Largo Agostino Gemelli, 8, Rome, RM 00168, Italy
e-mail: nekroma@yahoo.it; serafino.vanella@rm.unicatt.it; annacatu@hotmail.it; emanuela.traini@rm.unicatt.it; cp.lombardi@rm.unicatt.it; marcoraffaelli@rm.unicatt.it



C.P. Lombardi, R. Bellantone (eds.), *Minimally Invasive Therapies for Endocrine Neck Diseases*, DOI 10.1007/978-3-319-20065-1_19

(laser, ultrasound, electrocoagulation – monopolar and bipolar), ultrasonic coagulation (Ultracision, Harmonic scalpel; Ethicon Endo-Surgery, Cincinnati, OH), electroligation sealing using LigaSure (LigaSure Vessel Sealing System; Valleylab, Boulder, CO, USA).

## 19.2 Harmonic Scalpel

The development of ultrasonically activated coagulating shears in the early 1990s has provided an alternative to other methods of controlling blood vessels.

The role of harmonic scalpel in minimally invasive thyroid surgery is well defined and emphasized since its use allows an excellent hemostasis in small operative space. The HS coagulates and simultaneously cuts tissue using mechanical energy with ultrasonic frequency at 55.5 kHz. This avoids extreme temperatures that can hurt the surrounding important structures, producing less thermal damage and reducing the operative time.

This instrument was originally designed for laparoscopic surgery [2, 3] because of its remarkable advantages of simultaneous cutting and coagulation of medium-caliber vessels as well as the small amplitude of its waves, all of which make it a useful tool in surgical fields where proximity of vital structures does not permit the use of thermal devices. This early indication for cavity surgery was extended to other fields, such as video-assisted thyroidectomy (VAT) [4], parotidectomy [5, 6], and neck dissection [7].

Total thyroidectomy represented the ideal model to assess the effectiveness of ultrasonic scalpels because of the size of the vessel, the proximity of superior and recurrent laryngeal nerves, and the necessity of preserving parathyroid glands, which are susceptible to damage if thermal devices are used [8].

The harmonic scalpel setup consists of a generator, a hand piece, and a blade. The hand piece contains an ultrasonic transducer that consists of a stack of piezoelectric crystals sandwiched between two metal cylinders under pressure. The transducer is attached to the blade through a mount. The 110-volt generator is a high-frequency switching power supply controlled by a microprocessor that pulses the transducer in the hand piece with alternated current. This current allows the transducer to vibrate at its natural harmonic frequency of 55.5 kHz. The blade used most frequently in thyroid surgery looks like a curved paddle with a sharp inner beveled side for cutting and a blunt outer radius for contemporary coagulating. The generator can be adjusted from a level of 1–5 to increase cutting speed and decrease coagulation by increasing the blade's lateral excursion [9].

The waves are transferred to the active blade of the instrument, vibrating harmoniously at the same frequency. In addition to the direct cutting action of the vibrating blade, ultrasound waves cause cavitation fragmentation of tissues and additional cutting effect [10]. The coagulation effect occurs due to tissue protein denaturation [11]. In contrast to electrical or laser coagulation, working with harmonic scalpel is associated with a considerably lower production of thermal energy (up to 80 °C), thus causing significantly less damage to the adjacent tissue [12, 13].

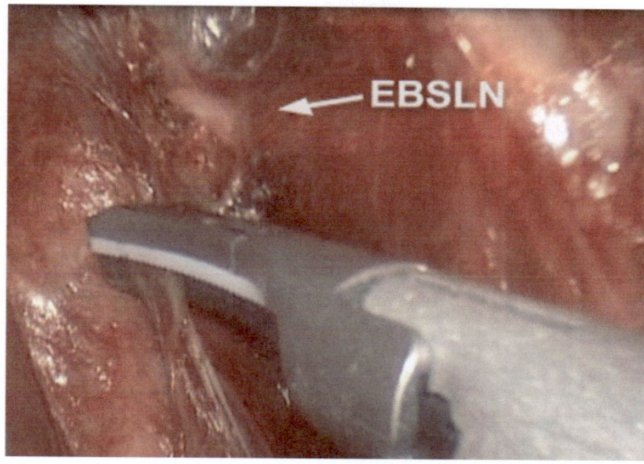


**Fig. 19.1** Superior pole dissection using harmonic scalpel during mini-invasive video-assisted thyroidectomy. *EBSLN* external branch of superior laryngeal nerve

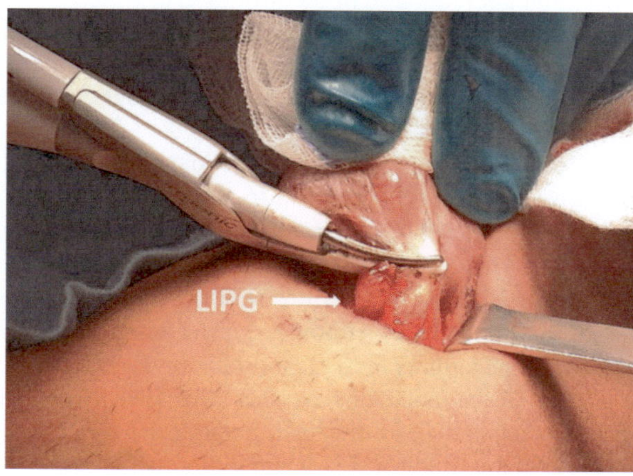


**Fig. 19.2** Inferior pole dissection using Harmonic Focus® during mini-invasive thyroidectomy. *LIPG* left inferior parathyroid gland

Among the ultracision system devices, the CS14C (ultracision harmonic scalpel) is the instrument most frequently used during both open and minimally invasive thyroidectomy (Fig. 19.1) [14–21], but some surgeons consider this tool to be large and cumbersome, especially for fine grasping and dissection capabilities. In this context, an innovative technical improvement of the device for thyroid surgery has recently been implemented and was made available in 2008: Harmonic FOCUS shears (Fig. 19.2). These very new, hand activated shears, keeping the same effective ultrasonic coagulation mechanism, were completely renewed in their design, reproducing the familiar "Kelly clamp" in shape, with very thin and delicate tips. This new tool allows the surgeon to easily dissect and coagulate and cut vessels in narrow spaces [22].

Many published, comparative and observational, studies have variably reported some significant advantages in terms of operative time [16, 23–25], complications rate [26, 27], and reductions in incision size [25, 27–29] with the use of HS (ultracision or focus) respect to the conventional techniques, as clamp-and-tie in thyroid surgery [30].

In our previous study, in 2008, besides confirming that HS utilization during total thyroidectomy allows for a significant reduction in operative time (about 30 %) when compared with the conventional CT technique, we extensively analyzed the influence of this element on costs; the authors assert that, since time spent in the operating room is expensive [31], this would counterbalance the cost of the HS hand piece and eventually result in a overall cost saving. The significantly higher cost of disposable materials in the HS group was counterbalanced by significant higher costs of drugs, personnel and operative room charges in the CT group related to the longer operative time, and operative room utilization time. Nonetheless, the shorter operative time implies the possibility to treat more patients in the same operative sessions. One could anticipate that with the utilization of the HS, surgeons could perform one conventional total thryoidectomy more every three or four procedures. This could mean at least one operation more for each operative session. Ultimately, this could result in a better utilization of health resources and, above all, in a potential significant reduction of the waiting list, which, at least in our health system, has a crucial role. Another potential additional advantage of the use of HS and consequent avoidance of manual tying could be the possible reduction of human resources in the operating room. In other words, surgeons could theoretically accomplish thyroidectomy without any assistant [30].

In 2010, Miccoli et al. conducted a randomized controlled trial about the utilization of Harmonic FOCUS compared to standard CT technique in thyroid surgery. They found a significant reduction of operative time in the FOCUS group (33.4 vs. 47.2 min). They assert that the significant reduction rate of operative time occurred because the FOCUS shears allow not only coagulation and cutting the vessels but also the dissection of planes without requiring any further tools; furthermore, the very low occurrence of failures in the hemostatic division of vessels (both veins and arterials) avoids the use of manual ligatures or clips, which is time consuming. One of the most important advantages of this instrument is the very rare occurrence of delayed bleeding [32]. In this study, a significant difference in the drainage output between the two groups in favor of the FOCUS group was observed. Postoperative pain was significantly lower after 12 h and also after 24 h. The explanation for such a significant difference might be found in the shorter operative time, the reduction of neck hyperextension due to the easier access to the upper pedicle [32], and consequent reduced stretching of the wound. Others also note that edema of the tissues is reduced because of the much lower temperature reached by the Harmonic shear [22, 33].

In 2008, Cirocchi et al. conducted a systematic review and meta-analysis to compare the surgical effectiveness of HS vs. CT in total thyroidectomy in patients with thyroid benign and/or malignant pathologies. They observed that the main significant advantages of HS are shorter operative duration, lower intraoperative blood loss, and lower overall drainage volume.

In this analysis, the reduction of operative time has the advantage to reduce significantly the costs of utilization of operating room. The cut and coagulation functions permit also to reduce lymphorrea depending on ligations and sections and the authors deduce that this leads to the opportunity of anticipated discharge and subsequent reduction of costs of permanence in the hospital.

The incidence of postoperative complications is similar in two groups (transient laryngeal nerve palsy, permanent laryngeal nerve palsy, transient hypocalcemia, permanent hypocalcemia) [34].

A meta-analysis conducted in 2010 by Ecker et al. confirmed the impact of the HS on operating time, with a reduction of nearly 25 % when compared with all other hemostatic methods. With regard to postoperative pain, the data show that patients in the harmonic scalpel group had a significantly less painful postoperative course when compared with patients with suture/clip ligation plus electrocoagulation [35].

Also Melck et al., in a meta-analysis realized in 2010, showed that the utilization of the HS for total and subtotal thyroidectomy significantly reduced operative time compared to CT by greater than 23 min. Furthermore, there was a 31 % decreased risk of transient postoperative hypocalcemia with HS utilization and there was also no statistically significant difference in the risk of transient postoperative nerve damage between the two groups. Authors speculate that use of the HS may facilitate dissection of the parathyroid glands in a plane farther away from the parathyroid gland capsule, thus reducing the chance of damaging their blood supply, directly or indirectly, with either mechanical forces or electrical currents [36].

## 19.3 LigaSure

The LigaSure vessel sealing system (Valleylab, Boulder, Colorado) is a hemostatic device primarily designed for abdominal operations. A bipolar, electrosurgical device, it seals vessels as large as 7 mm in diameter by denaturing collagen and elastin within the vessel walls and the surrounding connective tissue. When compared with unipolar cautery, LigaSure has a reduced energy spread profile (<2 mm) and a potentially decreased risk of injury to adjacent structures [37, 38].

The device is used in abdominal surgery and has proved suitable for use in thyroid surgery [39]. LigaSure, allowing vessel sealing and division with no dispersion of the electric power and with little or no heat production, has been widely used in diverse fields of surgery for its efficiency and safety. However, in thyroid surgery, where a considerable amount of minute vessels must be divided and hence microsurgical techniques required, LigaSure is also preferred for its further efficiency by shortening the duration of the operation (Fig. 19.3) [1].

A characteristic specific to the LigaSure is the possibility to modulate the quantity of energy by applying appropriate pressure to the grip [40, 41].

Some surgeons found the earlier LigaSure precise instrument to be time consuming (in comparison with the harmonic scalpel), especially because of the absence of an integrated cutting mechanism and the lack of dissection capabilities. In this context, the LigaSure LF1212 was introduced in 2010 as an innovative technical advance for open thyroid surgery. This device is also capable of cutting with an integrated mechanism, and it is suitable for both blunt dissection and grasping and dividing tissue [42].

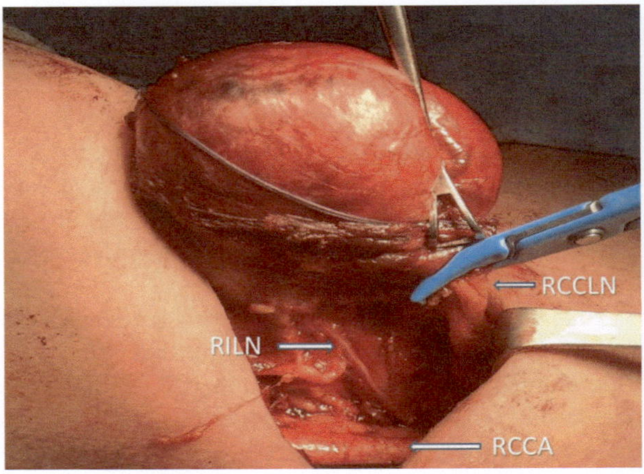


**Fig. 19.3** Central neck dissection using LigaSure Precise®. *RCCA* right common carotid artery, *RCCLN* right central compartment lymph nodes, *RILN* right inferior laryngeal nerve

As for HS, several studies analyzed the use of LigaSure in thyroid surgery in comparison with CT technique and quantified the advantages in terms of operative time, reduction of perioperative complications, and decrease in hospital stay.

In 2006, Franko et al., in their clinical trial, confirmed that operative time was significantly decreased by an average of 20 min through the use of LigaSure in thyroid surgery, but this procedure did not result in any increase or decrease in the incidence of clinically apparent RLN injury, bleeding necessitating reoperation, or postoperative hypocalcemia, whether transient or permanent [43].

In 2009, Yao et al. analyzed the results of thyroid surgery performed with LigaSure compared to the conventional operation and they found that LigaSure thyroidectomy took significantly less time to complete (mean, −11.97 min). They associated the reduced operative duration with LigaSure to better intraoperative hemostatic control and not needing to ligate the vessels.

The authors noticed no significant difference in the rates of overall and individual postoperative complications (transient and permanent hypocalcemia, transient and permanent nerve lesions, hematomas, wound infections) for patients undergoing conventional vs. LigaSure thyroidectomy. Moreover, because it is used solely during the entire procedure for vascular ligation of all thyroid vessels, no suture ligations are necessary, no foreign bodies (i.e., ligations or clips) are left behind; therefore, the risk of knot slipping and clip dislodgment is nearly eliminated.

Furthermore, the clarification that, after LigaSure thyroidectomy, the postoperative pain treatment and analgesic requirements were significantly reduced, and patients returned pain-free to normal work or social activity significantly earlier is remarked by different studies [38, 44].

A further study, conducted by Ignatjovic et al. in 2011, concludes that the effects of the LigaSure procedure are equivalent to the ligation technique [45], while the maximum temperatures, energy dissipation, and collateral damage are markedly less in comparison with other nonligature hemostasis methods [46, 47]. In addition, the blood pressure necessary to break the site of blood vessel sealing is four times higher than the maximum possible arterial pressure (850–900 mmHg), and more than twofold higher than the maximum venous pressure (200–250 mmHg) [48–50]. In this study, intraoperative blood loss is lower in LigaSure group and the duration of surgery is shorter, the economic effects was generally concluded to be irrelevant as compared to the total price of the surgery [51].

## 19.4 BiClamp

Bipolar thermofusion BiClamp 150 (ERBE Elektromedizin GmbH, Teubingen, Germany, www.erbe-med.com) is a tool specifically designed for thyroid surgery. It works on the principle of bipolar thermofusion of tissue. Low-voltage energy is strong enough to seal vessels of up to 7 mm in diameter on the basis of collagen fiber fusion [48]. The hand piece is shaped like forceps and is easily used to grasp and coagulate the vessel. It is useful for tissue preparation as well. After placing the hand piece into the proper position on the vessel and pushing the pedal, electrocoagulation starts. The process ends with acoustic signals from the processing unit, after the vessel is sealed and it is possible to cut it. An automatic stop function prevents heat injury from the surrounding tissues. Another advantage of the instrument is the possibility of resterilization. It should not be used in the area of the RLN due to the potential risk of injuring the nerve from the dispersion of heat. The tool is not suitable for coagulation of very small vessels because forceps tips of BiClamp are thicker than conventional bipolar coagulation tips. Encrusted coagulations could adhere to the forceps tips and there is danger of damaging the vessel when the forceps are withdrawn [52].

Some studies were conducted to prove the effectiveness of this device in thyroidectomy compared to other hemostatic techniques.

Pniak et al., in a review of 2014, assert that the bipolar thermofusion BiClamp is an effective and safe method for vessels sealing during thyroidectomy, including sealing of the main thyroid vessels. They demonstrated that BiClamp may achieve statistically significant reductions in the frequency of postoperative bleeding compared with conventional vessel ligature and it also leads to significant reductions in operative time [52].

## 19.5 Comparison Between Devices

Most studies comparing the LigaSure to HS have been performed on patients undergoing abdominal surgeries, such as hysterectomies, laparoscopic splenectomies, and laparoscopic colectomies [53, 54]. Studies have compared conventional knot tying to the LigaSure device or harmonic scalpel in total thyroidectomy, but few have done a comparison of both devices [24, 28, 55–59].

One of these studies was conducted in 2011 by Zarebczan et al. and it showed no difference in the rate of transient hoarseness, permanent recurrent laryngeal nerve injury, transient hypocalcemia, and hematoma formation between the two devices when used in total thyroidectomy. When comparing the two devices to one another, researchers found a significant decrease in operative time when the harmonic scalpel was used, with an average decrease in operative time of 15 min and similar findings in operative time were shown for patients who underwent thyroid lobectomy: cases in which the LigaSure was used took 7 min longer on average. They also illustrated a decrease in length of hospital stay for patients who underwent total thyroidectomy with the harmonic scalpel [60].

In 2008, Sartori et al. conducted a comparison study, in which they analyzed three groups of patients, who underwent thyroidectomy using CT, HS, or LigaSure. They showed that there was a significant difference in overall morbidity between patients in the CT group and the other two; HS and LigaSure groups had a higher complication rate but there was no difference between LigaSure and HS patients; in particular, there was a statistically significant difference in postoperative hypocalcemia rate between patients operated with conventional technique and those in the new technologies groups. When comparing LigaSure and HS patients, postoperative calcemia did not significantly differ, but patients in the HS group had a higher relative risk of postoperative hypoparathyroidism (RR = 3.75).

However, this had no impact on patient outcome since hypocalcemia was always transient and asymptomatic in more than two thirds of the patients and the length of hospital stay was not affected. Recurrent laryngeal nerve palsies, instead, were the same in the three groups.

HS patients had a mean operating time shortening of 24 min when compared to CT patients, while no advantage was noticed regarding operating time when using LigaSure. Intraoperative blood losses were similar among groups [61].

Oussoultzoglou et al., in a prospective study conducted in 2008, conclude that HS is associated with reduced postoperative hypocalcemia, reduced postoperative oral calcium supplementation requirement, and reduces operative time compared with the LigaSure device [62].

Dionigi et al., in their article written in 2011, assert that the only justified comparison is between the new LigaSure™ LF1212, which has an integrated cutting capability, and the FOCUS. In their study, they found no significant differences in the operative time between the two groups (LigaSure and FOCUS). The rate of nerve lesions, bleeding, drainage, and postoperative calcium concentration were the same for the two devices, with no significant differences. The use of FOCUS significantly increased the incidence of hypoparathyroidism; their working hypothesis was that the parathyroid glands are more likely to be injured because of the potential for greater thermal spread when using the Harmonic FOCUS. However, the postoperative calcium levels were not significantly different between the two groups. The only significant finding within this context was a significantly reduced early postoperative PTH value, which potentially indicates a need for supplementation, in the FOCUS group. At 24 h after surgery, the calcium levels were no longer different, but calcium supplementation was still significantly higher in the FOCUS group.

The authors affirm that thermal injury to the parathyroids is avoidable by having a larger distance of the energy-based dissecting tools from these vital anatomical structures (>3 mm), or with a sequential use and water-cool of the instruments [63, 64].

The authors noticed, also, a lower rate of pain experienced while swallowing in the LigaSure group, but overall patients' low analgesic requirement and extra doses of analgesics were the same; they explained this with the hypothesis that LigaSure delivers less energy because of the presence of active feedback control over the power output, limiting thermal spread to adjacent tissues. Furthermore, in this study it is noticed that the LigaSure LF1212 allowed the surgeon to dissect, coagulate and cut vessels in significantly narrower spaces than did the FOCUS. A possible explanation for this is given considering the longer tips of the LF1212 and the consequent reduced stretching of the wound [42].

Rahbari et al. realized a study, in 2011, that showed no significant difference in the operative cost or operative time in thyroidectomies performed with HS or with LigaSure. There was also no significant difference in complication rates between the two groups, and in the cost and the number of pain medications used as a surrogate measure of pain associated with the thyroidectomy [65].

More recently, in 2013, Contin et al., in a meta-analysis, demonstrated that using energized vessel sealing systems (LigaSure) can significantly reduce operation time. Additionally, the use of HS was associated with several small-scale benefits, that is, reduced intra- and postoperative blood loss, reduced rates of transient hypocalcemia and postoperative pain as well as a reduced duration of hospital stay. While these improvements were marginal and not observed for the use of LigaSure, the conventional technique was not superior in any outcome investigated. In particular, the clinically important safety outcomes of recurrent nerve palsy and rates of clinically symptomatic hypocalcemia were not negatively affected by using any of the energized vessel systems. Nevertheless, the detected differences between the devices could be due to the different spectrum of use the devices offer. While the LigaSure offers more time-consuming multiple-sealing approaches at the same vessel, the HS divides the tissue at the same time of coagulation.

Apart from that, reduction of operation time is surely a significant benefit for surgical practice. However, the saving of operation time has to be set in relation to higher material costs. Since personnel and material costs differ from country to country, every single institution has to evaluate the potential benefit of employing these devices [41].

## References

1. Çakabay B, Çaparlar A (2012) Chapter 13.New Technologies in Thyroid Surgery, Thyroid and Parathyroid Diseases - New Insights into Some Old and Some New Issues, Dr. Laura Ward (Ed.), ISBN: 978-953-51-0221-2, InTech, Available from: http://www.intechopen.com/books/thyroid-and-parathyroid-diseases-new-insightsinto-some-old-and-some-new-issues/new-tecnologies-n-thyroid-sugery
2. Kunde D, Welch C (2003) Ultracision in gynaecological laparoscopic surgery. J Obstet Gynaecol 23:347–352
3. Underwood RA, Dunnegan DL, Soper NJ (1999) Prospective, randomized trial of bipolar electrosurgery vs ultrasonic coagulation for division of short gastric vessels during laparoscopic Nissen fundoplication. Surg Endosc 13:763–768
4. Miccoli P, Berti P, Raffaelli M, Materazzi G, Conte M, Galleri D (2002) Impact of harmonic scalpel on operative time during videoassisted thyroidectomy. Surg Endosc 16:663–666

5. Jackson LL, Gourin CG, Thomas DS, Porubsky ES, Klippert FN, Terris DJ (2005) Use of the harmonic scalpel in superficial and total parotidectomy for benign and malignant disease. Laryngoscope 115:1070–1073
6. Markkanen-Leppanen M, Pitkaranta A (2004) Parotidectomy using the harmonic scalpel. Laryngoscope 114:381–382
7. Miccoli P, Materazzi G, Fregoli L, Panicucci E, Kunz-Martinez W, Berti P (2009) Modified lateral neck lymphadenectomy: prospective randomized study comparing harmonic scalpel with clamp-and tie technique. Otolaryngol Head Neck Surg 140:61–64
8. Kowalski LP, Sanabria A, Vartanian JG, Lima RA, de Mendonca UB, dos Santos CR, Boldrini D Jr, de Mello LE, Pinto FP, Lehn CN, Correa LA, Dedivitis RA, Guimarães AV, Pedruzzi PA, Ramos HA, Gonçalves AJ, Suehara AB, Kanda JL, Capuzzo R, de Oliveira JC, Maria Paula Curado MP, de Góis Filho JF, Fukuyama E, Beserra IM Jr, de Carvalho Neto PB, Carvalho AL (2012) Total thyroidectomy with ultrasonic scalpel: a multicenter, randomized controlled trial. Head Neck 34:805–812
9. Ferri E, Armato E, Spinato G, Spinato R (2011) Focus harmonic scalpel compared to conventional haemostasis in open total thyroidectomy: a prospective randomized trial. Int J Otolaryngol 2011:357195
10. Amaral JF (1994) Ultrasonic dissection. Endosc Surg Allied Technol 2:181–185
11. Wiatrak BJ, Willging JP (2002) Harmonic scalpel for tonsillectomy. Laryngoscope 112:14–16
12. Hambley R, Hebda PA, Abell E, Cohen BA, Jegasothy BV (1988) Wound healing of skin incisions produced by ultrasonically vibrating knife, scalpel, electrosurgery, and carbon dioxide laser. J Dermatol Surg Oncol 14:1213–1217
13. Prgomet D, Janjanin S, Bilić M, Prstacić R, Kovac L, Rudes M, Katić V (2009) A prospective observational study of 363 cases operated with three different harmonic scalpels. Eur Arch Otorhinolaryngol 266:1965–1970
14. Gertsch P, Pelloni A, Guerra A, Krpo A (2000) Initial experience with the harmonic scalpel in liver surgery. Hepatogastroenterology 47:763–766
15. Kang SK, Kunanandam T, Clark L (2008) Prospective, case–control study of surgical efficiency of ultrasonic shear ("harmonic scalpel") thyroidectomy compared with conventional thyroidectomy. J Laryngol Otol 19:1–3
16. Cordón C, Fajardo R, Ramírez J, Herrera MF (2005) A randomized, prospective, parallel group study comparing the harmonic scalpel to electrocautery in thyroidectomy. Surgery 137:337–341
17. Kilic M, Keskek M, Ertan T, Yoldas O, Bilgin A, Koc M (2007) A prospective randomized trial comparing the harmonic scalpel with conventional knot tying in thyroidectomy. Adv Ther 24:632–638
18. Manouras A, Markogiannakis H, Koutras AS, Antonakis PT, Drimousis P, Lagoudianakis EE, Kekis P, Genetzakis M, Koutsoumanis K, Bramis I (2008) Thyroid surgery: comparison between the electrothermal bipolar vessel sealing system, harmonic scalpel, and classic suture ligation. Am J Surg 195:48–52
19. Miccoli P, Berti P, Frustaci GL, Ambrosini CE, Materazzi G (2006) Video-assisted thyroidectomy: indications and results. Langenbecks Arch Surg 391:68–71
20. Miccoli P, Materazzi G (2004) Minimally invasive videoassisted thyroidectomy (MIVAT). Surg Clin North Am 84:735–741
21. Ikeda Y, Takami H, Sasaki Y, Takayama J, Niimi M, Kan S (2002) Comparative studies of thyroidectomies: endoscopic surgery vs conventional open surgery. Surg Endosc 16:1741–1745
22. Miccoli P, Materazzi G, Miccoli M, Frustaci G, Fosso A, Berti P (2010) Evaluation of a new ultrasonic device in thyroid surgery: comparative randomized study. Am J Surg 199:736–740
23. Voutilainen PE, Haglund CH (2000) Ultrasonically activated shears in thyroidectomies. A randomised trial. Ann Surg 231:322–328
24. Siperstein A, Berber E, Morkoyun E (2002) The use of the harmonic scalpel vs conventional knot tying for vessel ligation in thyroid surgery. Arch Surg 137:137–142
25. Ortega J, Sala C, Flor B, Lledo S (2004) Efficacy and cost- effectiveness of the UltraCision harmonic scalpel in thyroid surgery: an analysis of 200 cases in a randomised trial. J Laparoendosc Adv Surg Tech A 14(1):9–12

26. Meurisse M, Defechereux T, Maweja S, Degauque C, Vandelaer M, Hamoir E (2000) Evaluation de l'utilisation du dissecteur ultrasonique Ultracision en chirurgie thyroïdienne. Etude prospective randomisée. Ann Chir 125:468–472
27. Miccoli P, Berti P, Dionigi L, D'Agostino J, Orlandini C, Donatini G (2006) Randomized controlled trial of harmonic scalpel use during thyroidectomy. Arch Otolaryngol Head Neck Surg 132:1069–1073
28. Shemen L (2002) Thyroidectomy using the harmonic scalpel: analysis of 105 consecutive cases. Otolaryngol Head Neck Surg 127:284–288
29. Terris DJ, Seybt MW, Gourin CG, Chin E (2006) Ultrasonic technology facilitates minimal thyroid surgery. Laryngoscope 116:851–854
30. Lombardi CP, Raffaelli M, Cicchetti A, Marchetti M, De Crea C, Di Bidino R, Oragano L, Bellantone R (2008) The use of "harmonic scalpel" versus "knot tying" for conventional "open" thyroidectomy: results of a prospective randomized study. Langenbecks Arch Surg 393:627–631
31. Viapiano J, Wards DS (2000) Operating room utilization: the need for data. Int Anesthesiol Clin 38:127–140
32. Defechereux T, Meurisse M (2006) Hemostasis and ultrasonic shears for thyroid surgery. Ann Chir 131:154–156
33. Kos M, Engelke W (2007) Advantages of a new technique of neck dissection using an ultrasonic scalpel. J Craniomaxillofac Surg 35:10–14
34. Cirocchi R, D'Ajello F, Trastulli S, Santoro A, Di Rocco G, Vendettuoli D, Rondelli F, Giannotti D, Sanguinetti A, Minelli L, Redler A, Basoli A, Avenia N (2010) Meta-analysis of thyroidectomy with ultrasonic dissector versus conventional clamp and tie. World J Surg Oncol 8:112
35. Ecker T, Carvalho AL, Choe JH, Walosek G, Preuss KJ (2010) Hemostasis in thyroid surgery: harmonic scalpel versus other techniques – a meta-analysis. Otolaryngol Head Neck Surg 143(1):17–25
36. Melck AL, Wiseman SM (2010) Harmonic scalpel compared to conventional hemostasis in thyroid surgery: a meta-analysis of randomized clinical trials. Int J Surg Oncol 2010:396079
37. Heniford BT, Matthews BD, Sing RF, Backus C, Pratt B, Greene FL (2001) Initial results with an electrothermal bipolar vessel sealer. Surg Endosc 15(8):799–801
38. Yao HS, Wang Q, Wang WJ, Ruan CP (2009) Prospective clinical trials of thyroidectomy with LigaSure vs conventional vessel ligation: a systematic review and meta-analysis. Arch Surg 144(12):1167–1174
39. Cakabay B, Sevinç MM, Gömceli I, Yenidogan E, Ulkü A, Koç S (2009) LigaSure versus clamp-and-tie in thyroidectomy: a single-center experience. Adv Ther 26(11):1035–1041.
40. Slakey DP (2008) Laparoscopic liver resection using a bipolar vesselsealing device: LigaSure. HPB (Oxford) 10(4):253–255
41. Contin P, Gooßen K, Grummich K, Jensen K, Schmitz-Winnenthal H, Büchler MW, Diener MK (2013) ENERgized vessel sealing systems versus CONventional hemostasis techniques in thyroid surgery—the ENERCON systematic review and network meta-analysis. Langenbecks Arch Surg 398(8):1039–1056
42. Dionigi G, Boni L, Rausei S, Frattini F, Ferrari CC, Mangano A, Leotta A, Franchin M (2012) The safety of energy-based devices in open thyroidectomy: a prospective, randomised study comparing the LigaSure™ (LF1212) and the Harmonic® FOCUS. Langenbecks Arch Surg 397(5):817–823
43. Franko J, Kish KJ, Pezzi CM, Pak H, Kukora JS (2006) Safely increasing the efficiency of thyroidectomy using a new bipolar electrosealing device (LigaSure) versus conventional clamp-and-tie technique. Am Surg 72(2):132–136
44. Youssef T, Mahdy T, Farid M, Latif AA (2008) Thyroid surgery: use of the LigaSure vessel sealing system versus conventional knot tying. Int J Surg 6(4):323–327
45. Rajbabu K, Barber NJ, Choi W, Muir GH (2007) To knot or not to knot? Sutureless haemostasis compared to the surgeon's knot. Ann R Coll Surg Engl 89(4):359–362

46. Kim FJ, Chammas MF Jr, Gewehr E, Morihisa M, Caldas F, Hayacibara E, Baptistussi M, Meyer F, Martins AC (2008) Temperature safety profile of laparoscopic devices: Harmonic ACE (ACE), Ligasure V (LV), and plasma trisector (PT). Surg Endosc 22(6):1464–1469
47. Diamantis T, Gialikaris S, Kontos M, Gakiopoulou C, Felekouras E, Papalois A, Agrogiannis G, Patsouris E, Bastounis E (2008) Comparison of safety and efficacy of ultrasonic and bipolar thermal energy: an experimental study. Surg Laparosc Endosc Percutan Tech 18(4):384–390
48. Richter S, Kollmar O, Schilling MK, Pistorius GA, Menger MD (2006) Efficacy and quality of vessel sealing: comparison of a reusable with a disposable device and effects of clamp surface geometry and structure. Surg Endosc 20(6):890–894
49. Harold KL, Pollinger H, Matthews BD, Kercher KW, Sing RF, Heniford BT (2003) Comparison of ultrasonic energy, bipolar thermal energy, and vascular clips for the hemostasis of small-, medium-, and large-sized arteries. Surg Endosc 17(8):1228–1230
50. Kennedy JS, Stranahan PL, Taylor KD, Chandler JG (1998) High-burststrength, feedback-controlled bipolar vessel sealing. Surg Endosc 12(6):876–878
51. Ignjatović M, Kostić Z (2011) Thyroidectomy with LigaSure. Surg Today 41(6):767–773
52. Pniak T, Formánek M, Matoušek P, Zeleník K, Komínek P (2014) Bipolar thermofusion BiClamp 150 in thyroidectomy: a review of 1156 operations. Biomed Res Int 2014:707265
53. Kwok SY, Chung CC, Tsui KK, Li MK (2005) A double-blind, randomized trial comparing Ligasure and Harmonic Scalpel hemorrhoidectomy. Dis Colon Rectum 48(2):344–348
54. Campagnacci R, de Sanctis A, Baldarelli M, Lezoche G, Guerrieri M (2007) Electrothermal bipolar vessel sealing device vs. ultrasonic coagulating shears in laparoscopic colectomies: a comparative study. Surg Endosc 21(9):1526–1531
55. Lachanas V, Prokopakis E, Mpenakis A, Karatzanis AD, Velegrakis G (2005) The use of Ligasure Vessel Sealing System in thyroid surgery. Otolaryngol Head Neck Surg 132(3):487–489
56. Koh Y, Park J, Kim JW, Lee SW, Choi EC (2010) Clipless and sutureless endoscopic thyroidectomy using only the harmonic scalpel. Surg Endosc 24(5):1117–1125
57. Musunuru S, Schaefer S, Chen H (2008) The use of the LigaSure for hemostasis during thyroid lobectomy. Am J Surg 195(3):382–384
58. Sandonato L, Cipolla C, Graceffa G, Fricano S, Li Petri S, Prinzi G, Latteri S, Latteri MA (2003) Bipolar electrothermic coagulation (LigaSure bipolar vessel sealing system) in thyroid surgery. Chir Ital 55(3):411–415
59. McNally M, Agle S, Williams R, Pofahl WE (2009) A comparison of two methods of hemostasis in thyroidectomy. Am Surg 75(11):1073–1076
60. Zarebczan B, Mohanty D, Chen H (2011) A comparison of the LigaSure and harmonic scalpel in thyroid surgery: a single institution review. Ann Surg Oncol 18:214–218
61. Sartori PV, De Fina S, Colombo G, Pugliese F, Romano F, Cesana G, Uggeri F (2008) LigaSure versus Ultracision® in thyroid surgery: a prospective randomized study. Langenbecks Arch Surg 393:655–658
62. Oussoultzoglou E, Panaro F, Rosso E, Zeca I, Bachellier P, Pessaux P, Jaeck D (2008) Use of BiClamp decreased the severity of hypocalcemia after total thyroidectomy compared with LigaSure: a prospective study. World J Surg 32(9):1968–1973
63. Campbell PA, Cresswell AB, Frank TG, Cuschieri A (2003) Realtime thermography during energized vessel sealing and dissection. Surg Endosc 17(10):1640–1645
64. Smith CT, Zarebczan B, Alhefdhi A, Chen H (2011) Infrared thermographic profiles of vessel sealing devices on thyroid parenchyma. J Surg Res 170(1):64–68
65. Rahbari R, Mathur A, Kitano M, Guerrero M, Shen WT, Duh QY, Clark OH, Kebebew E (2011) Prospective randomized trial of ligasure versus harmonic hemostasis technique in thyroidectomy. Ann Surg Oncol 18:1023–1027

# Topical Hemostatic Agents

# 20

Luca Revelli, Serena Elisa Tempera, Chiara Bellantone, Marco Raffaelli, and Celestino Pio Lombardi

## 20.1 Introduction

Even when suitable anesthetics became available, many surgeons believed that operations on the thyroid gland were too hazardous to be attempted. Especially for the most serious complication of thyroidectomy: bleeding [1].

> Can thyroid gland be removed with a reasonable hope of saving the patient? Experience emphatically answers: no.
>
> Should the surgeon be so adventurous or foolhardy to undertake the enterprise …
>
> … every stroke of his knife will be followed by a torrent of blood and lucky will it be for him if his victim lives long enough to enable him to finish his horrid butchering …
>
> […] No honest and sensible surgeon would ever engage in it.
>
> Samuel D. Gross (1805–1884), Professor of Surgery, Jefferson Medical College, Philadelphia, *System of Surgery*

Appalling results of thyroid surgery led, in 1646, to the imprisonment of a surgeon for his work [2].

In 1850 – given the miserable outcomes of thyroidectomies – the French *Académie Royale de Médecine* forbade any operation on goiter [3, 4].

During the 1860s to the 1880s the introduction of improved anesthesia, new methods of infection prophylaxis, and improved hemostasis technique would provide the impetus for an important change.

The early history of hemostasis – as outlined beautifully by *Samuel Clark Harvey* in 1929 – starts with the use of crude ligatures, cautery, hot oil, and caustic substances to control hemorrhage [5].

L. Revelli (✉) • S.E. Tempera • C. Bellantone • M. Raffaelli • C.P. Lombardi
Unità Operativa di Chirurgia Endocrina e Metabolica,
Università Cattolica del Sacro Cuore, Roma, Largo Agostino Gemelli, 8,
Rome, RM 00168, Italy
e-mail: lucarevelli@rm.unicatt.it; serena.tempera@gmail.com; marcoraffaelli@rm.unicatt.it; cp.lombardi@rm.unicatt.it



C.P. Lombardi, R. Bellantone (eds.), *Minimally Invasive Therapies for Endocrine Neck Diseases*, DOI 10.1007/978-3-319-20065-1_20

It was only in 1600 that **Ambroise Parè**, a French surgeon, introduced vascular ligation as the preferable method to provide bleeding control.

The first effective hemostatic forceps were introduced only in 1874 by **Thomas Spencer Wells** (1818–1897) in London and by **Jules Emile Péan** (1830–1898) in Paris [5].

The use of such devices began much earlier in Europe than in the United States. **William Steward Halsted** (1852–1922) witnessed thyroid surgeries using dozens of hemostats while in Europe during 1879. His only prior experience with their use, during thyroid surgery in the United States, had occurred at the Roosevelt Hospital of New York under **Henry Berton Sands** (1830–1888). At that time, the entire American hospital had only two hemostats at their disposal [4]. Halsted championed the use of hemostats in his country upon his return to the United States late in 1879.

Forceps had a marked influence on outcomes of thyroid surgery [6].

Incidence of morbidity with thyroid surgery decreased significantly after standardization of the capsular dissection technique by Thompson in 1973 [7], and total thyroidectomy is increasingly accepted for the treatment of cancer and benign thyroid diseases.

New technologies for the prevention and control of bleeding were gradually introduced in surgical practice over the past century: electrical scalpel (1924), bipolar forceps (1940s), and recently the radio frequency and ultrasonic scalpel (2000s).

A critical problem for the surgeon in the operating room has been always oozing blood, where cautery and suture ligation are not feasible. For this reason, over the past decades, means such as lasers ($CO_2$, Argon, and Nd-YAG), and spray-electrocoagulation have been introduced. Topical agents have also been developed to promote hemostasis in a wide variety of surgical procedures where the control of bleeding may result particularly difficult or impossible (coagulopathies and platelets dysfunction, parenchymal tissues, bony surfaces, etc.). Most of these topical agents were originally developed to improve wound healing in soldiers with severe burn injuries during World War I, World War II, and Vietnam and Korea War [8].

Currently, hypoparathyroidism and recurrent laryngeal nerve palsy are the most frequent postoperative complications associated with thyroid surgery. In terms of severity, postoperative hemorrhage is a rare but potentially lethal complication, occurring in 0.3–2 % of cases [9–13].

Hemorrhage correlated with a thyroidectomy usually occurs within 24 h, and the most significant hematomas become apparent after 6–8 h [14].

More in detail, the time of occurrence of the postoperative hematoma would be in:

1. <1–2 % of cases, immediate/early
2. 43 % within 6 h
3. 38 % between 7 and 12 h
4. 8 % after 24 h [15]

The intraoperative bleeding hampers the vision of the operative field and of the delicate anatomical structures, complicating the surgical dissection: it can cause indirect morbidity related to injury of the recurrent nerves and lesions of the parathyroid glands.

## 20.2 Indications

Topical hemostatic agents (THA) are used when surgical hemostasis is inadequate or impractical. Electrocautery may not be useful for controlling bleeding in some surgical fields such as:

1. Around nerves (e.g., recurrent laryngeal nerve, vagus, spinal accessory, loop of the hypoglossal nerve)
2. Medullary bone surfaces (e.g., hyoid bone after *Sistrunk*'s procedure)
3. Needle-hole bleeding from vascular grafts
4. Raw areas on cut surfaces (e.g., muscle fibers, thyroid tissue, parenchyma of the salivary glands)

The majority of *routine*, elective operations are performed in patients with normal hemostasis and with minimal blood loss.

Patients who are anticoagulated and those with bleeding diatheses (e.g., factor deficiencies, disseminated intravascular coagulation), or have platelets dysfunction (e.g., aspirin therapy) can continue to ooze from surgical surfaces in spite of adequate surgical hemostasis [16].

Under ideal circumstances, patients with hemostatic abnormalities have their underlying defects corrected prior to proceeding with surgery; however, this is not always possible. Anticoagulated patients, patients receiving antiplatelet therapy, and those with congenital or acquired bleeding diatheses may require emergency surgical procedures to manage trauma or unrelated conditions or to manage hemorrhage that is a result of their disorder. Under these circumstances, correction of the hemostatic defect is undertaken *en route* to or simultaneously with the procedure [17].

Hemostatic abnormalities can also develop during the course of surgery (e.g., hypothermia, disseminated intravascular coagulation).

The newer oral anticoagulant drugs (*rivaroxaban* [Xarelto®], *apixaban* [Eliquis®], and *dabigatran* [Pradaxa®]), unlike *warfarin*, do not have a reversal agent. Biologically active topical hemostats may be effective in this setting [18].

## 20.3 Topical Hemostatic Agents

The four main categories of topical hemostatic agents (THA) are as follows:

1. **Physical passive agents (passive hemostatics)**, which promote hemostasis using a passive substrate, including collagen, gelatins, and regenerated oxidized cellulose. Their mechanism of action is to provide platelet activation and aggregation. They are of bovine, equine, swine, or vegetable origin and are available as sponge, sheets, gauze, fleece, and powder [8, 17].
2. **Biologically active agents (active hemostatics)**, which enhance coagulation at the bleeding site. Active agents participate at the end of the coagulation cascade

to form a fibrin clot. This group includes products containing fibrinogen and thrombin (fibrin sealants, adhesive sealants).

Products with purified fibrinogen and thrombin were first successfully used in the 1970s. The first fibrin sealants to be commercially available in Europe were, in the early 1980s, Tissucol® and Beriplast®, whereas in the United States the Food and Drug Administration (FDA) approved the licensing of fibrin sealants only in 1998 because of the presumed risk of viral hepatitis transmission. The lack of availability of these products in the United States until 1998 resulted in the production of fibrin glue from blood-bank cryoprecipitate ("home-made") with a lower concentration of fibrinogen [19]. At the moment, fibrin sealants are still the most effective hemostatic adhesive agents available for surgical purpose [8].

3. **Sealants (tissue adhesive)** and topical agents, which are not strictly hemostatic. They have adhesive and sealing properties that make them be useful in wound closure, vascular anastomosis protection, and prevention of leakages. They may be synthetic (cyanoacrylates and PEG – polyethylene glycol sealants) or semi-synthetic (glutaraldehyde-albumina) sealants [20].
4. **Combined THA**, products made by a combination of different THA or TA.

## 20.3.1 Passive Hemostatics

Passive hemostatics (PH) promote hemostasis through several effects. The matrix material provides a stimulus that activates platelets and the extrinsic pathway and provides a scaffold for thrombus deposition. The dry matrix also absorbs water and concentrates hemostatic factors at the site of bleeding, and tamponades bleeding vessels by exerting pressure.

Between the various PA, we may mention:

### 20.3.1.1 Cellulose-Based Hemostatic Agents

Cellulose-based hemostatic agents are vegetable-derived products, biodegradable and biocompatible. They are completely reabsorbed by hydrolysis with a low rate of foreign-body reactions and no immunologic risk. They also have antimicrobial activity and can be used for the prevention and treatment of surgical site infection. There are two formulations commercially available: oxidized regenerated cellulose obtained from wood pulp cellulose and oxidized cellulose obtained from cotton fiber.

**Oxidized regenerated cellulose** (ORC) is a dry, absorbable sterile mesh (Surgicel®) that can be applied directly to an area of bleeding. A single-layer sheet is fully absorbed in about 14 days. Results are optimal if bleeding is minimal (oozing) [21].

*In vitro* studies have found that ORC has bactericidal activity against a wide range of gram-positive and negative organisms because of its acidic pH. The low pH also inhibits proteases and elastase, which may be beneficial in chronic wounds; however, this same property may inhibit its resorption. Residual ORC may be associated with infection and adhesion formation.

#### 20.3.1.2 Gelatin-Based Hemostatic Agents

Gelatin-based hemostatic agents are prepared from purified pork skin gelatin or bovine derived gelatin. They provide a mechanical matrix that promotes clotting and can be combined with topical thrombin. Gelatin-based agents are available in sponge, powder, or granular forms.

**Gelatin Matrix** (GM) (Gelfoam®, Surgifoam®) is a hydrocolloid made from acid partial hydrolysis of porcine-derived collagen that is whipped into foam and then dried. It is available in sponge or powder form. Gelatin sponge absorbs blood or fluid up to 40 times its weight and it expands up to 200 % in its dimensions. The dry sponge form can be tailored to any shape and although rigid when dry, the sponge becomes pliable after moistening. Once in place, pressure is applied for several minutes to achieve hemostasis. The sponge can be left in place and is completely absorbed after 4–6 weeks. Because gelatin foam has a neutral pH, it does not inactivate thrombin, and thus, it is common practice to moisten it with topical thrombin to synergize the effects of these agents.

The disadvantages of gelatin include an increased incidence of infection, granuloma and fibrosis formation, and – similar to dry matrix product – the potential for disruption of the clot if the sponge is removed. Although all brands of gelatin matrix are derived from porcine connective tissue, it is not considered to be antigenic [17, 21].

#### 20.3.1.3 Collagen-Based Hemostatic Agents

Collagen-based hemostatic agents, bovine or equine derived, in addition to promoting hemostasis are useful as a scaffold upon which cells proliferate and migrate accelerating wound healing. Many agents are combined with thrombin in order to enhance the effectiveness. There are many formulations commercially available: sponge, powder, fiber, and sheet.

**Microfibrillar Collagen** (MC) is an absorbable acid salt obtained from bovine collagen (Avitene®). MC acts as a scaffold for clot formation and activates platelets. MC can be applied directly to the bleeding site as a powder, but foam sheet formulations (Avitene Ultrafoam®) are available. MC is fully absorbed within 3 months. MC remains effective with the use of heparin, but is less effective when platelet counts are below 20,000/mm$^3$.

**Microporous Polysaccharide Spheres** (MPS) (Arista®) are derived from potato starch, which accelerates clot formation by acting as a molecular sieve to absorb water and concentrate platelets and blood proteins. MPS are available in powder form and are used by first applying pressure to the bleeding site with a dry surgical sponge for 2 minutes to achieve a relatively dry surface, then liberally applying the powder with the bellows applicator. Gentle pressure is reapplied with a fresh surgical sponge for 1–2 minutes until hemostasis is achieved. The advantages of MPS include low cost, rapid absorption (within 48 h), and freedom from transmissible viruses or alloantigens. In addition, MPS does not act as a *nidus* for infection or cause foreign body reactions.

In the group of PH we can mention also **Bone Wax (BW)** used sometimes for blood oozing from the cut surface of medullary bone (e.g., in median sternotomy or in the hyoid bone resection in the *Sistrunk's* procedure). BW (composed of beeswax, paraffin, and wax-softening agents) physically occludes bleeding vessels within bone to stop bleeding. When using BW, a minimal amount should be used and it is rubbed across the surface of the bone surface without leaving a raised plug. BW is inexpensive and effective, but can lead to infection or granuloma formation which can interfere with bone healing [22].

**Ostene** is an effective alternative to BW. It is a wax-like compound of a water-soluble alkaline oxide copolymer that occludes bleeding vessels in bone, similar to BW, but it does not persist in the wound as a foreign body. In animal studies comparing Ostene with BW, Ostene did not remain in the wound beyond 3 weeks and bone healing was more pronounced in the Ostene group [17, 23].

## 20.3.2 Active Hemostatics

### 20.3.2.1 Fibrin Sealants (FS)

Fibrin sealants (FS) are involved at the end of the coagulation cascade to induce a clot at the site of bleeding. FS are a two-component system that includes a solution of concentrated fibrinogen and factor XII, and a solution of thrombin and calcium (Tisseel®, Vitagel®, Cryoseal®, Evicel®) When mixed together – just prior to use – a fibrin clot forms. The two components are applied simultaneously using a two-syringe technique. Commercially available preparations consist of a combination plunger, side-by-side syringes and a dual needle-tip to facilitate even application of each component.

Patches (TachoSil®, Veriset®, Evarrest®) and pads (FibrinPad®) composed of fibrin sealant combined with other hemostatic agents (*polyglactin*, oxidized regenerated cellulose) are in the early stages of clinical investigation [24].

A large number of commercial and blood bank prepared ("home-made") fibrin sealants are commonly used in a variety of surgical settings: these products are somehow similar in composition but actually vary widely as to components and preparation methods [8].

### 20.3.2.2 Thrombin-Based Hemostatic Agents

Topical thrombin (TT) is reconstituted from a lyophilized powder. It can be applied using a sprayer or applied with a needle and syringe to direct its application to a specific area of bleeding. TT can also be used in conjunction with a gelatin matrix agent (sponge or granules) that provides the thrombin with an immediate scaffold for clot formation. Due to its liquid nature, thrombin applied in combination with gelatin granules (FloSeal®, Surgiflo®) may control bleeding more quickly than thrombin-soaked pieces of gelatin foam. Human thrombin and a recombinant thrombin are available for use, largely replacing bovine thrombin.

## 20.3.3 Tissue Adhesive

Tissue adhesives (TA) are low viscosity liquids that polymerize in few seconds forming a solid film that connects the tissue surfaces. This property makes adhesives effective tissue sealants and effective hemostatic agents.

They can be divided in synthetic (*cyanoacrylates* and PEG – *polyethylene glycol* sealants) and semi-synthetic (*glutaraldehyde-albumina*) sealants.

**Cyanoacrylate** TA *octyl-2-cyanoacrylate* (Dermabond®) and *butyl-2-cyanoacrylate* (Histoacryl®) are liquid monomers that change to strong polymers with exposure to moisture. Cyanoacrylates have numerous surgical and medical applications such as: skin closure and wound repair (especially in pediatrics) with formation of an antimicrobial barrier, esophageal and gastric varices management, air leaks prevention in lung resection, lymphatic leaks, and reparation of peripheral nerves [8, 17, 20].

### 20.3.4 Combined THA

Between the various products made by a combination of different THA or TA we may mention:

**Collagen sponge** coated with human fibrinogen and thrombin (TachoSil®). The sponge is manufactured from horse tendons. TachoSil® reacts upon contact with blood, other body fluids or saline to form a clot that glues it to the tissue surface. Hemostasis is reached in a few minutes, and the sponge is absorbed within several weeks. Some patients experience hypersensitivity or allergic reactions.

**Porous collagen matrix + polyethylene glycol (PEG)** (Hemopatch®) is a new resorbable sealing hemostat that has a dual-method mechanism of action: two components interact to achieve hemostasis by sealing off the bleeding surface and initiating the body's own clotting mechanisms.

When in contact with tissue, NHS-PEG forms covalent bonds between the collagen pad and tissue proteins, which seals the tissue and induces hemostasis. In preclinical tests, it achieved fast and effective hemostasis (fully controlling bleeding at 2 minutes).

## 20.4 Adverse Effects and Complications

Adverse effects of THA and tissue adhesives are related to the composition and characteristics of the preparation, location of placement, and absorption time. Excessive amounts of a slowly degrading product can serve as a *nidus* for infection, and agents placed into a confined place can cause compression of surrounding structures, particularly if the product has a tendency to expand.

### 20.4.1 Impaired Wound Healing

Excess application of topical hemostatic agents can impede wound healing. Granuloma formation has been reported with the use of microfibrillar collagen, gelatin foam, and cyanoacrylate [21]. In addition, the metabolites of cyanoacrylates (e.g., *cyanoacetate* and *formaldehyde*) can cause an inflammatory response in the surrounding tissues.

### 20.4.2 Surgical Infection

There are many clinical reports of wound infections associated with the use of THA. Adverse factors such as emergency procedure, transfusion, and prolonged operative time are associated with an increased risk of surgical wound infection and frequently coexist with the need for hemostatic agents, and thus, any analysis of the risk of infection due to hemostatic agent is confounded. The risk of infection may be minimized by removing excess topical hemostatic agents from the wound after hemostasis is achieved, when possible.

### 20.4.3 Allergic Reactions

Allergic reactions (including anaphylaxis) are associated primarily with bovine-derived fibrin sealants. These products should not be used in patients with a history of prior anaphylactic reactions to plasma products or IgA deficiency [25].

### 20.4.4 Blood-Borne Disease

The potential transmission of infectious disease (e.g., hepatitis, HIV), even from screened and tested blood, is a risk of any product that contains blood components. The use of recombinant human thrombin should reduce the risk. Healthcare workers in the operating room should exercise extra caution when using thrombin-derived products, particularly if used in an aerosolized form.

### 20.4.5 Vascular Thrombosis

THA should not be injected into a blood vessel or within an opened vessel [17].

## 20.5 Choice of Topical Hemostatic Agent

The choice of THA to use depends upon:

1. Character, amount, and location of bleeding
2. Type of surgical procedure
3. The availability of a given agent
4. Cost considerations

5. Surgeon preference and habits

Biologically active agents (e.g., topical thrombin, fibrin seal) are more useful for brisk bleeding compared with dry matrix agents (e.g., gelatin matrix) and are more effective in the setting of coagulopathy.

Although more expensive, fibrin sealants have significantly higher rates of hemostatic control compared with thrombin-gelatin combinations. Fibrin sealant and bovine albumin-glutaraldehyde tissue adhesives (Bioglue®) are appropriate choices when moderate bleeding does not respond to other measures [26].

## 20.6 Cost Considerations

THA are generally prepackaged for one-time use in quantities that are generally sufficient to manage bleeding from a single site.

Although these preparations should not be used unnecessarily, they are cost-effective if they:

1. Save operative time
2. Reduce transfusions
3. Prevent a return to the operating room

The cost of these agents falls in the range between an electrosurgery pen and the handset of various tissue-sealing energy sources (e.g., ultrasonic scalpel).

Less expensive agents are frequently used in a routine or preventive setting to minimize blood loss. The more expensive agents (fibrin sealants and microfibrillar collagen) are often more effective in the setting of coagulopathy or anticoagulation and are frequently the preferred choice when bleeding is not easily controlled [17].

**Conclusions**

Accurate hemostasis during neck surgery plays a key role in achieving successful patient's outcome. Therefore, in addition to traditional hemostatic methods, several THA and TA have been developed to reduce time in operating room and complications.

THA may decrease intraoperative bleeding and facilitate modern surgical technologies such as minimally invasive surgery, video-assisted (MIVAP, MIVAT), endoscopic and robotic procedures.

THA are useful adjuncts to surgical hemostasis for controlling nonspecific bleeding.

A large number of commercial and blood bank prepared fibrin sealants are commonly used in a variety of surgical settings (biologically active agents, active hemostatics): these products are somehow similar in composition but actually vary widely as to components and preparation methods. Agents that enhance normal hemostatic mechanisms include thrombin-based products.

Adjunctive local hemostatic treatments include physical passive agents (passive hemostatics, such as cellulose-based hemostatic agents, gelatin-based hemostatic agents, collagen-based hemostatic agents), sealants (tissue adhesive, such as *cyanoacrylates*, PEG – *polyethylene glycol* hydrogels, *glutaraldehyde-albumina* sealants), and Combined THA and TA products.

The ideal hemostatic should be safe, effective, practical, and cost-effective.

Adverse effects and complications from THA and TA are generally uncommon. Most problems can be avoided by limiting the amount of agent remaining within the wound once hemostasis has been achieved.

Complications related to thrombin-based agents (which are blood products) include the potential for transmission of blood-borne disease and anaphylaxis with the bovine-derived agents.

Other problems that can arise include impaired wound healing and infection.

The choice of which THA to use depends upon the character, amount, and location of bleeding; type of surgical procedure; the availability of a given agent; cost considerations; and surgeon preference and habits.

Surgeons should be familiar with THA to ensure an optimal use in theater.

## References


1. Ellis H (2001) A history of surgery. Greenwich Medical Media, London
2. Giddings AEB (1998) The history of thyroidectomy. J R Soc Med 91(Suppl 33):3–6
3. Welbourn RB (1990) The thyroid. In: The history of endocrine surgery. Praeger, New York, pp 19–27
4. Halsted WS (1920) The operative story of goitre. The author's operation. Johns Hopkins Hosp Rep 19:71–257
5. Harvey SC (1929) The history of haemostasis. Hoeber, New York
6. Welbourn RB (1996) Highlights from endocrine surgical history. World J Surg 20:603–612
7. Thompson NW, Olsen WR, Hoffman GL (1973) The continuing development of the technique of thyroidectomy. Surgery 73:913–927
8. Masci E, Santoleri L, Belloni F et al (2011) Topical hemostatic agents in surgical practice. Transfus Apher Sci 45:305–311
9. Lacoste L, Gineste D, Karayan J et al (1993) Airway complications in thyroid surgery. Ann Otol Rhinol Laryngol 102:441–446
10. Shaha AR, Jaffe BM (1994) Practical management of post-thyroidectomy hematoma. J Surg Oncol 57:235–238
11. Shandilya M, Kieran S, Walshe P et al (2006) Cervical haematoma after thyroid surgery: management and prevention. Ir Med J 99:266–268
12. Testini M, Marzaioli R, Lissidini G et al (2009) The effectiveness of FloSeal matrix hemostatic agent in thyroid surgery: a prospective, randomized, control study. Langenbecks Arch Surg 394(5):837–842
13. Calò PG, Pisano G, Piga G et al (2010) Postoperative hematomas after thyroid surgery. Incidence and risk factors in our experience. Ann Ital Chir 81:343–347
14. Reeve T, Thompson NW (2000) Complications of thyroid surgery: how to avoid them, how to manage them, and observations on their possible effect on the whole patient. World J Surg 24:971–975
15. Rosato L, Avenia N, Bernante P et al (2004) Complications of thyroid surgery: analysis of a multicentric study on 14, 934 patients operated on in Italy over 5 years. World J Surg 28:271–276

16. Samudrala S (2008) Topical hemostatic agents in surgery: a surgeon's perspective. AORN J 88(3):S2–S11
17. Peralta E, Sanfey H, Collins KA (2014) Overview of topical hemostatic agents and tissues adhesives used in the operating room. http://www.uptodate.com, Topic 15069 Version 9.0
18. Lai A, Davidson N, Galloway SW et al (2014) Perioperative management of patients on new oral anticoagulants. Br J Surg 101(7):742–749
19. Spotnitz WD, Mintz PD, Avery N et al (1987) Fibrin glue from stored human plasma. An inexpensive and efficient method for local blood bank preparation. Am Surg 53:460–464
20. Lombardi CP, Bracaglia R, Revelli L et al (2011) Aesthetic result of thyroidectomy: evaluation of different kinds of skin suture. Ann Ital Chir 82(6):449–455; discussion 455–456
21. Mannucci PM (1998) Hemostatic drugs. N Engl J Med 339(4):245
22. Sudmann B, Bang G, Sudmann E (2006) Histologically verified bone wax (beeswax) granuloma after median sternotomy in 17 of 18 autopsy cases. Pathology 38:138
23. Vestergaard RF, Nielsen PH, Terp KA (2014) Effect of hemostatic material on sternal healing after cardiac surgery. Ann Thorac Surg 97:153
24. Spotnitz WD, Burks S (2008) Hemostats, sealants, and adhesives: components of the surgical toolbox. Transfusion 48:1502
25. Schoenecker JG, Johnson RK, Fields RC et al (2003) Relative purity of thrombin-based hemostatic agents used in surgery. J Am Coll Surg 197(4):580
26. Achneck HE, Sileshi B, Jamiolkowski RM et al (2010) A comprehensive review of topical hemostatic agents: efficacy and recommendations for use. Ann Surg 251:217

# Critical Appraisal

# 21

Randall P. Scheri and Julie Ann Sosa

## 21.1 Introduction

Over the last 20 years, new technologies have been developed which have dramatically changed the field of surgery. While meticulous surgical technique and attention to detail remain the hallmarks of thyroid surgery, many surgeons have incorporated several technologies to enable them to perform thyroidectomy safely and faster. The previous chapters have reviewed the most common technologies used by thyroid surgeons, including intraoperative stimulation and monitoring of the external branch of the superior laryngeal nerve and the recurrent laryngeal nerve, as well as utilization of hemostatic devices and agents. This chapter will critically appraise the literature regarding these new technologies and summarize our recommendations.

## 21.2 External Branch Superior Laryngeal Nerve Intraoperative Nerve Monitoring

Injury to the external branch of the superior laryngeal nerve (EBSLN) can occur during thyroidectomy, resulting in alterations in the patient's voice quality, projection, and ability to produce pitch in the highest ranges [1, 2]. These changes may be subtle, but are particularly significant for singers and other voice professionals. The standard techniques to minimize the risk of injury to the EBSLN are either direct visualization of the nerve before ligation of the superior thyroid vessels or ligation of superior thyroid vessels on the thyroid capsule without attempts to identify the nerve [3]. Nerve injury may still occur in up to 58 % of patients [4]. Identification and

R.P. Scheri • J.A. Sosa (✉)
Department of Surgery, Duke University, Durham, NC, USA
e-mail: r.scheri@duke.edu; julie.sosa@duke.edu



C.P. Lombardi, R. Bellantone (eds.), *Minimally Invasive Therapies for Endocrine Neck Diseases*, DOI 10.1007/978-3-319-20065-1_21

preservation of the EBSLN is often difficult because of its small caliber and variable anatomic pathway, particularly for patients with short necks, large goiters, and advanced cancers, where the anatomy is altered and the nerve is more intimately associated with the superior thyroid vessels [5]. Furthermore, the EBSLN cannot be identified in approximately 20 % of patients by direct visualization; this is generally the case when the nerve travels within the inferior constrictor muscle [6]. Because of the high rate of injury (as frequent as 58 %) [4] and increased difficulty identifying the EBSLN, intraoperative nerve stimulation and monitoring (IONM) have been employed as an adjunct to identify and minimize injury to the EBSLN.

There have been several studies that have evaluated IONM for EBSLN; however, the majority of these studies have been small, retrospective, nonrandomized, or single armed. To date, three randomized controlled trials [7–9] have evaluated the effect of IONM on EBSLN injury. Cernea et al. assessed EBSLN function with stimulation of the nerve followed by visual inspection for contraction of the cricothyroid muscle and a subsequent twitch. Seventy-six patients were randomized to three groups: IONM, dissection by a surgical resident without nerve identification, and dissection by a senior surgeon without nerve identification. Voice function was evaluated 1 week after surgery, and cricothyroid muscle function measured by percutaneous electromyograph 1 month after surgery. Both voice function and cricothyroid muscle electromyography were repeated at 6 months for patients with early EBSLN paralysis. The nerve identification rate was 93 % in the IONM group. There were no EBSLN injuries in the IONM group. However, 28 % of patients in the resident group and 12 % of patients who had surgery by the senior surgeon group had EBSLN injury ($p=0.01$) on early assessment. Voice function correlated with nerve injuries. At 6 months follow-up, 57 % of patients in the resident group and no patients in the senior surgeon group had persistent nerve injury. Due to the small number of patients, a statistical analysis between these groups was not performed. The study had several limitations. Many patients were lost to follow-up, and 26 % of patients were excluded during the course of the study for reasons not described. Accordingly, an intention to treat analysis was not performed, so potential bias in the results cannot be excluded.

Lifante et al. [8] assessed EBSLN function under regional anesthesia using electrodes placed directly into the cricothyroid muscle. Forty-seven patients were randomized either to visual identification of the EBSLN plus IONM, or to direct visual identification alone. Following surgery, patients were assessed with the Voice Handicap Index-10 [10] and the Reflux Symptom Index [11]. The nerve identification rate was 66 % in the IONM group compared to 21 % in the control group ($p=0.003$). Voice function 3 months after surgery was impaired in the control group compared to the IONM group ($p=0.034$). Long-term follow-up of voice function was not performed. Unfortunately, a blinded, objective assessment of EBSLN function was not performed with either laryngoscopy or cricothyroid muscle electromyography, thereby preventing a correlation between patients' perceived voice function and EBSLN function.

Barczynski et al. [9] performed the largest randomized controlled trial to date evaluating IONM of the EBSLN. Two hundred ten patients were randomized either to meticulous exploration for, and identification of, the EBSLN, or to fastidious exploration for, and identification of, the EBSLN with the aid of IONM. EBSLN function was assessed using endotracheal tube electrodes and direct visual contraction of a cricothyroid muscle twitch. The nerve identification rate was 84 % for the IONM compared to 34 % for the control group ($p<0.001$). The rate of temporary EBSLN palsy was 1 % for the IONM group compared to 5 % for the control group ($p=0.02$). Voice impairment and abnormal stroboscopy were more common in the control group than the IONM group 3 weeks after surgery ($p=0.03$), but after 3 months, these differences resolved ($p=0.57$). There was no difference in permanent EBSLN palsy rates ($p=0.57$).

In summary, studies evaluating IONM for EBSLN have been small and have employed different methodologies to identify the nerve. Data appear to support the concept that IONM is associated with increased identification of the EBSLN, with subsequent reduction in transient voice disturbance, and decreased frequency of temporary dysfunction in the EBSLN. Compared to visualization alone, IONM does not appear to be associated with alteration in long-term voice function or the rate of permanent EBSLN injury. The American Academy of Otolaryngology and Head and Neck Surgery guidelines for improving voice outcomes after thyroid surgery [12] evaluated the published evidence addressing protection of the EBSLN. Based on an intermediate level of evidence and a preponderance of benefit over harm, the guidelines recommended that surgeons should take steps to preserve the EBSLN when performing thyroid surgery. The role of IONM was not specifically addressed.

We feel that the evidence demonstrating the potential benefit of IONM of the EBSLN is still lacking; therefore, the technology cannot be recommended routinely, although the data to date are promising. The available studies are small, and the techniques used for nerve identification and measurement of patient outcomes have been inconsistent between studies. Further, there are to date no data to definitively demonstrate that IONM is associated with superior long-term voice function. While cost-effectiveness was not specifically evaluated in any of these studies, it is likely lower with IONM because long-term patient quality of life is not significantly compromised when IONM is not employed. We feel that additional studies are needed to provide adequate data to assess the value of EBSLN IONM; in particular, they should include evaluation of cost and cost-effectiveness.

## 21.3 Recurrent Laryngeal Nerve Intraoperative Nerve Monitoring

Recurrent laryngeal nerve (RLN) IONM was introduced in the 1990s [13] as an adjunct to the gold standard of RLN visualization. Recent studies have revealed that 53 % of general surgeons [14] and 65 % of otolaryngologists [15] in the United States employ IONM during thyroid surgery. The prevalence of IONM is even more common in Germany, where a recent survey of surgery departments was performed. The survey response rate was 53 %, and the respondents accounted for 75 % of all thyroid surgeries done in Germany. The survey revealed that IONM was used for 92 % of thyroidectomies in 2010 [16]. Despite the widespread use of IONM, there is considerable debate regarding its benefit in improving outcomes for thyroid surgery, and about whether the technology is cost-effective.

Numerous studies have evaluated the role of RLN IONM; however, the vast majority of studies have been observational in nature. In large series (greater than 100 nerves at risk), the average rate of nerve paralysis with IONM was 4.7 %, compared to 5.7 % without IONM. These two injury rates were not significantly different in any of the studies [12]. A study by Dralle et al. [17] reviewed 16,448 patients with 29,998 nerves at risk that underwent thyroid surgery recorded in a German registry of data from 63 hospitals. There was no significant difference ($p=0.97$) in the permanent RLN injury rate for IONM (0.80 %) compared to nerve visualization alone (0.89 %). Risk factors for permanent RLN injury were recurrent malignant goiter, recurrent benign goiter, and thyroid malignancy (Odds Ratio 6.66, $p<0.0001$, 4.67, $p<0.0001$, and 2.0, $p=0.002$, respectively). A nonrandomized study by Chan et al. [17] evaluating 1,000 nerves at risk revealed no difference in RLN injury rate as measured by laryngoscopy with IONM in primary surgery, but did show a significant benefit in the setting of remedial surgery (19 % vs. 7.8 %, $p=0.017$). There was also a trend towards lower RLN injury rates for patients with cancer and retrosternal goiters. A recent meta-analysis by Higgins et al. [18] of 44 studies (34 case series, seven comparative trials, and one randomized controlled trial) evaluated 64,699 nerves at risk and showed that the rate of transient and permanent RLN injury for visualization alone (3.12 % and 0.59 %, respectively) compared to IONM (3.52 % and 0.75 %, respectively) was not significantly different ($p=0.44$). This study did not specifically evaluate the potential value of IONM for remedial surgery. A significant weakness of this meta-analysis was the heterogeneity of the studies included, making a comparison of the data challenging. The methodology for IONM was different and included electrodes placed directly in the vocalis muscle as well as endotracheal tube electrodes. The method for IONM allocation included surgeon preference, consecutive allocation, and equipment availability. Surgeon experience and resident involvement were not evaluated. The timing of initial laryngoscopy ranged from immediately postoperative to 2 weeks after surgery. Persistent vocal cord paralysis was assessed at times ranging from 3 to 24 months after surgery.

Only two randomized controlled trials have compared RLN visualization and IONM. Dionigi et al. [19] assessed IONM for video-assisted thyroidectomy. Seventy-two patients were randomized to IONM or visualization alone. The incidence of RLN injury identified by direct laryngoscopy was 2.7 % (1 patient) for the IONM group compared to 8.3 % (3 patients) for the nerve visualization only group ($p=$NS). There were no permanent injuries to the RLN in either group. However, the study was small and underpowered to identify a significant difference between the study arms. A larger study by Barczynski et al. [20] randomized 1,000 patients to visualization alone or IONM. Nerve monitoring was performed using the Neurosign® system, where an electrode is placed directly into the vocalis muscle. Transient RLN injury was significantly higher in the visualization group compared to the IONM group (3.8 % versus 1.9 %, $p=0.011$). The permanent RLN injury rate was similar for both groups (1.2 % versus 0.8 %, $p=0.368$). A subgroup analysis of patients stratified by surgical risk revealed that for low-risk patients, there was no difference in transient RLN injury rates (2.8 % vs. 1.8 %), but injury to the RLN was more frequent in the high risk group (4.9 % vs. 2.0 %, $p=0.011$). There was no difference in permanent RLN injury rates based on risk stratification.

In addition to minimizing RLN injury, proponents of IONM have advocated that its use facilitates nerve identification, aids in nerve dissection, prognosticates post-operative nerve function, and can identify the site of nerve injury [21]. RLN identification rates using IONM and nerve mapping are between 98 and 100 %. In a study by Snyder et al. [22], IONM assisted with identification for 3 % of nerves with aberrant anatomy and 7 % of nerves during difficult dissections. Another study by Sari et al. [23] showed that time needed to identify the RLN was significantly shortened by 7 min ($p<0.005$) using IONM compared to nerve visualization alone, leading to shorter total operating room times with IONM ($p=0.001$). The experience of the participating surgeons was not stated for the study, bringing into question the generalizability of the findings.

After RLN identification, advocates of IONM suggest that it can aid in dissection of the nerve and determine the mechanism and site of injuries. In a study by Snyder et al. [24] of 666 RLNs at risk during thyroid and parathyroid surgery, IONM was helpful during the dissection of 7.5 % of patients, including patients with a bifurcated RLN, extensive scar tissue, and medial nerve displacement. The location and mechanism of nerve injury can also be determined with IONM. In the same study, the most common mechanism of RLN injury was a traction injury at the ligament of Berry. The injury location can be precisely identified using nerve mapping along the length of the nerve. If a ligature or clip is identified at the site of RLN injury, it can be removed, which theoretically should facilitate eventual nerve recovery.

Another perceived advantage of IONM is the ability to prognosticate nerve function at the conclusion of surgery. This is particularly important for bilateral surgery where injury to both RLNs is devastating and may lead to tracheostomy. While a RLN transection is readily apparent, blunt injury from stretch or compression is frequently not visibly detectable. Several studies have shown that surgeons are very poor visually judging RLN function intraoperatively and detect only 10–14 % of injuries [25, 26]. Furthermore, nerve injury was only suspected in one of six (16 %) patients with bilateral RLN injury [27]. In contrast, modern IONM using electromyography waveforms is highly specific and associated with a high negative predictive value, ranging from 92 to 100 % [28]. In a study by Goretzki et al. [29], 48 patients with planned total thyroidectomy using IONM lost signal during dissection of the first lobe. In 26 (55 %) patients, the surgical strategy was changed and the operation terminated after the first lobectomy, with completion thyroidectomy performed at a later date. For the remaining patients, either a total thyroidectomy with the assistance of a senior surgeon or a smaller bilateral surgery was performed. No patients in the delayed group had bilateral nerve injuries compared to 17 % in the nondelayed group.

While IONM intermittently assesses the integrity of the RLN, a new method using continuous IONM with vagal stimulation has been developed. This could potentially allow identification of an impending nerve injury and alert the surgeon to alter surgical technique to avoid injury. Early studies have revealed no adverse side effects from continuous vagal stimulation [30, 31]. To date, the studies evaluating continuous IONM are small, but do appear to identify neural changes prior to loss of nerve signal [32, 33]. We eagerly anticipate larger studies and further development of this technology to determine if this may be associated with decreased frequency of RLN injury. Investigations to date have largely consisted of adult patients, so application in the pediatric population is still under-studied.

Although IONM is widely used, there is little uniformity in nerve monitoring across centers with regard to technique and the technology/system employed [21]. With the goal of improving the quality of IONM, the multidisciplinary International Neural Monitoring Study Group has published guidelines in an effort to standardize IONM by providing recommendations for equipment set up, endotracheal tube placement, and troubleshooting algorithms for loss of signal. These guidelines assert that IONM is safe and not associated with neural injury or cardiac arrhythmias (from vagal stimulation). The International Neural Monitoring Study Group [21] makes its recommendations on evidence-based literature and experience of the study group. The guidelines state that neural monitoring should be a component of all thyroid surgeries, since technically difficult surgeries cannot always be predicted preoperatively. Even though IONM provides the greatest benefit in difficult surgeries, routine use enhances surgeon familiarity with, and intricate knowledge of, the machine setup, as well as interpretation of signals and troubleshooting of the system. The German practice guidelines [34] are based on critical analysis of the literature and consensus opinion of the multidisciplinary working group. The guidelines state that while IONM may be complimentary, it does not replace the gold standard of nerve visualization. It can be considered for all thyroid surgery because it may facilitate identification of the RLN, assess RLN function at the conclusion of surgery, and avoid bilateral RLN injury. The American Academy of Otolaryngology and Head and Neck Surgery (AAOHNS) has recently published guidelines for improving voice outcomes after thyroid surgery [12]. Based on an intermediate level of evidence from one randomized controlled trial, observational studies, and a preponderance of benefit over harm, the guidelines state that IONM may be considered for patients having thyroid surgery due to proven benefit in RLN identification time, complex and remedial cases, and avoidance of bilateral RLN paralysis. Accordingly, the guidelines recommend that surgeons may consider IONM for bilateral thyroid surgery, remedial thyroid surgery, and surgery in the setting of existing RLN paralysis. The guidelines from each of the three groups are different, reflecting differences in interpretation of the quality of the data and inconsistent results from published studies. The studies are small and likely underpowered to identify small potential incremental benefit for nerve monitoring. In addition, they have been inconsistent in design, in the relative complexity of included cases and perceived surgical risk, and surgeon experience, leading to difficulty in drawing firm conclusions that are generalizable to a large patient population.

## 21.4 Hemostatic Devices

Meticulous hemostasis is essential in thyroidectomy in order to maintain a dry surgical field and avoid an inadvertent injury to the RLN, parathyroid glands, and prevent a postoperative hematoma. Traditionally suture ligation, metal clip placement, bipolar cautery, and electrocautery accomplished these goals, but they can be time consuming. Over the last 15 years, new hemostatic devices have been developed that compliment traditional techniques. The most widely used devices are harmonic scalpel (HS) and LigaSure (LS). HS uses high frequency ultrasound energy to coagulate and cut tissue and vessels simultaneously. LS is a modified computer controlled bipolar dissecting and sealing device.

Lombardi et al. [35] conducted a randomized controlled trial of 200 patients comparing HS to conventional techniques. The mean operative time was significantly shorter by 22 min (30 %) in the HS group ($p<0.001$). There were no differences in RLN injury, hypoparathyroidism, or postoperative hematoma between the groups. Material costs were higher in the HS group, but this was balanced by higher operating room costs in the conventional treatment group, leading to similar overall hospital costs. Other studies have reported similar reduction in operative times, but conflicting results for other postoperative outcomes, including hypoparathyroidism and RLN injury [36, 37]. A meta-analysis comparing HS to conventional techniques by Melck et al. [38] included 9 randomized controlled trials that enrolled 822 patients. The mean operative time was significantly shorter by 23 min in the HS group ($p<0.001$). Transient hypoparathyroidism was significantly less frequent in the HS group (14.5 %) compared to the conventional group (21.5 %), $p=0.01$. The frequency of transient and permanent RLN injury, permanent hypoparathyroidism, and postoperative hematoma were similar for HS and conventional treatments.

Saint Marc et al. [39] conducted a randomized controlled trial of 200 patients comparing LS to conventional techniques. The mean operative time was significantly shorter by 7 min (14 %) in the LS group ($p<0.001$). There were no differences in RLN injury, hypoparathyroidism, or postoperative hematoma between the groups. A meta-analysis comparing LS to conventional techniques by Yao et al. [40] included four randomized and five nonrandomized trials enrolling 927 patients and revealed similar results. The mean operative time for the LS group was significantly shorter for total thyroidectomy by 20 min ($p<0.05$). The frequency of transient or permanent hypoparathyroidism, transient or permanent RLN injury, postoperative hematoma, and intraoperative blood loss were similar for LS and conventional thyroidectomy. A network meta-analysis comparing HS, LS, and conventional hemostatic techniques by Contin et al. [41] included 35 randomized controlled trials with 4, 061 patients. The majority of studies included in the meta-analysis (60 %) were performed by experienced surgeons; 6 % of studies were stratified by surgical experience, but the remaining studies (34 %) did not specify surgical experience. A matched pairwise meta-analysis was performed for the primary outcome with a subgroup analysis performed by surgical experience, type of surgery (thyroidectomy vs. thyroid lobectomy), and study sponsor (investigator vs. industry). The HS and LS were associated with significantly reduced operative time compared to conventional techniques, by 22.3 and 13.8 min, respectively ($p<0.001$). On subgroup analysis, HS and LS were associated with shorter operative times in all groups. In a direct comparison, operations with HS compared to LS were reduced by 8.4 min ($p=0.032$.). Subgroup analysis revealed LS was slower than HS by 7 min for thyroidectomy. Subgroup analysis could not be performed for surgical experience, as experienced surgeons performed five of the six studies. HS was associated with a slightly lower frequency of transient hypoparathyroidism compared to conventional techniques ($p=0.025$). There were no differences between HS, LS, or conventional techniques in the rate of RLN injury, permanent hypoparathyroidism, or postoperative hematoma. The authors note that LS and HS devices have evolved over time, and the differences in operative time between the groups may change. Cost was not evaluated in this meta-analysis, but has been evaluated in some small individual studies. One study compared the cost of HS to conventional techniques for thyroidectomy and found that HS dissection required 20 % less time resulting in 15 % lower total hospital fees than with conventional techniques [42]. Another study comparing LS to conventional techniques revealed that thyroidectomy with LS on average cost 10 % less than conventional thyroidectomy [43].

## 21.5 Hemostatic Agents

There is little data in the literature on the use of hemostatic agents in thyroid surgery. Some of the agents that are available include oxidized cellulose, fibrin, and thrombin. They are easy to apply, readily available, and have few side effects, but they are not a replacement for meticulous hemostasis. Amit et al. [44] performed a randomized controlled trial of 190 patients comparing Surgicel (oxidized cellulose) vs. thyroidectomy without the use of any hemostatic agents. Four patients in the Surgicel group developed postoperative hematoma and required surgical exploration for bleeding. No patients in the control group developed hematoma, but the difference was not significant. Drain volume (133 ml vs. 93 ml), time to drain removal (1.4 vs. 1.9 days), and length of hospital stay (1.8 vs. 2.7 days) were longer in the Surgicel group ($p<0.001$). Multivariate analysis was not performed to evaluate for other possible explanations for the differences in length of hospital stay between the groups. They could have included patient demographic, clinical, and pathologic characteristics, as well as surgeon-related factors. A randomized controlled trial of 150 patients by Testini et al. [45] compared Floseal (collagen/thrombin agent), Fibrillar (surgicel collagen patch), and conventional surgery. The mean operating time was shortest in the Floseal group (105 min) compared to fibrillar (122 min) and conventional surgery without utilization of hemostatic agents (133 min), $p=0.006$. Time to drain removal was shorter in the Floseal group, and this was associated with shorter hospital stay. There was no difference between the groups in the rates of postoperative complications. The frequency of postoperative bleeding and hematoma are infrequent in experienced hands. There is a scarcity of studies evaluating hemostatic agents, and the studies have been small, leaving them underpowered to identify a difference between the study groups. Accordingly, more data need to be obtained to evaluate if any hemostatic agents are beneficial for optimizing patient outcomes following thyroid surgery.

## Conclusion

New technology is available in the operating room that can be incorporated by surgeons to perform thyroidectomy and potentially reduce operative time and minimize postoperative complications. The current literature regarding RLN IONM does not yet demonstrate that routine monitoring is superior to the "gold standard" nerve visualization. The frequency of RLN injury in expert hands is very low, and studies have been unable to demonstrate a significant difference in long-term patient outcomes. There have been inconsistencies in methodology, patient selection, and surgeon experience across studies, which may confound comparison of results. Inconsistency in interpretation of the published data is reflected in differences in recommendations across published practice guidelines. Guidelines have generally suggested that RLN IONM may be considered, but they stop short of asserting that it is necessary or standard of care. Certainly, IONM should not be used as a "crutch" for inexperienced surgeons to tackle challenging thyroid operations, and it should not be used as a criterion for determining which surgeons are most able to perform thyroidectomy. More data, particularly in the arena of cost-effectiveness, are necessary.

While the authors do not believe that IONM or hemostatic devices and agents must be used during thyroidectomy, we do routinely use them at our institution. In our complex endocrine surgery practice of three high-volume surgeons, we feel that IONM can speed RLN identification and thereby expedite dissection; it is most helpful for difficult and remedial cases, and also can assist postoperatively when communicating with patients about prognosis of RLN function. If signal is lost during lobectomy, it can prevent bilateral RLN injury. We feel that if IONM is used, it should be used regularly, since it is critical to be able to troubleshoot loss of signal during a case. Hemostatic devices allow us to be more efficient in the operating room, and they are especially useful in our training environment, particularly when the first assistant is relatively junior and less able to operate efficiently.

While new technologies are helpful, they do not replace meticulous technique and attention to detail. In addition, experience of the surgeon as measured by the volume of cases performed is clearly associated with enhanced patient outcomes [17, 46]. New technologies might enhance, but certainly cannot replace, the eyes and skills of a high-volume thyroid surgeon.

## References


1. Dackiw AP, Rotstein LE, Clark OH (2002) Computer-assisted evoked electromyography with stimulating surgical instruments for recurrent/external laryngeal nerve identification and preservation in thyroid and parathyroid operation. Surgery 132(6):1100–1106; discussion 7–8. Epub 2002/12/20
2. Sulica L (2004) The superior laryngeal nerve: function and dysfunction. Otolaryngol Clin North Am 37(1):183–201, Epub 2004/04/06
3. Barczynski M, Randolph GW, Cernea CR, Dralle H, Dionigi G, Alesina PF et al (2013) External branch of the superior laryngeal nerve monitoring during thyroid and parathyroid surgery: International Neural Monitoring Study Group standards guideline statement. Laryngoscope 123(Suppl 4):S1–S14, Epub 2013/07/09

4. Jansson S, Tisell LE, Hagne I, Sanner E, Stenborg R, Svensson P (1988) Partial superior laryngeal nerve (SLN) lesions before and after thyroid surgery. World J Surg 12(4):522–527, Epub 1988/08/01
5. Cernea CR, Ferraz AR, Nishio S, Dutra A Jr, Hojaij FC, dos Santos LR (1992) Surgical anatomy of the external branch of the superior laryngeal nerve. Head Neck 14(5):380–383, Epub 1992/09/11
6. Lennquist S, Cahlin C, Smeds S (1987) The superior laryngeal nerve in thyroid surgery. Surgery 102(6):999–1008, Epub 1987/12/01
7. Cernea CR, Ferraz AR, Furlani J, Monteiro S, Nishio S, Hojaij FC et al (1992) Identification of the external branch of the superior laryngeal nerve during thyroidectomy. Am J Surg 164(6):634–639, Epub 1992/12/01
8. Lifante JC, McGill J, Murry T, Aviv JE, Inabnet WB 3rd (2009) A prospective, randomized trial of nerve monitoring of the external branch of the superior laryngeal nerve during thyroidectomy under local/regional anesthesia and IV sedation. Surgery 146(6):1167–1173, Epub 2009/12/05
9. Barczynski M, Konturek A, Stopa M, Honowska A, Nowak W (2012) Randomized controlled trial of visualization versus neuromonitoring of the external branch of the superior laryngeal nerve during thyroidectomy. World J Surg 36(6):1340–1347, Epub 2012/03/10
10. Rosen CA, Lee AS, Osborne J, Zullo T, Murry T (2004) Development and validation of the voice handicap index-10. Laryngoscope 114(9):1549–1556, Epub 2004/10/12
11. Belafsky PC, Postma GN, Koufman JA (2002) Validity and reliability of the reflux symptom index (RSI). J Voice 16(2):274–277, Epub 2002/08/02
12. Chandrasekhar SS, Randolph GW, Seidman MD, Rosenfeld RM, Angelos P, Barkmeier-Kraemer J et al (2013) Clinical practice guideline: improving voice outcomes after thyroid surgery. Otolaryngol Head Neck Surg 148(6 Suppl):S1–S37, Epub 2013/06/14
13. Eisele DW (1996) Intraoperative electrophysiologic monitoring of the recurrent laryngeal nerve. Laryngoscope 106(4):443–449, Epub 1996/04/01
14. Sturgeon C, Sturgeon T, Angelos P (2009) Neuromonitoring in thyroid surgery: attitudes, usage patterns, and predictors of use among endocrine surgeons. World J Surg 33(3):417–425, Epub 2008/09/02
15. Singer MC, Rosenfeld RM, Sundaram K (2012) Laryngeal nerve monitoring: current utilization among head and neck surgeons. Otolaryngol Head Neck Surg 146(6):895–899, Epub 2012/03/09
16. Dralle H, Sekulla C, Lorenz K, Nguyen Thanh P, Schneider R, Machens A (2012) Loss of the nerve monitoring signal during bilateral thyroid surgery. Br J Surg 99(8):1089–1095, Epub 2012/06/15
17. Dralle H, Sekulla C, Haerting J, Timmermann W, Neumann HJ, Kruse E et al (2004) Risk factors of paralysis and functional outcome after recurrent laryngeal nerve monitoring in thyroid surgery. Surgery 136(6):1310–1322, Epub 2005/01/20
18. Higgins TS, Gupta R, Ketcham AS, Sataloff RT, Wadsworth JT, Sinacori JT (2011) Recurrent laryngeal nerve monitoring versus identification alone on post-thyroidectomy true vocal fold palsy: a meta-analysis. Laryngoscope 121(5):1009–1017, Epub 2011/04/27
19. Dionigi G, Boni L, Rovera F, Bacuzzi A, Dionigi R (2009) Neuromonitoring and video-assisted thyroidectomy: a prospective, randomized case–control evaluation. Surg Endosc 23(5):996–1003, Epub 2008/09/23
20. Barczynski M, Konturek A, Cichon S (2009) Randomized clinical trial of visualization versus neuromonitoring of recurrent laryngeal nerves during thyroidectomy. Br J Surg 96(3):240–246, Epub 2009/01/30
21. Randolph GW, Dralle H, Abdullah H, Barczynski M, Bellantone R, Brauckhoff M et al (2011) Electrophysiologic recurrent laryngeal nerve monitoring during thyroid and parathyroid surgery: international standards guideline statement. Laryngoscope 121(Suppl 1):S1–S16, Epub 2010/12/25

22. Snyder SK, Sigmond BR, Lairmore TC, Govednik-Horny CM, Janicek AK, Jupiter DC (2013) The long-term impact of routine intraoperative nerve monitoring during thyroid and parathyroid surgery. Surgery 154(4):704–711; discussion 11–13. Epub 2013/09/07
23. Sari S, Erbil Y, Sumer A, Agcaoglu O, Bayraktar A, Issever H et al (2010) Evaluation of recurrent laryngeal nerve monitoring in thyroid surgery. Int J Surg 8(6):474–478, Epub 2010/07/06
24. Snyder SK, Lairmore TC, Hendricks JC, Roberts JW (2008) Elucidating mechanisms of recurrent laryngeal nerve injury during thyroidectomy and parathyroidectomy. J Am Coll Surg 206(1):123–130, Epub 2007/12/25
25. Lo CY, Kwok KF, Yuen PW (2000) A prospective evaluation of recurrent laryngeal nerve paralysis during thyroidectomy. Arch Surg 135(2):204–207, Epub 2000/02/11
26. Patow CA, Norton JA, Brennan MF (1986) Vocal cord paralysis and reoperative parathyroidectomy. A prospective study. Ann Surg 203(3):282–285, Epub 1986/03/01
27. Bergenfelz A, Jansson S, Kristoffersson A, Martensson H, Reihner E, Wallin G et al (2008) Complications to thyroid surgery: results as reported in a database from a multicenter audit comprising 3,660 patients. Langenbecks Arch Surg 393(5):667–673, Epub 2008/07/18
28. Dralle H, Sekulla C, Lorenz K, Brauckhoff M, Machens A (2008) Intraoperative monitoring of the recurrent laryngeal nerve in thyroid surgery. World J Surg 32(7):1358–1366, Epub 2008/02/29
29. Goretzki PE, Schwarz K, Brinkmann J, Wirowski D, Lammers BJ (2010) The impact of intraoperative neuromonitoring (IONM) on surgical strategy in bilateral thyroid diseases: is it worth the effort? World J Surg 34(6):1274–1284, Epub 2010/02/10
30. Ulmer C, Friedrich C, Kohler A, Rieber F, Basar T, Deuschle M et al (2011) Impact of continuous intraoperative neuromonitoring on autonomic nervous system during thyroid surgery. Head Neck 33(7):976–984, Epub 2011/06/16
31. Lamade W, Ulmer C, Seimer A, Molnar V, Meyding-Lamade U, Thon KP et al (2007) A new system for continuous recurrent laryngeal nerve monitoring. Minim Invasive Ther Allied Technol 16(3):149–154, Epub 2007/06/19
32. Schneider R, Randolph GW, Sekulla C, Phelan E, Thanh PN, Bucher M et al (2013) Continuous intraoperative vagus nerve stimulation for identification of imminent recurrent laryngeal nerve injury. Head Neck 35(11):1591–1598, Epub 2012/11/22
33. Phelan E, Schneider R, Lorenz K, Dralle H, Kamani D, Potenza A et al (2014) Continuous vagal IONM prevents recurrent laryngeal nerve paralysis by revealing initial EMG changes of impending neuropraxic injury: a prospective, multicenter study. Laryngoscope 124(6):1498–1505, Epub 2013/12/07
34. Musholt TJ, Clerici T, Dralle H, Frilling A, Goretzki PE, Hermann MM et al (2011) German Association of Endocrine Surgeons practice guidelines for the surgical treatment of benign thyroid disease. Langenbecks Arch Surg 396(5):639–649, Epub 2011/03/23
35. Lombardi CP, Raffaelli M, Cicchetti A, Marchetti M, De Crea C, Di Bidino R et al (2008) The use of "harmonic scalpel" versus "knot tying" for conventional "open" thyroidectomy: results of a prospective randomized study. Langenbecks Arch Surg 393(5):627–631, Epub 2008/07/16
36. Miccoli P, Berti P, Dionigi G, D'Agostino J, Orlandini C, Donatini G (2006) Randomized controlled trial of harmonic scalpel use during thyroidectomy. Arch Otolaryngol Head Neck Surg 132(10):1069–1073, Epub 2006/10/18
37. Defechereux T, Rinken F, Maweja S, Hamoir E, Meurisse M (2003) Evaluation of the ultrasonic dissector in thyroid surgery. A prospective randomised study. Acta Chir Belg 103(3):274–277, Epub 2003/08/14
38. Melck AL, Wiseman SM (2010) Harmonic scalpel compared to conventional hemostasis in thyroid surgery: a meta-analysis of randomized clinical trials. Int J Surg Oncol 2010:396079, Epub 2010/01/01
39. Saint Marc O, Cogliandolo A, Piquard A, Fama F, Pidoto RR (2007) LigaSure vs clamp-and-tie technique to achieve hemostasis in total thyroidectomy for benign multinodular goiter: a prospective randomized study. Arch Surg 142(2):150–156; discussion 7. Epub 2007/02/21

40. Yao HS, Wang Q, Wang WJ, Ruan CP (2009) Prospective clinical trials of thyroidectomy with LigaSure vs conventional vessel ligation: a systematic review and meta-analysis. Arch Surg 144(12):1167–1174, Epub 2009/12/23
41. Contin P, Goossen K, Grummich K, Jensen K, Schmitz-Winnenthal H, Buchler MW et al (2013) ENERgized vessel sealing systems versus CONventional hemostasis techniques in thyroid surgery – the ENERCON systematic review and network meta-analysis. Langenbecks Arch Surg 398(8):1039–1056, Epub 2013/11/19
42. Ortega J, Sala C, Flor B, Lledo S (2004) Efficacy and cost-effectiveness of the UltraCision harmonic scalpel in thyroid surgery: an analysis of 200 cases in a randomized trial. J Laparoendosc Adv Surg Tech A 14(1):9–12, Epub 2004/03/24
43. O'Neill CJ, Chang LY, Suliburk JW, Sidhu SB, Delbridge LW, Sywak MS (2011) Sutureless thyroidectomy: surgical technique. ANZ J Surg 81(7–8):515–518
44. Amit M, Binenbaum Y, Cohen JT, Gil Z (2013) Effectiveness of an oxidized cellulose patch hemostatic agent in thyroid surgery: a prospective, randomized, controlled study. J Am Coll Surg 217(2):221–225, Epub 2013/07/23
45. Testini M, Marzaioli R, Lissidini G, Lippolis A, Logoluso F, Gurrado A et al (2009) The effectiveness of FloSeal matrix hemostatic agent in thyroid surgery: a prospective, randomized, control study. Langenbecks Arch Surg 394(5):837–842, Epub 2009/05/08
46. Sosa JA, Bowman HM, Tielsch JM, Powe NR, Gordon TA, Udelsman R (1998) The importance of surgeon experience for clinical and economic outcomes from thyroidectomy. Ann Surg 228(3):320–330, Epub 1998/09/22

# Part V

# Key-Points

# How to Avoid and Manage Post-operative Complications

22

David Scott-Coombes

## 22.1 Recurrent Laryngeal Nerve/Voice Injury

### 22.1.1 Pre-operative Considerations

The patient should be aware about the risk to the voice and the consequences of such an injury, temporary and/or permanent. It is important that surgeons know their own results in order to be able to offer accurate consent. The risk is particularly increased in re-operative surgery. Thyroid surgery for extended procedures and malignancy also carry a higher risk. It is important to know that the vocal cords are functioning prior to surgery by means of laryngoscopy.

### 22.1.2 Operation

The strategies to identify and preserve the nerves together with intra-operative adjuncts are described in earlier chapters.

### 22.1.3 Post-operative Management

All patients should undergo a post-operative vocal cord inspection. It will allow the surgeon to accurately know his/her results. There are a number of reasons why the voice might be hoarse after surgery and laryngoscopy will give the surgeon greater confidence in managing hoarseness. The timing of the laryngoscopy is debatable – the earlier one looks, the more temporary palsies will be identified. Treatment is

D. Scott-Coombes
Department of Endocrine Surgery, University Hospital of Wales, Cardiff, UK
e-mail: david.scott-coombes@wales.nhs.uk



C.P. Lombardi, R. Bellantone (eds.), *Minimally Invasive Therapies for Endocrine Neck Diseases*, DOI 10.1007/978-3-319-20065-1_22

divided into management of aspiration and improvement of the voice and patients should be managed by an expert in this field in a multidisciplinary setting that involves input from speech and language therapists.

## 22.2 Haemorrhage/Haematoma

Post-operative haemorrhage occurs in about 1 % of all neck operations and can be life-threatening. The resulting haematoma compresses local (small) veins in the neck that leads to oedema. The oedema most favourably collects in the submucosa of the vocal folds (owing to the potential space), which in turn causes the glottis to close, and results in an obstructed airway.

### 22.2.1 Pre-operative Considerations

Anti-platelet medication (aspirin; Clopidogrel) should be stopped at least 7 days prior to the date of surgery. Warfarin should be stopped and alternative modes of anticoagulation should be adopted according to local protocols. Patients with hypervascular goitre, such as Graves' disease are theoretically at greater risk, but the surgeon must be vigilant to minimize haemorrhage during every neck operation.

### 22.2.2 Operation

The surgeon should be obsessive about preventing haemorrhage – dissecting in precise tissue planes and methodically ligating vessels. Whilst there are a number of technological aids to haemostasis, there is no evidence that they reduce the risk of post-operative bleeding. At the end of surgery, efforts should be made to identify any potential venous haemorrhage. This can either be achieved by asking the anaesthetist to simulate a valsalva manoeuvre or to place the patient in the head-down (Trendelenburg) position. Both of these techniques increase venous pressure and seek to reveal previously unidentified sources of haemorrhage [1]. There is no evidence that insertion of a drain either prevents the development of a haematoma or reliably alerts staff to post-operative haemorrhage.

When closing the strap muscles, many surgeons leave a space at the inferior (caudal) end to allow egress of any bleeding into the superficial space and to facilitate insertion of a finger into the wound to unfasten the strap muscle suture in an emergency (see below).

### 22.2.3 Post-operative Management

The anaesthetist is an important ally. Every attempt should be made to avoid a rise in central venous pressure in the early post-operative period – minimizing coughing, vomiting and crying out in pain. Most bleeds occur within the first 2 h of

**Table 22.1** Management of post-operative haemorrhage

| |
|---|
| 1. High flow oxygen |
| 2. Call for doctor skilled in airway management |
| 3. Either |
| (a) Intubate |
| (b) Evacuate haematoma |
| (i) Attempt aspiration with large bore needle/syringe |
| (ii) Remove skin and strap sutures and manually evacuate haematoma |
| 4. Once airway stabilized – return to theatre to explore neck |

surgery, but there are reports of significant haemorrhage up to and beyond 24 h post surgery [2]. For this reason many surgeons are unwilling to deliver a day-case thyroidectomy service [3]. If day surgery is considered, patient selection is very important – taking into account the proximity of the patient's home to the hospital and the presence of a carer who is able to return the patient.

Every unit should have a protocol for managing this event and there should be regular instruction courses for all members of staff (medical and nursing) (Table 22.1). Signs of a significant bleed include neck swelling, increased respiratory rate and effort followed by stridor and reduced oxygen saturation. The purpose of any intervention is to remedy the airway obstruction at the site of the haematoma. If the anaesthetist is on the unit, most effective strategy is to re-intubate and return the patient to theatre. In the absence of such skilled staff it is important to remember that the problem is the haematoma, which should be evacuated. One might try to aspirate the haematoma with a wide-bore cannula, but often the haematoma is clotted. The next step is to open the wound 'there and then' by removing the skin sutures and perhaps the sutures to the strap muscles. As soon as the haematoma has been evacuated there is an immediate improvement in the airway. At the same time the surgeon and anaesthetist should be called and the patient is then returned to theatre to deal with the bleeding. Great care must be given to avoiding injury to the recurrent laryngeal nerves and parathyroid glands [4]. Often the site of the bleeding cannot be identified. The wound is washed out and closed again – typically with a drain.

## 22.3 Hypoparathyroidism

This results from insufficient functioning parathyroid tissue at the end of surgery. In the era of targeted parathyroid surgery, it is rarely seen after parathyroidectomy for single gland disease. It is also very rare after a hemithyroidectomy suggesting that it occurs when three or more parathyroid glands are injured/excised.

### 22.3.1 Pre-operative Considerations

Making patients aware is very important because hypoparathyroidism is the commonest complication of bilateral thyroid surgery. It may be temporary or permanent. Rates of hypoparathyroidism vary hugely in the literature, partly due to a lack of standardization of definitions. Outcomes from national audits are probably a better reflection of the true incidence. In Scandinavia 16 % of patients take calcium 6 weeks after surgery. In the UK, nearly 30 % are taking calcium at discharge and rates are even higher for those with Graves' disease and those who underwent a central nodal dissection. At long-term follow-up between 4 % (Scandinavia) and 7 % (UK) are taking calcium/Vitamin D at long-term follow-up. These rates are much higher than reported series and may be over reporting as patients may be taking Vitamin D or calcium for other reasons. Nevertheless this presents a challenge to thyroid surgeons.

### 22.3.2 Operation

The best approach to post-operative hypoparathyroidism is prevention. Surgical technique is of utmost importance whereby the surgeon must make every effort to identify the parathyroid glands prior to dissection and ligation of the branches of the inferior thyroid artery (see Part III). In circumstances when the blood supply cannot be preserved, autotransplantation should be undertaken. This involves excising the parathyroid gland, mincing it into 1 mm cubes and either directly placing it in a pocket of muscle or making a suspension of parathyroid cells in normal saline and then inoculating the fluid directly into muscle.

### 22.3.3 Post-operative Management

Hypocalcaemia is the consequence of this complication and is associated with paraesthesiae of extremities (face, hands, toes) exacerbated by compression of the limbs (such as crossing one's legs, sitting on the toilet). In profound hypocalcaemia patients will suffer with tetany manifest as carpopedal spasm, altered mental state, chest pain, bronchospasm and heart failure. In extreme cases there can be seizures and cardiac arrhythmia. Physical signs of hypocalcaemia include Chvostek's and Trousseau's. Whilst the severity of the symptoms often mirrors the degree of hypocalcaemia, this is not always the case.

All Units should have a written protocol for the management of post-operative hypocalcaemia (Table 22.2). Essentially this involves prescribing doses of calcium and/or Vitamin D titrated against the severity of the hypocalcaemia and symptoms. Blood calcium tests should be regularly repeated until a stable state of normocalcaemia has been achieved. When intravenous calcium is delivered, it is essential that extravasation is avoided and cardiac monitoring is needed to identify arrhythmias.

## 22.4 Pain

Most endocrine neck surgery is tolerated very well by patients and pain is relieved by simple analgesics/anti-inflammatory drugs. Locoregional anaesthesia (See Chap. 12) provides an excellent adjunct to analgesia and helps to avoid the use of opiates

**Table 22.2** Management of post-operative hypocalcaemia

| Plasma calcium (corrected) mmol/l (NR: 2.20–2.60) | Symptomatic | Asymptomatic |
|---|---|---|
| >2.15 | Milk | Nil |
| 2.00–2.15 | Calcichew 1 g *tds* | Nil |
| 1.90–2.00 | Calcichew 1 g *tds*<br>1-alfacalcidol 1 μg *od* | Calcichew 1 g *tds* |
| 1.80–1.90 | Calcichew 1 g *tds*<br>1-alfacalcidol 1 μg *bd* | Calcichew 1 g *tds*<br>1-alfacalcidol 1 μg *bd* |
| <1.80 | Tetany – 10–30 ml i.v. calcium gluconate over 10–15 min<br>Repeat blood calcium measurement after 30 min | Calcichew 1 g *tds*<br>1-alfacalcidol 1 μg *tds* |

*od* once daily, *tds* three times per day, *NB* intravenous calcium should be administered in a well-sited large peripheral vein and extravasation should be avoided to prevent tissue necrosis

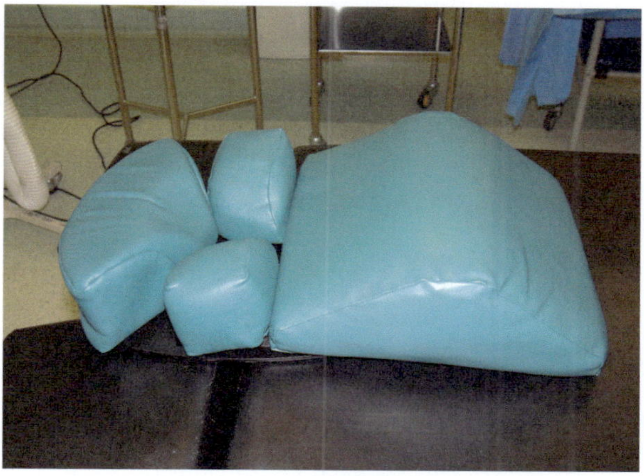

**Fig. 22.1** Padded shoulder/neck/head support for neck extension

(and their side effects). In addition to the surgical trauma, neck extension can cause headaches and arm pain/paraesthesiae. This can be minimized by using a specially designed support (Fig. 22.1).

## 22.5 Wound Complications

Wound infection – is a rare complication of (clean) neck surgery. There is no indication for prophylactic antibiotics. Patients present with the classical symptoms and signs of inflammation. Cellulitis is treated with antibiotics. If there is a deep infection, injury to the airway should be suspected and may be associated with surgical emphysema (see below). In such cases the wound should be explored, drained and the trachea inspected.

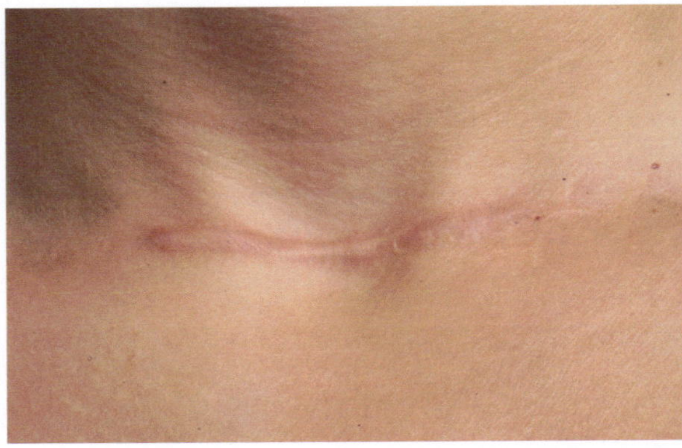

**Fig. 22.2** Hypertrophic scar positioned close to the sternal notch

Hypertrophy and keloid scar – are rare complications. Most neck wounds heal with excellent cosmetic outcome especially when the incision is sited in a skin crease at least two finger-breadths cephalic to the sternal notch. Incisions placed nearer to the sternal notch are at risk of hypertrophic healing [5] (Fig. 22.2). Care must be taken to avoid excessive stretching of the wound edges (especially in a short wound) and inadvertent thermal injury from electrocautery/haemostatic devices. Care must be taken when closing the skin to ensure that the edges are accurately opposed. Despite these precautions some patients may still develop hypertrophy of the wound. This is best managed with the cooperation of dermatologists.

## 22.6 Rare Complications

**Hypothyroidism** This is an inevitable consequence of a total thyroidectomy. However, it may occur in up to one-third of patients following hemithyroidectomy and should be discussed with the patient prior to surgery. The risk factors for requiring thyroxine are an elevated pre-operative TSH, increasing age and the presence of a background thyroiditis [6, 7]. In the absence of any risk factors the rate of hypothyroidism is approximately 3 %. For the management of hypothyroidism – see Chap.24.

**Horner's Syndrome** This arises as a result of dividing the sympathetic trunk, which is most at risk during nodal dissection. This injury results in partial ptosis; miosis and anhidrosis. Occasionally there may be ipsilateral facial flushing due to capillary vasodilatation. When suspected, patients should be referred to an ophthalmologist. The diagnosis is confirmed with the application of alpha-agonist apraclonidine to both eyes and an increased mydriatic effect is observed on the affected side (Fig. 22.3a, b). Corrective surgery may be indicated if the ptosis is severe.

**Tracheal Injury** This is a rare complication in thyroid surgery. When identified at the time of surgery a primary repair is done with absorbable sutures. In such circumstances a drain may be placed and antibiotics prescribed. Occasionally a patient may present a few days after surgery. The patient presents with neck swelling and

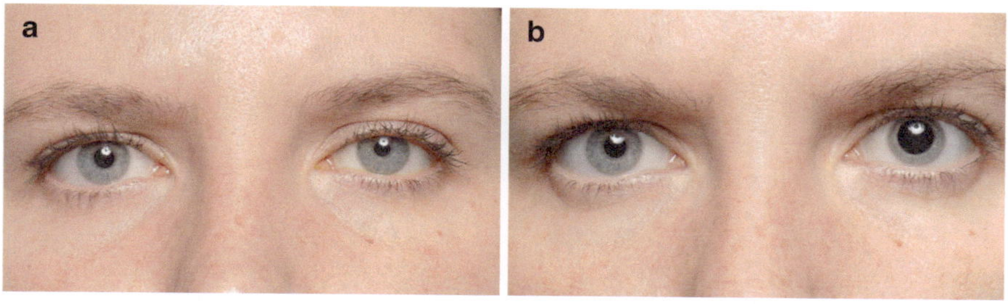

**Fig. 22.3** Horner's syndrome. (**a**) Ptosis and miosis on the left. (**b**) Reactive mydriasis on the left after application of alpha agonist

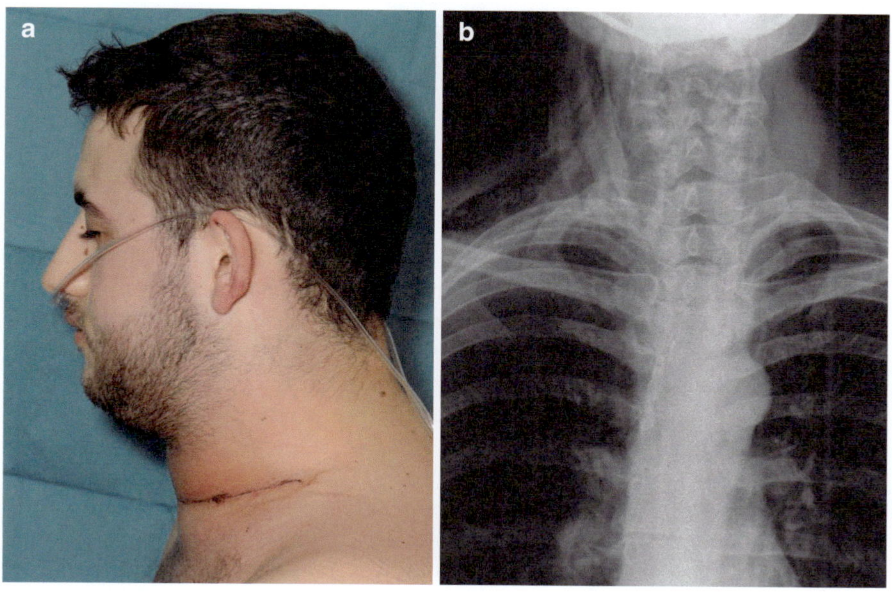

**Fig. 22.4** (**a**) Swollen neck in a man with tracheal injury following thyroidectomy. (**b**) Surgical emphysema on plain X-ray

on examination there is surgical emphysema. This can be confirmed with a plain X-ray (Fig. 22.4a, b). This can be occult or present a few days after primary closure of an inadvertent injury closed the clot on the inside of the trachea lifts off and initiates a fit of coughing which forces air out through a tiny breach in the trachea. This is managed by admission for observation, reassurance and antibiotics. This usually spontaneously resolves. In severe cases the wound may need to be re-explored, lavaged and drained. ENT assistance should be sought.

**Chylothorax** This develops following injury to the thoracic duct, usually sited on the left side of the neck. This complication is most likely to occur during nodal dissection. Patients display symptoms of respiratory distress and a chest X-ray will

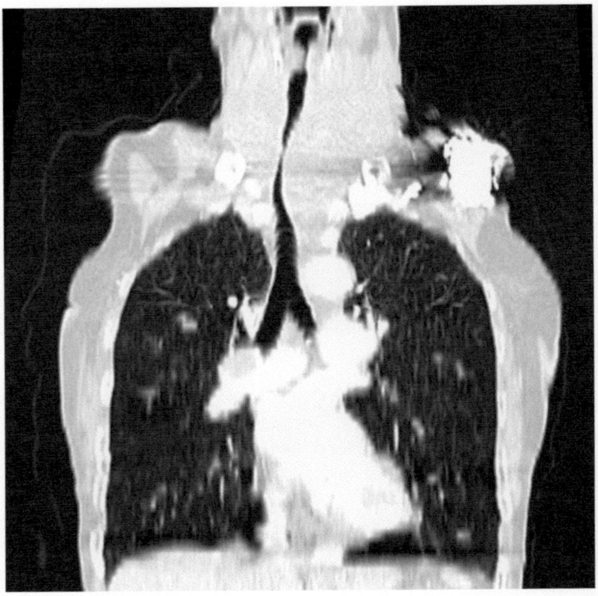

**Fig. 22.5** Coronal CT demonstrating pronounced tracheal compression

reveal evidence of a pleural effusion. In circumstances when a drain was placed – it will reveal a milky discharge. Most patients can be managed conservatively. This involves drainage (if a drain has not been placed) and strategies to minimize the flow of chyle. Non-operative strategies include TPN; octreotide therapy or a short-chain fatty acid (very low fat) diet [8]. Surgery is contemplated on the rare occasions when conservative treatment fails.

**Tracheomalacia** This is the phenomenon of a weakness in the cartilaginous tracheal wall resulting in collapse of the lumen with consequent loss of airway. It is very rarely seen in the western world and is more commonly reported in areas such as Asia [9, 10] (most post-thyroidectomy airway problems are due to recurrent laryngeal nerve injury). Tracheomalacia is associated with long-standing massive goitre often associated with retro sternal extension and tracheal compression (Fig. 22.5). It can be predicted intra-operatively as the trachea is soft and collapsible on palpation. When anticipated, the patient is kept intubated overnight and the endotracheal tube cuff is deflated the next morning. If there is a good air leak the patient can then be extubated. A tracheostomy is performed whenever there is doubt about the integrity of the airway.

**Thyroid Storm** This is a rare and life-threatening complication of thyroid surgery in patients with thyrotoxicosis. Patients develop a constellation of symptoms and signs secondary to the high circulating levels of free T3 and T4. Prevention is the best philosophy and is achieved from ensuring that patients are biochemically euthyroid prior to surgery. Antithyroid drugs are the mainstay of treatment and an endocrinologist should be involved. When side effects or patient compliance are an issue – patients are treated with iodine prior to surgery, with or without beta-blockers.

Despite these efforts, thyrotoxic storm may arise and is then an emergency with mortality as high as 10–50 % [11] that should be managed in critical care. It is important to consider the diagnosis as it may be confused with sepsis. The mainstay of treatment is propylthiouracil, beta-blockade and intravenous corticosteroids.

## 22.7 Complaints and Litigation

Prevention is better than the cure! Prior to surgery there are many opportunities to identify problems before they arise. It is important to manage patients' expectations and make them fully aware of the possible complications and their consequences.

Does the patient use their voice professionally? If so – for what reason and to what level? This information may well influence a decision about surgery.
Is it clear why the thyroid/parathyroid surgery is being offered? Are both doctor and patient confident that an operation will improve symptoms?
Have you told the patient about the risks to the parathyroid glands and the likelihood of needing calcium supplements temporarily or permanently?
Have you discussed the possibility of needing levothyroxine after a hemithyroidectomy?
Does the patient understand the lack of precision of imaging and biopsy in the pre-operative diagnosis of thyroid cancer?
Does the patient understand that not all patients with primary hyperparathyroidism are cured at the first attempt – and why?
If tracheostomy is a possibility – is the patient aware?

Thorough counselling pre-operatively is likely to reduce complaints post-operatively.

## References

1. Moumoulidis I, Del Pero MM, Brennan L, Jani P (2010) Haemostasis in head and neck surgical procedures: Valsalva manoeuvre versus Trendelenberg tilt. Ann R Coll Surg Engl 92:292–294
2. Leyre P, Desurmont T, Lacoste L, Odasso C, Bouche G, Beaulieu A, Valagier A, Charalambous C, Gibelin H, Debaene B, Kraimps JL (2008) Does the risk of compressive hematoma after thyroidectomy authorize 1-day surgery? Langenbecks Arch Surg 393:733–737
3. Doran HE, Palazzo FF (2012) Questionable safety of thyroid surgery with same day discharge. Ann R Coll Surg Engl 94:543–547
4. Harding J, Sebag F, Sierra M, Palazzo FF, Henry JF (2006) Thyroid surgery: postoperative hematoma–prevention and treatment. Langenbecks Arch Surg 391:169–173
5. Kim JH, Sung JY, Kim YH, Lee YS, Chang HS, Park CS, Roh MR (2012) Risk factors for hypertrophic surgical scar development after thyroidectomy. Wound Repair Regen 20: 304–310
6. Tomoda C, Ito Y, Kobayashi K, Miya A, Miyauchi A (2011) Subclinical hypothyroidism following hemithyroidectomy: a simple risk-scoring system using age and preoperative thyrotropin level. ORL J Otorhinolaryngol Relat Spec 73:68–71

7. Said M, Chiu V, Haigh PI (2013) Hypothyroidism after hemithyroidectomy. World J Surg 37:2839–2844
8. McCray S, Parrish CR (2004) When chyle leaks: nutrition intervention. Pract Gastroenterol 28:60
9. Findlay JM, Sadler GP, Bridge H, Mihai R (2011) Postthyroidectomy tracheomalacia: minimal risk despite significant tracheal compression. Br J Anaesth 5:16
10. Agarwal A, Mishra AK, Gupta SK, Arshad F, Tripathi M, Singh PK (2007) High incidence of tracheomalacia in longstanding goiters: experience from an endemic goitre region. World J Surg 31:832–837
11. Akamizu T, Satoh T, Isozaki A, Wakino S, Iburi T et al (2012) Diagnostic criteria, clinical features, and incidence of thyroid storm based on nationwide surveys. Thyroid 22:661–679

# Perioperative Medical Treatment

# 23

Salvatore M. Corsello, Vincenzo Di Donna,
and Rosa Maria Paragliola

## 23.1 Preoperative Medical Management

Before proceeding to surgery an accurate evaluation of the patient's anesthesiological risk is necessary and any major medical conditions and risk factors should be addressed.

Within few days or weeks before a thyroidectomy, at least a dosage of thyroid stimulating hormone (TSH) and serum calcium should be performed in order to exclude the presence of thyrotoxicosis and identify patients who may have parathyroid disease in conjunction with thyroid disease. Preoperative serum calcitonin should be obtained for patients with nodular pathology in order to exclude the presence of a medullary thyroid cancer. If this suspicion is confirmed, a screening of the type 2 multiple endocrine neoplasia (MEN) syndrome is necessary, particularly of pheochromocytoma and primary hyperparathyroidism; the analysis for a RET proto-oncogene mutation and the possible genetic counseling can also be performed after surgery [1].

A high-quality diagnostic thyroid ultrasound should be performed in all patients in order to correctly program the surgical strategy [2], while further imaging exams such as computed tomography (CT) or magnetic nuclear resonance are not routinely needed. However, it is important to note that the high iodine load in CT contrast may delay the subsequent administration of postoperative radioactive iodine in patients with thyroid cancer.

If hyperthyroidism or thyrotoxicosis are present, particular attention is needed in order to prevent the possibility of the so-called thyroid storm, a rare potentially life-threatening condition which usually occurs during surgery or in the first 18 h after the procedure. It may be precipitated by the stress of surgery, anesthesia, or thyroid manipulation and may be prevented by pretreatment with anti-thyroid drugs and

S.M. Corsello (✉) • V. Di Donna • R.M. Paragliola
Unit of Endocrinology, Università Cattolica del Sacro Cuore, Rome, Italy
e-mail: md5368@mclink.it



C.P. Lombardi, R. Bellantone (eds.), *Minimally Invasive Therapies for Endocrine Neck Diseases*, DOI 10.1007/978-3-319-20065-1_23

achievement of a functional euthyroidism [3]. Both anti-thyroid drugs methimazole (MMI) or propylthiouracil and beta-adrenergic blockers can be used for such aim. After euthyroidism is reached, patients with Graves' hyperthyroidism may also be given inorganic iodine; Lugol's solution or a saturated solution of potassium iodide (SSKI) should be administered. Potassium iodide can be given as 5–7 drops (0.25–0.35 mL) Lugol's solution (8 mg iodide/drop) or 1–2 drops (0.05–0.1 mL) SSKI (50 mg iodide/drop) three times daily mixed in water or juice for 10 days before surgery (Bahn *Thyroid* 2011). This treatment induces an involution of the gland and decreases its vascularity and intraoperative blood loss during thyroidectomy. The iodide should be given only while the patient is under the effect of full doses of the antithyroid drug; otherwise, the iodide may permit an exacerbation of the thyrotoxicosis [4]. Preoperative iodine is less likely to benefit patients with toxic multinodular goiter or toxic adenoma, whose thyroid glands tend to be less hypervascular than in patients with Graves' disease. Corticosteroids have been used in conjunction with beta-blockers and iopanoic acid to prepare thyrotoxic patients for emergent surgery [5]. Patients who are intolerant or unable to take thionamides should be pretreated with beta-adrenergic blockers alone, whereas patients with Graves' hyperthyroidism can be treated with beta-blockers and iodine too. However, if the problem with anti-thyroid drugs is a minor rash or low-grade fever, the drug is continued or a change is made to a different thionamide. More severe reactions (severe fever or rash, leukopenia, jaundice, or serum sickness) necessitate a withdrawal of thionamide with a shift to another form of therapy. When thyroidectomy is indicated in amiodarone-induced thyrotoxicosis (AIT) the preoperative management may be difficult although mandatory. Type 1 AIT (occurring in patients with an underlying thyroid pathology such as autonomous nodular goiter or Graves' disease) is best treated with MMI to prevent new hormone synthesis usually adding potassium perchlorate (800–1000 mg/day). Type 2 AIT (a destructive thyroiditis that results in excess release of preformed $T_4$ and $T_3$ into the circulation) is better treated with anti-inflammatory therapy such as prednisone with improvement usually within a few weeks. Propranolol or atenolol are the usual drugs used for preparation of patients with AIT going to surgery. Antithyroid drugs should be stopped at the time of thyroidectomy, and beta-adrenergic blockers should be stopped gradually after surgery.

In patients affected by primary hyperparathyroidism before proceeding to parathyroidectomy, a careful evaluation to exclude MEN1 and MEN2A association should be performed. If necessary, patient should be treated preoperatively with medical therapy to control hypercalcemia (furosemide, bisphosphonate, corticosteroids, cinacalcet).

## 23.2 Medical Treatment of Postsurgical Hypothyroidism

Postsurgical hypothyroidism is a permanent condition requiring a long-life therapy, except for cases of relapsing goiter or hyperthyroidism in patients who underwent less than near-total thyroidectomy. The gold standard therapy is L-thyroxine ($LT_4$)

monotherapy per os, as for all other causes of hypothyroidism [6]. In fact, since the peripheral conversion of $T_4$ to biologically active triiodothyronine ($T_3$) was documented in 1970, $T_4$ monotherapy has become the mainstay of treating hypothyroidism, replacing desiccated thyroid and other forms of $T_4$ and $T_3$ combination therapy (Fig. 23.1).

A number of studies, following observations about the benefit of $T_4$ and $T_3$ combination therapy, have largely failed to confirm an advantage of this approach to improve cognitive or mood outcomes in hypothyroid individuals treated with $T_4$ alone [7]. Furthermore, there is no evidence to support using desiccated thyroid hormone in preference to $LT_4$ monotherapy and therefore it should not be used for the treatment of hypothyroidism [8]. Finally, patients taking dietary supplements and nutraceuticals for hypothyroidism should be advised that commercially available thyroid-enhancing products are not a remedy for hypothyroidism and should be counseled about the potential side effects of various preparations, particularly those containing iodine or sympathomimetic amines as well as those marked as "thyroid support" since they could be adulterated with large amounts of thyroid hormones. However, it cannot be excluded that in the future the development of new more effective thyroid hormone analogues or new insights about the individual $T_4$ and $T_3$ requirement will modify the therapeutic strategy in some special populations such as patients with polymorphisms of type 2 deiodinase.

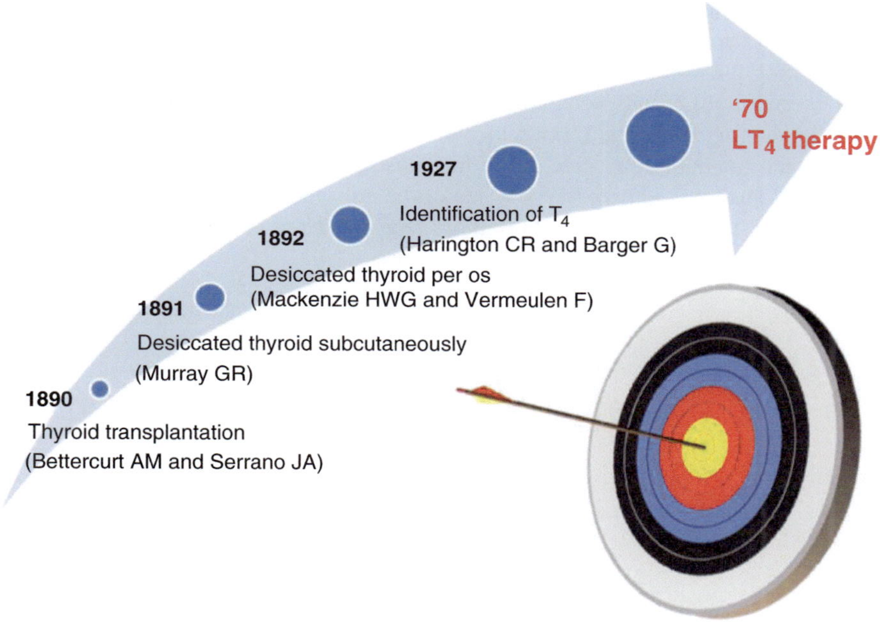


**Fig. 23.1** Historical evolution of treatment of hypothyroidism

Different formulations of $LT_4$ are currently available and their bioequivalence is still debated. In particular there are solid tablets, soft gel capsules, and oral solutions in drops or monodose vials. The soft gel capsules, recently available in a wide range of strengths, markedly increase the compliance for the patients. Furthermore, liquid oral formulations (drops, vials, and more handy soft gel capsules) offer advantages in patients with difficult swallowing, such as children and elderly patients, and conditions interfering with $LT_4$ absorption (Table 23.1) [9].

In fact oral absorption of drugs from solid tablets is dependent upon the release of the drug from the formulation, the dissolution of the drug, and the permeability of the drug across the gastrointestinal tract. In particular the dissolution is pH sensitive with a higher $T_4$ dose requirement in patients with higher gastric pH. Soft gel capsules containing $T_4$ dissolved in glycerin show the most consistent dissolution pattern and the less pH dependency. This is particularly useful in patients concurrently on $T_4$ and gastric pH altering drugs, such as proton pump inhibitors.

It is worthwhile to note that 6–8 weeks after the formulation or brand of $LT_4$ has been changed A check of thyroid function tests is appropriate, because there may be subtle differences in bioavailability of $T_4$ formulations.

The current approach to calculate the starting dose of $LT_4$ after total thyroidectomy is mainly based on the patient's body weight (BW). In patients who do not present with cardiac symptoms or malabsorption, the most common recommended starting dose of $LT_4$ ranges from 1.6 to 1.7 μg/kg/day [3, 6]. Since it is an acute hypothyroidism, a gradual titration of the dosage is not needed. However, the mean substitutive $LT_4$ dosage in adults can vary between 1 and 2.2 or more μg/kg per day depending on the type of intervention and possible individual malabsorption. These values are obviously physiologically greater during childhood.

Reaching the optimal $LT_4$ replacement dose in the shortest time after thyroidectomy is important but also challenging. Indeed, in the literature this time is highly variable, ranging from 2 to 120 weeks, with a median of 3.6 months, and only about 30 % reach the euthyroid state at the first postsurgery follow-up [10]. This is not surprising since it is known that BW is not the only factor which predicts the optimal dose of $LT_4$. In fact, several authors suggested the correlation between $LT_4$

**Table 23.1** Principal causes of altered absorption of $LT_4$

| | |
|---|---|
| Transient | Different bioequivalence of $LT_4$ |
| | Poor compliance |
| | Interfering drugs |
| | *Helicobacter pylori* |
| | Parasitosis |
| Permanent | Atrophic gastritis |
| | Celiac disease |
| | Lactose intolerance |
| | Inflammatory bowel diseases |
| | Gastroparesis |
| | Short bowel syndrome |
| | Gastrointestinal surgery |

requirement and other factors, such as body mass index (BMI) or body surface, gender and menopause, age, and disease causing hypothyroidism. The role of these variables could be explained by the differences in lean body mass (LBM) [11] considering that most metabolic processes, including $T_4$ and $T_3$ deiodination, occur within this body compartment. Moreover, several authors noted that LBM correlates with thyroid and liver size, another important site of $T_4$ conversion. Weaker evidence supports the independent role of gender, age, and BMI [12–14] that also seem to be more likely related to the differences in LBM. However, from a practical point of view, an accurate calculation of LBM requires the use of formulas or techniques that are not cost-effective in the clinical setting, such as, the dual energy X-ray absorptiometry (DEXA). Based on these findings, in the literature few alternative methods are described to calculate the $LT_4$ starting dose after thyroidectomy (Table 23.2) [15–17]. However, no formula has been shown to have a better predictive value than the classic method based only on the patient's body weight.

In a recent study (Di Donna et al.) we readdressed the major predicting factors for the $LT_4$ requirement in order to elaborate a new strategy which could increase the accuracy of the $LT_4$ starting dose after total thyroidectomy. To validate our strategy, we compared it with the different methods currently proposed in the literature. In the first part of the study, a retrospective review of 92 patients (retrospective cohort) who underwent total thyroidectomy for benign disease and started $LT_4$ therapy with a starting dose of about 1.6 μg/kg per day approximated to the nearest marketed formulation was performed; the results obtained by this retrospective analysis were used to formulate a nomogram for the calculation of the $LT_4$ dosage. In the second part of the study, this nomogram was prospectively applied in 31 consecutive patients after total thyroidectomy (prospective cohort). In particular, the patients in the prospective cohort began treatment with $LT_4$ with a recommended dose calculated by the nomogram and approximating to the nearest marketed formulation. The performance of this new strategy has been subsequently confirmed also in larger clinical records (Corsello S.M., personal data, 2015).

Exclusion criteria for both cohorts were: malignancy at histological examination, presence of symptoms or signs of malabsorption, assumption of drugs interfering with $LT_4$ absorption within 4 h following the ingestion of $LT_4$, suspected poor

**Table 23.2** Principal strategies proposed in the literature for the prediction of $LT_4$ requirement after total thyroidectomy for benign disease

| Author | Algorithm or formula | |
|---|---|---|
| Olubowale et al. [15] Chesterfield, UK | Weight (kg) | $LT_4$ dose (μg/day) |
| | <53 | 100 |
| | 54–86 | 125 |
| | 87–108 | 150 |
| | >108 | 175 |
| Mistry et al. [16] Hull, UK | $LT_4$ dose (μg/day) = (0.943 × Weight) + (−1.165 × Age) + 125.8<br>(simplified) $LT_4$ dose (μg/day) = Weight − Age + 125 | |
| Ojomo et al. [17] Madison, USA | $LT_4$ dose (μg/kg/day) = (− 0.018 × BMI + 2.13) × Weight | |

patient's compliance or eating or drinking anything, except water within 30 min following the assumption of $LT_4$, switch of formulation or brand of $LT_4$. Inclusion criteria for both cohort were: euthyroid state before thyroidectomy, start of $LT_4$ therapy within three days after thyroidectomy, use of the solid formulation and same brand of $LT_4$, check of serum TSH level at 6–8 weeks after thyroidectomy and subsequent checks until the achievement of the euthyroidism, showed by a serum TSH within the range of 0.4–2.5 µUI/mL.

At the first follow-up after 51 ± 16 (mean ± SD) days, only 37 patients in the retrospective cohort were euthyroid (40 %), while 55 required a dose adjustment, 31 because overdosed (34 %) and 24 because underdosed (26 %). Univariate analysis indicated that the strongest correlation with optimal $LT_4$ starting dose was with BW. The other correlations were with BMI, height, age, and preoperative $FT_3$. Based on these observations from the retrospective cohort, an analysis was performed to determine the optimal daily weight-related $LT_4$ dose (expressed as µg/kg/day) in different subgroups based on BMI and age. A univariate analysis revealed that the $LT_4$ dose requirement was inversely related to age and BMI. The comparison between the mean values of the optimal $LT_4$ dose in µg/kg/day in the different age and BMI subgroups revealed that this relationship was statistically significant for both age and BMI. Finally, the $LT_4$ dose in µg/kg was calculated in the 9 subgroups obtained by the combination of previous age and BMI groups. Optimal dose ranged from 1.8 µg/kg/day in patients with lower BMI and younger age to 1.4 µg/kg/day in patients with higher BMI and older age.

Based on these findings a user-friendly nomogram was developed (Fig. 23.2) and then used in the prospective cohort, in which it allowed at the first post-thyroidectomy follow-up (mean ± SD: 50 ± 19 days) to reach the euthyroidism in 21 (68 %) patients, while 6 (20 %) were underdosed and 4 (12 %) overdosed. Moreover, at the first post-thyroidectomy follow-up, overtreatment occurred in the group of elderly patients (age >65 years) in the retrospective cohort in 37 % and in the prospective cohort in no elderly patients.

| AGE \ BMI | <23 | 23–28 | >28 |
|---|---|---|---|
| <40 | 1.8 | 1.7 | 1.6 |
| 40–55 | 1.7 | 1.6 | 1.5 |
| >55 | 1.6 | 1.5 | 1.4 |

*$LT_4$*

**Fig. 23.2** Nomogram for the prediction of $LT_4$ pro kilogram starting dose after total thyroidectomy (Di Donna et al.). *BMI* kg/m², *age* years, *$LT_4$ dose* µg/kg/day

An analysis of how the different strategies proposed in the literature would have performed in the retrospective cohort showed that most effective of them would have predicted the correct $LT_4$ starting dose only in 38 of our patients (41 %), and would have been over-replacing in 40 (43.5 %) and under-replacing in 14 (15.5 %).

These data could be explained by the reduction in LBM observed with aging, in addition to the increased prevalence of obesity in elderly patients. Indeed the correlation with age remains significant also in the subgroups analysis by BMI. Perhaps this correlation could be also explained by a possible reduction of thyroxin metabolism in the older age. In regard to gender no statistical difference between women and men was found, while a correlation between height, but not body surface area, and the $LT_4$ optimal dose was reported. The interesting direct correlation between the optimal $LT_4$ dose and the presurgical level of $FT_3$ could be explained by the correlation between the level of the $T_3$ thyroidal production and the rate of conversion of $T_4$ to $T_3$ due to type 1 deiodinase. Also a different sensitivity of thyroid hormones receptor could be involved. More studies to investigate this matter are required.

Serum TSH (and possibly $FT_4$) should be tested in about 6 weeks after starting the replacement therapy. The TSH should be kept in a normal range for patients with benign disease, while a suppressive therapy should be considered in patients with thyroid cancer depending on prognostic risk. An annual TSH or less is sufficient long-term if patients are well clinically. Since its long half-life (about 1 week), $LT_4$ can be started within a week after surgery and it is essential to consider that the steady state of TSH and $FT_4$ is reached after at least 6 weeks and this is the minimum interval after which to evaluate the effect of changes in dosage. The dosage of thyroid hormones and TSH must be performed at fasting in the morning and before to assume $LT_4$, because it can increase $FT_4$ levels also of 20 % about 3 h after assumption and they can remain higher for about 9 h [18]. In special populations, such as elderly patients, pregnant women, patients with heart disease, assuming dugs interfering with $LT_4$ kinetics, undergoing major surgical interventions, poorly compliant, affected by conditions reducing $LT_4$ absorption, and patients with thyroid cancer, a targeted therapy performed by an expert endocrinologist is essential in order to avoid significant oscillations of serum levels of thyroid hormones able to worsen the patient's outcome.

Finally, it is essential to assume correctly the $LT_4$ therapy, preferably in the morning, at least half an hour before coffee and breakfast, particularly if rich in soy or fiber, and 4–6 h after possible interfering drugs. Also assumption in the evening before sleep and 2 h after last meal is possible, but this approach is less used in clinical practice [19].

## 23.3 Medical Treatment of Postsurgical Hypoparathyroidism

Hypocalcemia represents a common problem after parathyroidectomy and may be present after thyroidectomy. The reduction of serum calcium is due to hypoparathyroidism, with consequent reduction in bone reabsorption, increased calcium inflow into bone, increased calcium excretion, and decreased intestinal calcium absorption caused by reduced parathyroid hormone (PTH)-mediated renal 1,25-dihydroxycholecalciferol [1,25(OH)$_2$D] synthesis [20]. Hypoparathyroidism represents the most common complication of thyroid surgery, occurring transiently or permanently in 8.3 and 1.7 % of cases respectively [21].

Permanent hypoparathyroidism, defined as continuing need of replacement therapy 6 months after surgery, is an important tool for endocrinologist and it is more common when the goiter is extensive and anatomic landmarks are displaced and obscured. Standard treatment, based on oral calcium and vitamin D supplementation, should normalize serum calcium avoiding side effects such as nephrocalcinosis and nephrolithiasis.

Many authors have studied how to predict postsurgical hypocalcemia. Traditionally, the prediction of hypocalcemia is based on the evaluation after thyroidectomy of serum calcium trends every 6–12 h for 24–48 h, after which levels generally plateau [22]; serum calcium values that suggest treating postsurgical hypocalcemia are under 8 mg/dl [23]. For this reason, patients have to be observed for this period before they can be discharged in order to prevent development of hypocalcemia at home. Postoperative serum calcium less than 7.6 mg/dl on day 1 after thyroidectomy has 95 % specificity in predicting hypocalcemia [24]. Several studies have demonstrated that also PTH assay, performed after completing surgery, is an excellent predictor for the risk of hypocalcemia [25] and multiple algorithms have been offered. In the past, intraoperative PTH monitoring at 5, 10, and 20 min after the excision was proposed as useful to identify patients who will require postoperative calcium supplementation following thyroidectomy [26]. Other authors proposed that a PTH levels reduction of 65 % 6 h after thyroidectomy compared with preoperative values, shows sensitivity and specificity of 96.4 and 91.4 % respectively to predict postoperative hypocalcemia [27]. Specificity and sensibility of 100 % can be reached considering a decrease in PTH of 60 %, coupled with a simultaneous decrease in calcium of 10 %, 5–6 h postoperatively [28]. An unmeasurable PTH one day after surgery (<6.6 pg/ml) predicts a high risk to develop permanent hypoparathyroidism [29]. Recently, also the use of quick-intraoperative intact PTH (QiPTH) performed 15 min after total thyroidectomy (QiPTH 15) has been considered. QiPTH 15 > 15 pg/ml should be able to exclude a postoperative hypoparathyroidism, even if about 30 % of these patients develop transient and mild hypocalcemia within the first postoperative 18 h [30].

The development of hypocalcemia after thyroid surgery can be dependent on several factors. Hyperthyroidism has been shown to have significant effect on bone turn over even after restoring euthyroidism [31]. In fact, patients with Graves' disease have a dysregulation in calcium homeostasis, because they present lower postoperative serum calcium compared with patients with multinodular goiter, lower calcium/PTH set point, and a significantly increased release of PTH to hypocalcemic stimulus compared with controls [32]. In the first 24 h after total thyroidectomy for hyperthyroidism, transient biochemical hypocalcemia is common, occurring in 60 to 90% of patients [33–36]. Longer period of Graves' disease and low vitamin D levels represent additional factors contributing to hypocalcemia [37]. The role of vitamin D concentration in affecting calcium kinetics after thyroidectomy is still debated. In fact, it has been shown that low vitamin D levels are associated with 28-fold increase in chances of post total thyroidectomy clinically significant hypocalcemia [38]. On the other hand, some authors exclude that preoperative 25-hydroxycholecalciferol status significantly affects the overall perioperative calcium kinetics [39]. Elderly patients have significant risk factor for postoperative hypocalcemia [38], probably because of decreased intestinal calcium absorption, decreased renal 1α hydroxylation, and decreased cutaneous synthesis of vitamin D. Finally, transient hypoparathyroidism occurs in up to 20 % of patients after surgery for thyroid cancer [40].

Hypocalcemia, evaluated after correction for albumin values, may be associated with a wide field of clinical manifestation, ranging from no or few symptoms (cramps, paresthesia) if hypocalcemia is mild or chronic, to severe life-threatening conditions in case of severe or acute hypocalcemia. In particular, the severity of related symptoms (paresthesias, spasm, tetany, seizures) and signs (Chvostek's or Trousseau's signs, impaired cardiac contractility, prolonged QT interval) depends upon both the absolute level of calcium and the rate of decrease. Postsurgical hypocalcemia developing within few hours or few days after surgery ("acute" hypocalcemia), represents a condition in which serum calcium abruptly decreases starting from a condition of normocalcemia or hypercalcemia (primary hyperparathyroidism). For this reason, patients with acute hypocalcemia will be symptomatic at serum calcium values that would not cause symptoms in patients with chronic hypocalcemia.

In patients with acute and symptomatic hypocalcemia, intravenous calcium gluconate therapy will be required, while chronic or mild hypocalcemia can be treated with oral vitamin D and/or oral calcium. Calcitriol (1,25-dihydroxyvitamin D), which is the most active metabolite of vitamin D, is the most used in hypoparathyroidism because PTH should be requested for the renal conversion of calcidiol (25-hydroxyvitamin D) to the active metabolite calcitriol. It has a rapid onset of action (hours), and a biologic half-life of about 4–6 h. However, only few studies evaluated the optimal therapy of hypocalcemia and recommendations are often based on clinical experience.

Neuromuscular irritability with hypocalcemia requires prompt management in hospital and treatment with intravenous calcium. In particular, for symptomatic patients presenting with carpopedal spasm, tetany, seizures, ECG alterations and for asymptomatic patients with an acute decrease in serum corrected calcium to ≤7.5 mg/dL, intravenous calcium therapy is recommended [41]. The preferred form of intravenous calcium is calcium gluconate, because calcium chloride can cause local irritation [42]. One or two 10 ml vials of 10 % calcium gluconate (equivalent to 90–180 mg elemental calcium) should be diluted in 50–100 ml of 5 % dextrose and infused slowly over 10 min [43]. Electrocardiographic monitoring is recommended because dysrhythmias can occur in case of too rapid modification of serum calcium values. This treatment can be repeated until symptoms have cleared and often continuous administration of calcium may be needed to prevent recurrence of hypocalcemia. Patients should also receive oral calcium supplements and calcitriol [42]. The goal of the therapy is to maintain serum calcium at the lower end of the reference range (8 mg/dl). This can be obtained by administering ten 10 ml vials of 10 % calcium gluconate (equivalent to 900 mg of elemental calcium) in 1 l of 5 % dextrose or 0.9 % saline at an initial infusion rate of 50 ml/h. It is important to consider that calcium must be diluted in dextrose or saline to avoid vein irritation and that intravenous solution should not contain bicarbonate or phosphate, because they can form insoluble calcium salts [42]. Intravenous calcium should be continued until the patient is receiving an effective regimen of oral calcium and vitamin D. Moreover, concurrent hypomagnesemia can worse hypocalcemia, by inducing a resistance to PTH action and reducing its secretion. For this reason, if hypomagnesemia occurs, magnesium repletion must be considered. Persistent hypomagnesemia requires oral supplementation (300–400 mg day).

Patients with symptomatic hypocalcemia or a serum calcium concentration below 7.8 mg/dL should be treated with calcitriol 0.5 mcg twice daily and oral calcium 500 mg four times daily. The matter about the utility of a routine supplementation therapy with oral calcium and vitamin D in preventing symptomatic postsurgical hypocalcemia and allowing for a safe early discharge [44] has been confirmed by several studies, recently revised in a systematic review and meta-analysis [45]. However, there are also questions of whether prophylactic therapy should be considered. Recently, an algorithm for a selective supplementation protocol based on both postoperative PTH 4 h (4 h PTH) after total thyroidectomy and serum calcium levels in the first postoperative day (1 PO Ca) [46] has been offered. Authors proposed:

- to avoid treatment in patients with 4 h-PTH >10 pg/ml and 1PO-Ca ≥8.5 mg/dl
- to treat patients with 4 h-PTH >10 pg/ml and 1PO-Ca <8.5 mg/dl with oral calcium (3 g/day)
- to treat patients with 4 h-PTH <10 pg/ml and 1PO-Ca <8.5 mg/dl with oral calcium (3 g/day) and oral calcitriol (1 mcg/day)

This supplementation protocol is able to prevent symptomatic hypocalcemia and to avoid frequent evaluation of serum calcium concentration. Moreover, in patients with normal PTH and only subnormal serum calcium levels, treatment with oral calcium has been discontinued within 1 month, while after about 1 year of follow-up, only 8 % of patients with subnormal PTH and calcium were still in treatment. However, if calcitriol and oral calcium cannot be tapered until their discontinuation into few weeks, the hypoparathyroidism may be permanent. It is important to underline that long-term management of postsurgical hypoparathyroidism requires the addition of calcitriol, because of calcium alone can be often only transiently effective.

The aim of therapy in patients with permanent hypoparathyroidism is to relieve symptoms and to raise and maintain the serum calcium concentration in the low-normal range (8.0–8.5 mg/dl). This cut off can avoid the development of hypercalciuria due to the loss of renal calcium retaining effects of PTH [47]. The initial dose of oral calcium should be 1.0–1.5 g of elemental calcium daily [48]. The percentage of element content of the most used calcium salt forms is reported in Table 23.3.

**Table 23.3** Percentage of elemental calcium content of the most used calcium salt forms

| Salt | Element content (%) | Element content (1 g) | Milligrams of salt needed in order to obtain 1 g of elementary calcium (approximately) |
|---|---|---|---|
| Calcium carbonate | 40 | 400 mg | 2500 |
| Calcium phosphate | 38 | 380 mg | 2600 |
| Calcium chloride | 27 | 273 mg | 3700 |
| Calcium acetate | 25 | 253 mg | 4000 |
| Calcium citrate | 21 | 211 mg | 4800 |
| Calcium lactate | 13 | 130 mg | 770 |
| Calcium gluconate | 9 | 93 mg | 11,100 |

Modified from: Maeda et al. [55]

Although calcium carbonate is more often used, it may be less absorbed in older patients and those who have achlorhydria, who can be treated with another preparation, such as calcium citrate or calcium acetate. In fact, calcium carbonate dissolves only at an acid pH, and in patients with advanced renal failure or achlorhydria or taking $H_2$-blockers may be less adsorbed. Calcium citrate and mainly calcium acetate, on the contrary are soluble in both acid and alkaline environments.

Among all vitamin D formulations (Table 23.4), calcitriol is considered the treatment of choice [48]. In fact it acts more rapidly (hours) and the duration of action is short, allowing an easier management of a possible hypercalcemia due to overdosage. It can be administered starting from 0.25 mcg twice daily, with dose increments to achieve a low-normal serum calcium. Many patients require up to 2 mcg daily. The major side effects of calcitriol are risk of hypercalcemia and chronic hypercalciuria, the latter causing nephrolithiasis, nephrocalcinosis, and renal failure [49]. Hypercalciuria is the first sign of toxicity and can develop even in the absence of hypercalcemia. This is the reason why both serum and urinary calcium should be measured frequently (2-week intervals) initially and then every 6 months to 1 year once a stable dose is achieved. Calciuria should be maintained below 300 mg/day.

Replacement therapy with PTH is a viable option, as it corrects hypercalciuria and potentially reduces the risk of nephrocalcinosis, nephrolithiasis, and renal insufficiency. However, the long-term safety of PTH has not been established.

Patients affected by primary hyperparathyroidism undergoing parathyroidectomy have a rapid serum calcium fall after successful surgery. Postsurgical hypocalcemia is generally transient because normal parathyroid tissue recovers its function quickly (usually within 1 week). On the other hand, the persistence of hypocalcemia after parathyroidectomy can be due to intentional or accidental removal of all parathyroid glands, devascularization or trauma to residual parathyroid glands, but also to long-term suppression of residual non-pathological parathyroid glands by the previous excess of inappropriately secreted PTH. This phenomenon, called "hungry bone syndrome" [50], is defined as a prolonged (longer than 4th day

**Table 23.4** Vitamin D preparations for treatment of hypocalcemia

| Name | Daily dose | Time for normocalcemia | Duration of action |
|---|---|---|---|
| Vitamin $D_2$ (Ergocalciferol) | 400 units | 4–8 weeks | 2–6 months |
| Vitamin $D_3$ (Cholecalciferol) | 400 units | 4–8 weeks | 2–6 months |
| 25(OH)$D_3$ (Calcidiol) | 1–5 mcg | 2–5 weeks | 1–2 months |
| 1,25(OH $_2$)$D_3$ (Calcitriol) | 0.25–0.5 mcg | 2–5 days | 1–2 days |

From Endotext: http://www.endotext.org/chapter/hypocalcemia-diagnosis-and-treatment/

postoperatively) hypocalcemia (serum calcium <8.4 mg/dl) following parathyroidectomy for severe hyperparathyroidism. In addition to reduced serum calcium, also reduced serum phosphate and increased serum potassium levels can be observed. Moreover, the hypomagnesemia can contribute to the development of refractory hypocalcemia inducing a reduced PTH secretion and PTH resistance.

The syndrome most often occurs in patients who have developed a presurgical bone disease due to a chronic increase in bone reabsorption induced by high levels of PTH (osteitis fibrosa and/or "brown tumors") [50]. This phenomenon is probably due to the great increase of calcium usage by skeleton, occurring as result of removal of high PTH levels on bone, with arrest of bone reabsorption and rise of bone formation. Hungry bone syndrome has also been reported after thyroidectomy in patients affected by hyperthyroidism, because of the increase of bone turnover induced by thyroid hormone excess.

Risk factors associated to the development of hungry bone syndrome after parathyroidectomy are the volume of resected parathyroid adenoma, the preoperative blood urea nitrogen concentration, preoperative alkaline phosphatase concentration and older age, while preoperative serum calcium and PTH levels do not have predictive value [50]. A possible association between low preoperative vitamin D status and hungry bone syndrome has been proposed [51] while the causal relationship between preoperative treatment of hypercalcemia with bisphosphonate and hungry bone syndrome is still debated [52–54]. Therapy of hungry bone syndrome is aimed to correct hypocalcemia. Oral calcium supplementation (2–4 g of elemental calcium per day) should be started as soon as the patient is able to swallow. Calcium should be administered between meals to maximize intestinal absorption and minimize phosphate binding. Intravenous calcium is required in cases of rapid and progressive reduction in serum calcium or symptoms related to hypocalcemia (tetany, seizures, cardiac arrhythmias, laryngeal spasm) or if total serum calcium is below 7.5 mg/dL. Vitamin D supplementation is also useful. Even if there are no studies comparing the efficacy of intravenous vs. oral calcitriol administration, it is a common practice to administer calcitriol intravenously at increased doses. Once the serum calcium has stabilized at a safe concentration, intravenous therapy can be switched to oral calcitriol. Oral calcitriol should in turn be continued until the serum calcium normalization. Another method of correcting the hypocalcemia is dialysis. The administration of phosphate for hypophosphatemia is generally avoided in hungry bone syndrome (unless in cases of extremely low serum phosphate concentrations) because phosphate can combine with calcium reducing plasma calcium concentration.

## References

1. American Thyroid Association Guidelines Task Force, Kloos RT, Eng C, Evans DB, Francis GL, Gagel RF, Gharib H, Moley JF, Pacini F, Ringel MD, Schlumberger M, Wells SA Jr (2009) Medullary thyroid cancer: management guidelines of the American Thyroid Association. Thyroid 19:565–612
2. Wang LY, Palmer FL, Thomas D, Shaha AR, Shah JP, Patel SG, Tuttle RM, Ganly I (2014) Preoperative neck ultrasound in clinical node negative differentiated thyroid cancer. J Clin Endocrinol Metab 99:3686–3693
3. Bahn Chair RS, Burch HB, Cooper DS, Garber JR, Greenlee MC, Klein I, Laurberg P, McDougall IR, Montori VM, Rivkees SA, Ross DS, Sosa JA, Stan MN, American Thyroid Association, American Association of Clinical Endocrinologists (2011) Hyperthyroidism and other causes of thyrotoxicosis: management guidelines of the American Thyroid Association and American Association of Clinical Endocrinologists. Thyroid 21:593–646
4. Erbil Y, Ozluk Y, Giriş M, Salmaslioglu A, Issever H, Barbaros U, Kapran Y, Ozarmağan S, Tezelman S (2007) Effect of Lugol solution on thyroid gland blood flow and microvessel density in the patients with Graves' disease. J Clin Endocrinol Metab 92:2182–2189
5. Baeza A, Aguayo J, Barria M, Pineda G (1991) Rapid preoperative preparation in hyperthyroidism. Clin Endocrinol (Oxf) 35(5):439–442
6. Garber JR, Cobin RH, Gharib H, Hennessey JV, Klein I, Mechanick JI, Pessah-Pollack R, Singer PA, Woeber KA, American Association of Clinical Endocrinologists and American Thyroid Association Taskforce on Hypothyroidism in Adults (2012) Clinical practice guidelines for hypothyroidism in adults: cosponsored by the American Association of Clinical Endocrinologists and the American Thyroid Association. Endocr Pract 18:988–1028
7. Wiersinga WM, Duntas L, Fadeyev V, Nygaard B, Vanderpump MP (2012) 2012 ETA guidelines: the use of L-$T_4$+L-$T_3$ in the treatment of hypothyroidism. Eur Thyroid J 1:55–71
8. Hoang TD, Olsen CH, Mai VQ, Clyde PW, Shakir MK (2013) Desiccated thyroid extract compared with levothyroxine in the treatment of hypothyroidism: a randomized, double-blind, crossover study. J Clin Endocrinol Metab 98:1982–1990
9. Cellini M, Santaguida MG, Gatto I, Virili C, Del Duca S, Brusca N, Capriello S, Gargano L, Centanni M (2014) Systematic appraisal of lactose intolerance as cause of increased need for oral thyroxine. J Clin Endocrinol Metab 99:E1454–E1458
10. Di Donna V, Giannotti Santoro M, de Waure C, Ricciato MP, Paragliola RM, Pontecorvi A, Corsello SM (2014) A new strategy to estimate levothyroxine requirement after total thyroidectomy for benign thyroid disease. Thyroid 24:1759–1764
11. Santini F, Pinchera A, Marsili A, Ceccarini G, Castagna MG, Valeriano R, Giannetti M, Taddei D, Centoni R, Scartabelli G, Rago T, Mammoli C, Elisei R, Vitti P (2005) Lean body mass is a major determinant of levothyroxine dosage in the treatment of thyroid diseases. J Clin Endocrinol Metab 90:124–127
12. Jonklaas J (2010) Sex and age differences in levothyroxine dosage requirement. Endocr Pract 16:71–79
13. Devdhar M, Drooger R, Pehlivanova M, Singh G, Jonklaas J (2011) Levothyroxine replacement doses are affected by gender and weight, but not age. Thyroid 21:821–827
14. Jin J, Allemang MT, McHenry CR (2013) Levothyroxine replacement dosage determination after thyroidectomy. Am J Surg 205:360–363
15. Olubowale O, Chadwick DR (2006) Optimization of thyroxine replacement therapy after total or near total thyroidectomy for benign thyroid disease. Br J Surg 93:57–60
16. Mistry D, Atkin S, Atkinson H, Gunasekaran S, Sylvester D, Rigby AS, England RJ (2011) Predicting thyroxine requirements following total thyroidectomy. Clin Endocrinol (Oxf) 74:384–387
17. Ojomo KA, Schneider DF, Reiher AE, Lai N, Schaefer S, Chen H, Sippel RS (2013) Using of body mass index to predict optimal dosing after thyroidectomy. J Am Coll Surg 216:454–460
18. Ain KB, Pucino F, Shiver TM, Banks SM (1999) Thyroid hormone levels affected by time of blood sampling in thyroxine-treated patients. Thyroid 3:81–85

19. Bolk N, Visser TJ, Nijman J, Jongste IJ, Tijssen JG, Berghout A (2010) Effects of evening vs morning levothyroxine intake: a randomized double-blind crossover trial. Arch Intern Med 170:1996–2003
20. De Sanctis V, Soliman A, Fiscina B (2012) Hypoparathyroidism: from diagnosis to treatment. Curr Opin Endocrinol Diabetes Obes 19:435–442
21. Rosato L, Avenia N, Bernante P, De Palma M, Gulino G, Nasi PG, Pelizzo MR, Pezzullo L (2004) Complications of thyroid surgery: analysis of a multicentric study on 14,934 patients operated on in Italy over 5 years. World J Surg 28:271–276
22. Husein M, Hier MP, Al-Abdulhadi K, Black M (2002) Predicting calcium status post thyroidectomy with early calcium levels. Otolaryngol Head Neck Surg 127:289–293
23. Sabour S, Manders E, Steward DL (2009) The role of rapid PACU parathyroid hormone in reducing postthyroidectomy hypocalcemia. Otolaryngology 141:727–729
24. Pfleiderer AG, Ahamd N, Draper MR, Vrotsou K, Smith WK (2009) The timing of calcium measurements in helping to predict temporary and permanent hypocalcemia in patients having completion and total thyroidectomies. Ann R Coll Surg Engl 91:140–146
25. Stein DJ, Noordzij JP, Kepchar J, McLeod IK, Brietzke S, Calò PG (2013) Use of parathyroid hormone assay after thyroidectomy: a survey of US and European surgeons. Clin Med Insights Endocrinol Diabetes 6:39–45
26. Higgins KM, Mandell DL, Govindaraj S, Genden EM, Mechanick JI, Bergman DA, Diamond EJ, Urken ML (2004) The role of intraoperative rapid parathyroid hormone monitoring for predicting thyroidectomy-related hypocalcemia. Arch Otolaryngol Head Neck Surg 130:63–67
27. Noordzij JP, Lee SL, Bernet VJ, Payne RJ, Cohen SM, McLeod IK, Hier MP, Black MJ, Kerr PD, Richards ML, Lo CY, Raffaelli M, Bellantone R, Lombardi CP, Cohen JI, Dietrich MS (2007) Early prediction of hypocalcemia after thyroidectomy using parathyroid hormone: an analysis of pooled individual patient data from nine observational studies. J Am Coll Surg 205:748–754
28. Jumaily JS, Noordzij JP, Dukas AG, Lee SL, Bernet VJ, Payne RJ, McLeod IK, Hier MP, Black MJ, Kerr PD, Raffaelli M, Bellantone R, Lombardi CP, Dietrich MS (2010) Prediction of hypocalcemia after using 1- to 6-hour postoperative parathyroid hormone and calcium levels: an analysis of pooled individual patient data from 3 observational studies. Head Neck 32:427–434
29. Almquist M, Hallgrimsson P, Nordenström E, Bergenfelz A (2014) Prediction of permanent hypoparathyroidism after total thyroidectomy. World J Surg 38:2613–2620
30. Huang SM (2012) Do we overtreat post-thyroidectomy hypocalcemia? World J Surg 36:1503–1508
31. Pantazi H, Papapetrou PD (2000) Changes in parameters of bone and mineral metabolism during therapy for hyperthyroidism. J Clin Endocrinol Metab 85:1099–1106
32. Annerbo M, Hultin H, Stålberg P, Hellman P (2014) Left-shifted relation between calcium and parathyroid hormone in Graves' disease. J Clin Endocrinol Metab 99:545–551
33. Palit TK, Miller CC 3rd, Miltenburg DM (2000) The efficacy of thyroidectomy for Graves' disease: a meta-analysis. J Surg Res 90(2):161–165
34. Hughes OR, Scott-Coombes DM (2011) Hypocalcaemia following thyroidectomy for treatment of Graves' disease: implications for patient management and cost-effectiveness. J Laryngol Otol 125:849–852
35. Welch KC, McHenry CR (2011) Total thyroidectomy: is morbidity higher for Graves' disease than nontoxic goiter? J Surg Res 170:96–99
36. Pesce CE, Shiue Z, Tsai HL, Umbricht CB, Tufano RP, Dackiw AP, Kowalski J, Zeiger MA (2010) Postoperative hypocalcemia after thyroidectomy for Graves' disease. Thyroid 20:1279–1283
37. Erbil Y, Ozbey NC, Sari S, Unalp HR, Agcaoglu O, Ersöz F, Issever H, Ozarmagan S (2011) Determinants of postoperative hypocalcemia in vitamin D-deficient Graves' patients after total thyroidectomy. Am J Surg 201:685–691

38. Erbil Y, Barbaros U, Temel B, Turkoglu U, Issever H, Bozbora A (2008) The impact of age, vitamin D(3) level, and incidental parathyroidectomy on postoperative hypocalcemia after total or near total thyroidectomy. Am J Surg 197:439–446
39. Lang BH, Wong KP, Cheung CY, Fong YK, Chan DK, Hung GK (2013) Does preoperative 25-hydroxyvitamin D status significantly affect the calcium kinetics after total thyroidectomy? World J Surg 37:1592–1598
40. Flynn MB, Lyons KJ, Tarter JW, Ragsdale TL (1994) Local complications after surgical resection for thyroid carcinoma. Am J Surg 168:404–407
41. Murphy E, Williams GR (2009) Hypocalcaemia. Medicine 37:465–468
42. Tohme JF, Bilezikian JP (1996) Diagnosis and treatment of hypocalcemic emergencies. Endocrinologist 6:10–18
43. Cooper MS, Gittoes NJ (2008) Diagnosis and management of hypocalcaemia. BMJ 336:1298–1302
44. Bellantone R, Lombardi CP, Raffaelli M, Boscherini M, Alesina PF, De Crea C, Traini E, Princi P (2002) Is routine supplementation therapy (calcium and vitamin D) useful after total thyroidectomy? Surgery 132:1109–1113
45. Alhefdhi A, Mazeh H, Chen H (2013) Role of postoperative vitamin D and/or calcium routine supplementation in preventing hypocalcemia after thyroidectomy: a systematic review and meta-analysis. Oncologist 18:533–542
46. Raffaelli M, De Crea C, Carrozza C, D'Amato G, Zuppi C, Bellantone R, Lombardi CP (2012) Combining early postoperative parathyroid hormone and serum calcium levels allows for an efficacious selective post-thyroidectomy supplementation treatment. World J Surg 36:1307–1313
47. Kurokawa K (1987) Calcium-regulating hormones and the kidney. Kidney Int 32:760–771
48. Shoback D (2008) Clinical practice. Hypoparathyroidism. N Engl J Med 359:391
49. Bell NH, Stern PH (1978) Hypercalcemia and increases in serum hormone value during prolonged administration of 1alpha,25-dihydroxyvitamin D. N Engl J Med 298:1241–1243
50. Brasier AR, Nussbaum SR (1988) Hungry bone syndrome: clinical and biochemical predictors of its occurrence after parathyroid surgery. Am J Med 84:654–660
51. Silverberg SJ (2007) Vitamin D, deficiency and primary hyperparathyroidism. J Bone Miner Res 22(2):V100–V104
52. Lee IT, Sheu WH, Tu ST, Kuo SW, Pei D (2006) Bisphosphonate pretreatment attenuates hungry bone syndrome postoperatively in subjects with primary hyperparathyroidism. J Bone Miner Metab 24:255–258
53. Whitson HE, Lobaugh B, Lyles KW (2006) Severe hypocalcemia following bisphosphonate treatment in a patient with Paget's disease of bone. Bone 39:954–958
54. Corsello SM, Paragliola RM, Locantore P, Ingraudo F, Ricciato MP, Rota CA, Senes P, Pontecorvi A (2010) Post-surgery severe hypocalcemia in primary hyperparathyroidism preoperatively treated with zoledronic acid. Hormones (Athens) 9:338–342
55. Maeda SS, Fortes EM, Oliveira UM, Borba VC, Lazaretti-Castro M (2006) Hypoparathyroidism and pseudohypoparathyroidism. Arq Bras Endocrinol Metabol 50:664–673

# Patient Counselling and Patients' Involvement in Health Policy

# 24

Dominique Van Doorne and Moreno Busolin

## 24.1 For Physicians

The relationship between doctors and patients in 2014 is a matter that raises several complex and intriguing issues. The interaction between health care providers, physicians, patients, care givers, pharmaceutical and device companies solicits the attention of both public and private stakeholders. Opinions and recommendations coming from different parties should not be considered as an undesired interference but as a possible dialogue between stakeholders with increased transparency.

### 24.1.1 Informed Patients

Patients can gather medical information through books and specialized journals; they can follow TV and radio programmes, but what makes the difference with the early 1990s is the Internet. In matter of seconds they can receive a comprehensive picture regarding the specific illness, the potential remedies (drugs and/or surgery), the most specialized medical centres and who are the most skilled physicians. Of course, all information should be accurately verified but, in general, patients do not have the scientific know-how to discriminate good from bad quality information. When you search for "thyroid" on the web, you can get up to 41,700,000 results in 0.18 s! The amount of information is unmanageable by patients and therefore, most of the time the attention is focused on the first results where reliable sources can be found (such as Wikipedia and websites managed by scientific organizations or patients organizations) but also other less neutral sources, often sponsored by profit stakeholders.

D. Van Doorne, MD (✉) • M. Busolin
EUPATI National Liaison Team,
Rome, Italy
e-mail: dominique.vandoorne@gmail.com


C.P. Lombardi, R. Bellantone (eds.), *Minimally Invasive Therapies for Endocrine Neck Diseases*, DOI 10.1007/978-3-319-20065-1_24

How to cope with Internet-informed patients is a new challenge for physicians. More than 30 years ago most patients would solely trust their doctor and had no choice (little medical information and no travelling possibilities). They would never question medical issues and would just "let it be" or "cross fingers" or "pray God". Nowadays patients want to know more about the disease and its symptoms. They appreciate doctors willing to explain the treatment options and the expected effects and side effects. Sometimes they match the information coming from their doctor with the web.

The 2012 annual report of the European Patients Forum states that: "An effective empowerment strategy starts with promoting health literacy. This will equip patients with the knowledge and skills needed to take an active role in managing their health. It will help patients to get better information from health professionals to drive better and more cost-effective health outcomes. EPF believes that there is a need for a strategy on information to patients at EU level. High quality information on health, diseases and therapy options is vital to patient safety and empowerment"

More than ever it is crucial to take the time to give correct, transparent, patient-adapted explanations that reinforce the patient's confidence and empower the patient-doctor relationship.

Informed patients are more responsible and compliant with treatment and physician's advice therefore ultimately leading to improved health outcomes, quality of life and patient satisfaction.

> Most medical liability lawsuits are not about bad medicine; they are about poor communication and strained interpersonal relationship. A strong doctor-patient relationship, exemplified by the physician's presence to explain the proposed procedure and to answer pertinent questions, can be key in avoiding medical-legal issues [1].

Yet, doctor-patient communication is far from being good: in 2000 Britten et al. [2] identified 14 categories of misunderstanding, including: patient information unknown to the doctor (and vice versa); conflicting information given by different doctors and failures to communicate the reasons behind doctors' decision making in 20 general practices in England.

A complication issue may definitely compromise the patient trust if there is a lack of communication. The patients can understand complications but they cannot accept negligence, misinformation and refusal of discussion.

On the other hand, pressure on surgeons is very high, strained between patients' needs and counselling, surgical quality, error managing, lawsuits, defensive medicine and last but not least, spending reviews.

Patients' awareness has grown and the contingency of suing doctors is much higher and this is also affecting the health care system, given that the so-called defensive medicine is a bad practice for everybody: doctors look at patients as potential plaintiffs, health care costs are rising given the insurance premiums and over-treatment, while over-treatment and over-diagnosis are not the best care for the patient. In a US physicians' survey by Jackson Healthcare, 75 % of doctors say that they order more tests, procedures and medicines than are medically necessary in an attempt to avoid lawsuits. "Defensive medicine and the broken malpractice system are two of the major reasons that healthcare costs are soaring out of control" state Hal Scherz, MD and Wayne Oliver (Forbes 2013).

A no blame administrative compensation system is proposed by different patient-led non-profit organizations like "Patients for Fair Compensation".

## 24.2 Informed Consent

Before surgery or any invasive alternative or any new technology procedure, an "informed consent" has to be signed by the patient proving he has received the correct information from his physician. It has been a long journey starting last century, when Judge Benjamin Cardoso (1914, New York Appeal Court) noted that "every human being has a right to decide what shall be done with his or her body", thus establishing the concept of consent, where the patient has the right to accept or refuse treatment. In 1955, two cases arose where physicians had the duty to disclose potential surgical risks to patients: therefore, the concept of informed consent was established, requiring that patients freely consent to treatment and were fully informed about procedure's risk, benefits and alternatives. In the following years, informed consent has become "the process by which the treating health care provider discloses appropriate information to a competent patient so that the patient may make a voluntary choice to accept or refuse treatment" [3].

This definition of informed consent says that we are facing a kind of contract where the two parties sign an agreement based on appropriate information and patient's competency.

The appropriate information includes the following:

- The nature of the medical treatment and procedure
- Possible alternatives to the proposed intervention
- The risks, benefits and uncertainties related to each procedure
- Assessment of patient understanding
- The acceptance of the intervention by the patient [4]

Informed consents are written by doctors, which is questionable: patient advocates and physicians could work towards a better and friendlier informed consent with less medical jargon [5]. Patient advocates should be involved because they are more informed than doctors, not only to what the patient needs to know, but how he wants it to be explained and ultimately written.

### 24.2.1 New Technology and Innovative Surgical Treatments

Patient–physician communication is extremely important when a new surgical technique is proposed: more than ever the patient has to trust his doctor and feel confident.

The surgeon and the patient are both taking a higher risk compared to a well assessed surgical procedure because little data exist on efficacy and safety of the new procedure.

The clinical trials for new medicines guarantees a certain control by a third party, the ethic committee, while there is no such system when a new surgical procedure is adopted.

Who establishes the correct amount of risk to take? Ethic committees are involved only when a new technology is to be applied. Assessing the risk-benefit profile of innovative medicines and new technologies in western countries is a long and difficult process that may hinder pharmaceutical and surgical device companies from developing new technologies or medicines. Most of the new technologies are first being tested on patients in South America and Asia. Those small clinical data collected, together with the animal and laboratory data will be an essential part of documents forwarded to the western health regulating authorities for approval. Indeed our western approval system for new technologies needs to be questioned for ethical issues and discussed with all stakeholders involved. We may consider putting in place a patient and consumer working group for new medical devices as stated by the European Patients Forum: "Patients' unique perspective on the risks-benefits balance needs to be taken into account."

### 24.2.2 Patients Organizations and Patients Advocates Role in Health Care Decision-Making Process

The International Alliance for Patients Organizations IAPO states that "Healthcare policy decisions, at whatever level they are made, will ultimately affect patients' lives. Therefore patients have a moral and ethical right to play a meaningful role in developing health care policies. Engaging patients in health policy decision-making helps to ensure that policies reflect patient and caregiver needs, preferences and capabilities, making it an appropriate and cost-effective way to address the needs of the growing number of people with chronic conditions. But the influence of patient involvement and the impact of the patients' voice on policy-making can be restricted by numerous factors including practical and financial structures, differing knowledge bases, cultural barriers and personal attitudes".

To address some of these problems, EUPATI (European Patients' Academy on Therapeutic Innovation), was launched in February 2012 to increase the capabilities of patients and patient organizations to be effective advocates and advisors when new medicines are being developed. EUPATI will develop and disseminate objective, credible, correct and up-to-date public information about medicines research and development for the lay public. The Patients' Academy will build experts among patient advocates by administering them a full certificate training programme, and will also enhance competencies among patients and the public by creating a web educational toolbox and a public library on medicines R&D on the Internet. EUPATI will furthermore facilitate patient involvement by partnering up with academia, authorities, industries and ethics committees and through the creation of good practice guidelines. The educational modules will focus on the following areas: medicines development process from research to approval; personalized and predictive medicine; safety and risk/benefit assessment of medicines; pharmacoeconomics, health economics and health technology assessment; design and objectives of clinical trials, including involved stakeholders; patients' roles and responsibilities in medicines development.

This project represents a paradigm shift in empowering patients in medicines R&D.

Patients should also be involved in any health care innovation process, health-related policy, systems and delivery decisions to ensure that resources are invested in the right areas and properly address the needs of patients.

## 24.3 For Patients

### 24.3.1 Some Hints for Patients to Retrieve Correct Information from the Internet

In a few seconds you can get a comprehensive picture about any illness and potential remedies (drugs and/or surgery) on the web. When you open the web searching for "thyroid nodules" you get 1,830,000 results in 0.36 s. You can find some good and reliable information or you can end up in some strange or unreliable sites. So, what to do? You open the first webpages appearing on the screen?

### 24.3.2 How Can I Check the Quality of the Information I Find on the Web?

Here are a few recommendations to follow when searching for medical information on the web. Check the transparency and motivation of the webpage creators. Here are some useful hints once you enter the webpage:

1. Click on the "about us" button. This will give you an idea of who is writing the information on the webpage and why:
   - Is it a scientific society with a patient dedicated page?
   - Is it a university or a hospital or a clinic?
   - Is it Wikipedia?
   - Is it a patients' organization with a scientific committee?
   - Is it a patients' organization with no scientific committee?
   - Is it a single doctor webpage for his own promotion?
   - Is it a pharma industry sponsored webpage?
   - Is it a web forum or a personal blog?

The first four possibilities are usually more reliable because they are written by a group of health care professionals. The others are less neutral sources because their purpose is to promote profit stakeholders like single doctors or pharma industry but this does not mean the information is incorrect.

It is safe to compare different sources in order to obtain more reliable information.

### 24.3.3 How Can I Choose my Surgeon?

Obviously the experience of the surgeon is very important. Many studies suggest that surgical outcomes tend to be better when the surgeon performs a high number of operations each year (called surgical volume). The minimum surgical volume to consider a surgeon as a thyroid expert has not yet been determined but most agree that 50 thyroidectomies per year is the minimum number and more than 100 would be much better. We can say the same for the operating room nurses and staff. You may feel uncomfortable asking a surgeon about his surgical volume but surgeons are used to it, so don't hesitate!

This is even more important when a new alternative technology is suggested. You need to make sure that you are treated in a thyroid specialized centre with highly qualified thyroid experts.

Another important concern is about hospital rankings. Patients choose doctors not only on the basis of their experience and capabilities but also on the hospital reputation.

### 24.3.4 Alternative Options for Benign Nodule Treatment

Most thyroid nodules are discovered incidentally during other imaging exams, like carotid ultrasound. Luckily most of them are benign and will never cause symptoms, requiring a simple yearly follow-up. Nodule characteristics at ultrasound help your endocrinologist decide which nodule needs a fine needle aspiration (FNA) to determine whether the nodule is benign or malignant. All malignant nodules need surgery. Asymptomatic benign nodules usually do not have to be removed except in certain circumstances:

- Large nodules compressing nearby organs like the windpipe, the oesophagus or the nerve that controls the vocal cords and causing symptoms like breathing difficulty, swallowing problems or hoarseness.
- Large nodules responsible for an excess of thyroid hormone production (hyperfunctioning nodules) have to be removed, while small hyperfunctioning nodules can be "burned" with radioactive iodine and do not need to be removed.

Although thyroid surgery is considered by most doctors a simple procedure, the concern of temporary or permanent complications, and the effect on quality of life, however, remains relevant.

Therefore, various minimally invasive treatments, directed towards office-based management of symptomatic nodules, without requiring general anaesthesia, and with negligible damage to the skin and cervical tissues, have been proposed during the past two decades.

Today, ultrasound-guided percutaneous ethanol injection for large relapsing thyroid cysts is a well-established, safe and effective alternative to surgery. The cyst liquid is first aspirated and examined to exclude rare cancerous thyroid cysts. In case of cyst relapse the liquid is again aspirated and ethanol is injected into the cyst to "dry" the cyst's walls. Ultrasound-guided percutaneous ethanol injection is now considered the first choice treatment for large relapsing cysts because the efficacy rate, considered as a volume decrease of at least 50 % of the volume, is around 90 % with one or multiple ethanol injections and the complications rate is very low. Major complications are exceptional and most are temporary (transient vocal cord palsy). As the volume shrinkage induced is maintained over a prolonged period of time, treatment with ethanol should be considered the most cost-effective approach to benign thyroid cysts that recur after aspiration. Ultrasound-guided percutaneous ethanol injection is not a safe option for solid nodules because ethanol leakage in adjacent cervical soft tissues may cause a vocal cord nerve palsy with hoarseness, severe cervical pain and cervical tissue fibrosis (firm scar tissue).

Thermal ablation with laser or radiofrequency may represent a valid alternative to surgery for growing benign solid nodules. Specialized centres have now been treating quite a large number of patients for whom general anaesthesia or surgery were contraindicated. Trained operators may safely induce, with a single session of laser or radiofrequency ablation, a 50 % volume decrease and, in parallel, improve local symptoms. These outcomes seem stable for a prolonged period. Side effects and complications in less than 3 % of patients have been described, such as vocal cord palsy, cervical haematoma, nodule rupture and skin burns. It is then essential to choose a specialized centre with skilled operators.

### 24.3.5 Thyroid Surgery

Because laser or radiofrequency ablation techniques are still considered as innovative technologies to be performed only by highly specialized centres, thyroid surgery is still indicated in all patients with:

- A thyroid cancer (high suspicion on nodule FNA)
- Very large or growing nodules and goitres
- Symptomatic nodules (patients with hoarseness or swallowing difficulty or breathing discomfort)
- Hyperfunctioning large nodules, when radioiodine is contraindicated

In the last 20 years, technical progress has been made in thyroid surgical procedures: the minimally invasive approach has become the gold standard in surgery, allowing the thyroid surgeon to transform traditional surgery thyroidectomy into MIVAT (minimally invasive video-assisted thyroidectomy). MIVAT is not indicated for all patients and very large thyroid nodules, large goitres or certain thyroid cancer still require the classic thyroidectomy. The two techniques are equal in terms of efficacy and complications but, from the patient's perspective, the cosmetic impact of MIVAT, with a small surgical scar, is making the difference.

Total thyroidectomy complications are not frequent, haemorrhage and infection in less than 1 % in the first days following surgery, permanent hypoparathyroidism in 2 % of patients and monolateral vocal cord palsy in less than 1 %.

In conclusion, less invasive treatments are now available as an alternative to thyroid surgery for benign nodules volume reduction. To make a good choice, remember to ask your doctors which are the results and the complications of the treatment they suggest and what is the experience of the doctors performing the surgical procedure or the new nodule ablation techniques because, as already said, the complication rate decreases as the invasive procedure is performed by skilled doctors in highly specialized centres.

## References

1. Fleeter TB. Informed consent: more than just a signature. AAOS No. 2010.
2. Britten N et al (2000) Misunderstandings in prescribing decisions in general practice: qualitative study. BMJ 320(7233):484–488
3. Appelbaum PS (2007) Assessment of patients' competence to consent to treatment. N Engl J Med 357:1834–1840
4. De Bord J (2014) Informed Consent. Ethics in medicine. University of Washington School of Medicine
5. Farrington C (2011) Reconciling managers, doctors, and patients: the role of clear communication. J R Soc Med 104:231–236

MIX
Papier aus verantwortungsvollen Quellen
Paper from responsible sources
FSC® C105338

If you have any concerns about our products,
you can contact us on
**ProductSafety@springernature.com**

In case Publisher is established outside the EU,
the EU authorized representative is:
**Springer Nature Customer Service Center GmbH**
**Europaplatz 3, 69115 Heidelberg, Germany**

Printed by Libri Plureos GmbH
in Hamburg, Germany